Green Extraction and Formulation of Antioxidants Derived from Food and Agricultural Waste

Green Extraction and Formulation of Antioxidants Derived from Food and Agricultural Waste

Guest Editors

Dubravka Vitali Čepo
Kristina Radić

MDPI

Basel • Beijing • Wuhan • Barcelona • Belgrade • Novi Sad • Cluj • Manchester

Guest Editors

Dubravka Vitali Čepo
Department of Nutrition and Dietetics
University of Zagreb
Zagreb
Croatia

Kristina Radić
Department of Nutrition and Dietetics
University of Zagreb
Zagreb
Croatia

Editorial Office
MDPI AG
Grosspeteranlage 5
4052 Basel, Switzerland

This is a reprint of the Special Issue, published open access by the journal *Antioxidants* (ISSN 2076-3921), freely accessible at: https://www.mdpi.com/journal/antioxidants/special_issues/food_agricultural_waste.

For citation purposes, cite each article independently as indicated on the article page online and as indicated below:

Lastname, A.A.; Lastname, B.B. Article Title. *Journal Name* **Year**, *Volume Number*, Page Range.

ISBN 978-3-7258-5247-5 (Hbk)
ISBN 978-3-7258-5248-2 (PDF)
https://doi.org/10.3390/books978-3-7258-5248-2

Cover image courtesy of Dubavka Vitali Čepo

Contents

About the Editors

Dubravka Vitali Čepo

Dubravka Vitali Čepo is a full professor and head of the Department of Nutrition and Dietetics at the Faculty of Pharmacy, University of Zagreb. She leads multiple courses in the integrated undergraduate, graduate, and postgraduate programs in Pharmacy and Medical Biochemistry, focusing on food chemistry, nutrition therapy, food–drug interactions, and environmental health. Her scientific interests lie at the intersection of sustainability, nutrition, and public health, with a particular emphasis on re-evaluating industrial and food waste as secondary raw materials, especially in the development of nutraceuticals. Currently, she leads three scientific projects and has published over 70 scientific papers in this field. To date, she has mentored 7 PhD theses and more than 50 final student theses. She is an active member of the "Scientists for Climate Croatia" initiative and frequently participates in informal educational programs promoting sustainability and climate change awareness in various public institutions.

Kristina Radić

Kristina Radić is an Assistant Professor at the Department of Nutrition and Dietetics, Faculty of Pharmacy, University of Zagreb, where she actively contributes to teaching within the integrated undergraduate and graduate university programs in Pharmacy and Medical Biochemistry. She is involved in courses such as Physiological and Biochemical Aspects of Nutrition, Biochemistry of Nutrition, Nutrition Therapy, and Climate Change and Health. Her research focuses on the development of environmentally sustainable methods for extracting bioactive compounds from food waste, with particular emphasis on the formulation of nutraceuticals and the optimization of in vitro models for studying the bioavailability of biologically active food components. She has contributed to seven scientific projects and authored over 20 publications in the field. To date, she has supervised more than 10 graduate theses.

antioxidants

MDPI

Editorial

Advances in Green Extraction and Formulation of Antioxidants Derived from Food and Agricultural Waste

Kristina Radić and Dubravka Vitali Čepo *

Department of Nutrition and Dietetics, Faculty of Pharmacy and Biochemistry, University of Zagreb, 10000 Zagreb, Croatia; kristina.radic@pharma.unizg.hr
* Correspondence: dubravka.vitali@pharma.unizg.hr

Food and agricultural waste streams are increasingly recognized as abundant, underutilized sources of valuable bioactive compounds, particularly antioxidants. Their recovery and reuse align closely with the principles of the circular economy and sustainable nutrition, offering both environmental and economic benefits. However, several key limitations hinder the more widespread utilization of this concept, including variable composition and availability of raw material: economic and infrastructural challenges related to developing green extraction technologies at the industrial scale and undefined regulatory frameworks for the use of bioactive compounds from waste in foods.

Antioxidants have garnered significant attention in recent decades for their potential applications in functional foods and nutraceuticals. However, their particulate physicochemical properties—such as poor stability, low solubility, undesirable sensory characteristics, and limited bioavailability—pose major challenges for their effective use [1].

To address these limitations, the development of tailored extraction and formulation strategies is essential. Green technologies that use less energy and minimize the need for toxic solvents, and reduce the use of lipids, surfactants, and biopolymers in extraction/formulation processes are especially promising. These approaches aim not only to improve yields and maintain antioxidant stability but also to ensure their safe and efficient delivery to end products [2].

This Special Issue addresses the most recent development of technological processes that face the above-mentioned challenges and limitations enabling the efficient recovery and stabilization of antioxidants from waste biomass. The general aim is to showcase novel approaches that are not only scientifically robust but also aligned with green chemistry principles—favoring minimal energy consumption, reduced environmental impact, and obtaining safe end products.

The specific objectives of this Special Issue are as follows:

- present cutting-edge research on green extraction techniques for isolating antioxidants from food and agricultural waste materials;
- highlight the innovative formulation strategies that enhance antioxidant stability, solubility, and bioavailability;
- evaluate the functional, physicochemical, and safety characteristics of newly developed antioxidant-rich products;
- foster interdisciplinary dialog between food scientists, chemists, process engineers, and sustainability experts working at the intersection of waste utilization and bioactive compound delivery.

By compiling recent advances and emerging insights, this Special Issue aims to contribute meaningfully to the transition toward more sustainable and health-oriented food systems.

In the following overview, we synthesized the key insights and advancements presented across the ten contributions, identifying overarching trends, shared challenges, and emerging opportunities in the green extraction and formulation of antioxidants from food and diverse agricultural byproducts—from shrimp shells and wine lees to citrus peels, olive leaves, and sorghum stalks. This offers a comprehensive overview of the innovations driving the future of green antioxidant recovery and formulation.

Studies within this Special Issue demonstrated how green solvents, novel adsorbents, and nanostructured carriers could transform waste into high-value ingredients for food, pharmaceutical, and nutraceutical applications. A significant portion of the research was dedicated to the development and optimization of green extraction methods aiming to maximize the recovery of antioxidant compounds while minimizing the environmental impact. Ultrasound-assisted extraction (UAE), microwave-assisted extraction (MAE), supercritical fluid extraction (SFE), and deep eutectic solvents (DESs) are among the most promising approaches featured.

For example, wine lees from various grape cultivars were subjected to UAE using ethanol-water mixtures, yielding extracts rich in phenolic acids and flavonoids. Chemometric tools such as principal component analysis and partial least squares regression were employed to correlate extract composition with antioxidant activity, demonstrating the effectiveness of data-driven optimization [Contribution 1]. Similarly, aloe vera rind byproducts were processed using UAE combined with DESs, achieving high phenolic yields and excellent solvent recyclability, thus reinforcing the sustainability of the method [Contribution 2].

MAE was applied in a two-step biorefinery strategy to extract polyphenols, carotenoids, and pectin from mandarin peels [Contribution 3]. This approach not only improved extraction efficiency but also reduced energy consumption compared to conventional methods. In another study, SFE was used to recover bioactive compounds from apple peels, with extracts showing promising effects on mitochondrial Complex I activity, suggesting potential pharmacological applications [Contribution 4].

These studies align with broader trends in green chemistry, where novel solvents and low-energy processes are increasingly favored for their environmental and functional advantages [3].

Beyond extraction, several contributions focused on the formulation of antioxidant compounds into stable, bioavailable, and functional systems recognized for their ability to protect sensitive bioactives, improve solubility, and enable targeted delivery, particularly in food and cosmetic products [4].

One study developed nanostructured lipid carriers (NLCs) incorporating natural deep eutectic solvents (NaDESs) to encapsulate antioxidants from tapereba peel, a Brazilian Cerrado byproduct. The resulting formulation demonstrated strong antioxidant activity in cellular assays, significantly reducing reactive oxygen species levels [Contribution 5]. Another investigation combined cellulose-based edible films with liposome-based encapsulation of grape seed tannins. These films exhibited improved flexibility, wettability, and controlled release properties, making them suitable for food packaging applications [Contribution 6].

Another practical and impactful application of waste-derived bioactives is the integration of antioxidant-rich extracts into food matrices [5]. Several studies in this Special Issue demonstrated how such incorporation could enhance the nutritional and functional properties of food products.

Mandarin peel extracts were used to enrich wheat bread, resulting in increased flavonoid content and antioxidant activity. Although most polyphenols degraded during digestion, hesperidin remained bioaccessible, highlighting the importance of evaluating compound stability during post-processing [Contribution 7]. Similarly, sorghum byproduct extracts were used to fortify bread, extending its shelf life by approximately five days without compromising its sensory attributes [Contribution 8].

These findings support the growing interest in functional foods that deliver health benefits while contributing to waste reduction and resource efficiency [6].

At the core of this Special Issue was the principle of waste valorization—the transformation of low-value byproducts into high-value functional ingredients. This concept is best exemplified by studies on shrimp shell waste and olive leaf extracts.

Shrimp shell waste from Palaemon species was characterized by its antioxidant and antimicrobial properties, suggesting potential use as natural preservatives and colorants in the food industry [Contribution 9]. In another study, olive leaf polyphenols were selectively adsorbed onto biochar derived from grapevine pruning residues. This approach not only recovered valuable compounds but also demonstrated the utility of agricultural residues as functional materials [Contribution 10].

These examples illustrate how integrated biorefinery concepts and circular economy models can be applied to food systems, reducing waste and creating new economic opportunities [7].

The collection of studies presented in this Special Issue underscores the growing sophistication and interdisciplinary nature of green antioxidant recovery and formulation. Across the ten contributions, a clear trend emerges: the successful valorization of food and agricultural waste into high-value antioxidant ingredients hinges on both efficient extraction technologies and advanced formulation strategies. Green extraction methods—such as UAE, MAE, SFE, and DESs—demonstrate robust potential to recover bioactives from diverse byproducts while reducing environmental footprints. The adoption of chemometric tools further enhanced the process optimization, enabling data-driven improvements in yield and antioxidant efficacy.

On the formulation front, advanced delivery systems like NLCs and liposomes are increasingly used to overcome the common limitations of antioxidants—poor stability, solubility, and bioavailability. These systems not only protect the functional integrity of antioxidants but also broaden their applicability in food, pharmaceutical, and cosmetic contexts. In addition, incorporating antioxidant-rich extracts into food matrices illustrates a practical route for delivering health-promoting compounds to consumers while simultaneously extending shelf life and improving nutritional profiles.

The studies also highlight the importance of post-processing evaluation, particularly regarding compound bioaccessibility and sensory impact [8]. Furthermore, several contributions extend beyond individual compound recovery, embracing circular economy principles by developing integrated biorefinery models and exploring the dual utility of both bioactive extracts and their supporting materials—such as biochar and edible films. This approach maximizes the use of waste streams and aligns closely with sustainable development goals.

This Special Issue showcases vibrant and evolving research focused on the green recovery and application of antioxidants from food and agricultural waste. Collectively, the contributions affirm that sustainable extraction technologies and innovative formulation strategies are essential for unlocking the full potential of waste-derived bioactives [9]. These advancements not only mitigate environmental impact but also open new avenues in the development of functional foods, nutraceuticals, and eco-friendly packaging solutions.

At the core of these advancements is the principle of waste valorization—the conversion of discarded biomass into functional and commercially valuable ingredients. The integration of interdisciplinary expertise—from food science and chemistry to engineering and sustainability—emerges as a critical driver of innovation. As the demand for natural, health-enhancing products continues to grow, the insights and approaches detailed in this Special Issue offer a new insight for building circular, resilient, and health-oriented food systems.

Author Contributions: Conceptualization, D.V.Č. and K.R.; writing—original draft preparation, K.R.; writing—review and editing, D.V.Č. All authors have read and agreed to the published version of the manuscript.

Funding: This research received no external funding.

Acknowledgments: We wish to thank all the authors who contributed to the research topic of this Special Issue and the reviewers for their perceptive suggestions and comments. In particular, we acknowledge all of the Editorial staff from the *Antioxidants* journal for their support in the preparation of this Special Issue.

Conflicts of Interest: The authors declare no conflicts of interest.

Abbreviations

The following abbreviations are used in this manuscript:

DES	Deep eutectic solvent
MAE	Microwave-assisted extraction
NaDES	Natural deep eutectic solvent
NLC	Nanostructured lipid carrier
SFE	Supercritical fluid extraction
UAE	Ultrasound-assisted extraction

List of Contributions:

1. De Luca, M.; Restuccia, D.; Spizzirri, U.G.; Crupi, P.; Ioele, G.; Gorelli, B.; Clodoveo, M.L.; Saponara, S.; Aiello, F. Wine Lees as Source of Antioxidant Molecules: Green Extraction Procedure and Biological Activity. *Antioxidants* **2023**, *12*, 622. https://doi.org/10.3390/antiox12030622.
2. Ioannou, G.D.; Ioannou, K.A.; Christou, A.; Stavrou, I.J.; Kapnissi-Christodoulou, C.P. The Utilization of an Aloe Vera Rind By-Product: Deep Eutectic Solvents as Eco-Friendly and Recyclable Extraction Media of Polyphenolic Compounds. *Antioxidants* **2024**, *13*, 162. https://doi.org/10.3390/antiox13020162.
3. Jurić, M.; Golub, N.; Galić, E.; Radić, K.; Maslov Bandić, L.; Vitali Čepo, D. Microwave-Assisted Extraction of Bioactive Compounds from Mandarin Peel: A Comprehensive Biorefinery Strategy. *Antioxidants* **2025**, *14*, 722. https://doi.org/10.3390/antiox14060722.
4. Aresta, A.; De Vietro, N.; Cotugno, P.; Pierri, C.L.; Trisolini, L.; Zambonin, C. Supercritical Fluid Extraction of Bioactive Components from Apple Peels and Their Modulation of Complex I Activity in Isolated Mitochondria. *Antioxidants* **2024**, *13*, 307. https://doi.org/10.3390/antiox13030307.
5. Mello, V.C.; de Brito, G.O.; Radicchi, M.A.; Florêncio, I.; Piau, T.B.; Ferreira, E.A.; de Azevedo Chang, L.F.; Silveira, A.P.; Simões, M.M.; de Paiva, K.L.R.; et al. Advanced Solubilization of Brazilian Cerrado Byproduct Extracts Using Green Nanostructured Lipid Carriers and NaDESs for Enhanced Antioxidant Potentials. *Antioxidants* **2025**, *14*, 290. https://doi.org/10.3390/antiox14030290.
6. Vidal, C.; Lopez-Polo, J.; Osorio, F.A. Physical Properties of Cellulose Derivative-Based Edible Films Elaborated with Liposomes Encapsulating Grape Seed Tannins. *Antioxidants* **2024**, *13*, 989. https://doi.org/10.3390/antiox13080989.

7. Gómez-Mejía, E.; Sacristán, I.; Rosales-Conrado, N.; León-González, M.E.; Madrid, Y. Valorization of Citrus reticulata Blanco Peels to Produce Enriched Wheat Bread: Phenolic Bioaccessibility and Antioxidant Potential. *Antioxidants* **2023**, *12*, 1742. https://doi.org/10.3390/antiox12091742.
8. Amoriello, T.; Mellara, F.; Ciorba, R.; Ceccarelli, D.; Amoriello, M.; Taddei, F.; Ciccoritti, R. Phenols Extraction from Sorghum Byproducts: Upcycling Strategies and Food Applications. *Antioxidants* **2025**, *14*, 668. https://doi.org/10.3390/antiox14060668.
9. Maia, M.L.; Grosso, C.; Barroso, M.F.; Silva, A.; Delerue-Matos, C.; Domingues, V.F. Bioactive Compounds of Shrimp Shell Waste from Palaemon serratus and Palaemon varians from Portuguese Coast. *Antioxidants* **2023**, *12*, 435. https://doi.org/10.3390/antiox12020435.
10. Prelac, M.; Major, N.; Cvitan, D.; Anđelini, D.; Repajić, M.; Ćurko, J.; Kovačević, T.K.; Goreta Ban, S.; Užila, Z.; Ban, D.; et al. Valorization of Olive Leaf Polyphenols by Green Extraction and Selective Adsorption on Biochar Derived from Grapevine Pruning Residues. *Antioxidants* **2024**, *13*, 1. https://doi.org/10.3390/antiox13010001.

References

1. Khan, M.K.; Paniwnyk, L.; Hassan, S. *Polyphenols as Natural Antioxidants: Sources, Extraction and Applications in Food, Cosmetics and Drugs*; Springer: Singapore, 2019; ISBN 9789811338106.
2. Cheriyan, B.V.; Karunakar, K.K.; Anandakumar, R.; Murugathirumal, A.; Kumar, A.S. Eco-friendly extraction technologies: A comprehensive review of modern green analytical methods. *Sustain. Chem. Clim. Action* **2025**, *6*, 100054. [CrossRef]
3. Shi, L.; Zhao, W.; Yang, Z.; Subbiah, V.; Suleria, H.A.R. Extraction and characterization of phenolic compounds and their potential antioxidant activities. *Environ. Sci. Pollut. Res.* **2022**, *29*, 81112–81129. [CrossRef] [PubMed]
4. Elmowafy, M.; Al-Sanea, M.M. Nanostructured lipid carriers (NLCs) as drug delivery platform: Advances in formulation and delivery strategies. *Saudi Pharm. J.* **2021**, *29*, 999–1012. [CrossRef] [PubMed]
5. Caleja, C.; Barros, L.; Antonio, A.L.; Oliveira, M.B.P.P.; Ferreira, I.C.F.R. A comparative study between natural and synthetic antioxidants: Evaluation of their performance after incorporation into biscuits. *Food Chem.* **2017**, *216*, 342–346. [CrossRef] [PubMed]
6. Radić, K.; Galić, E.; Vinković, T.; Golub, N.; Vitali Čepo, D. Tomato Waste as a Sustainable Source of Antioxidants and Pectins: Processing, Pretreatment and Extraction Challenges. *Sustainability* **2024**, *16*, 9158. [CrossRef]
7. Nguyen, T.H.; Wang, X.; Utomo, D.; Gage, E.; Xu, B. Circular bioeconomy and sustainable food systems: What are the possible mechanisms? *Clean. Circ. Bioecon.* **2025**, *11*, 100145. [CrossRef]
8. Teixeira, J.L.d.P.; Baptista, D.P.; Orlando, E.A.; Gigante, M.L.; Pallone, J.A.L. Effect of processing on the bioaccessibility of essential minerals in goat and cow milk and dairy products assessed by different static in vitro digestion models. *Food Chem.* **2022**, *374*, 131739. [CrossRef] [PubMed]
9. Voss, M.; Valle, C.; Calcio Gaudino, E.; Tabasso, S.; Forte, C.; Cravotto, G. Unlocking the Potential of Agrifood Waste for Sustainable Innovation in Agriculture. *Recycling* **2024**, *9*, 25. [CrossRef]

antioxidants

MDPI

Article

Wine Lees as Source of Antioxidant Molecules: Green Extraction Procedure and Biological Activity

Michele De Luca [1,†], Donatella Restuccia [1,†], Umile Gianfranco Spizzirri [1,*], Pasquale Crupi [2], Giuseppina Ioele [1], Beatrice Gorelli [3], Maria Lisa Clodoveo [2], Simona Saponara [3] and Francesca Aiello [1]

1 Department of Pharmacy, Health and Nutritional Sciences, University of Calabria, 87036 Rende, Italy
2 Interdisciplinary Department of Medicine, University of Bari "Aldo Moro", 70124 Bari, Italy
3 Department of Life Sciences, University of Siena, Via Aldo Moro 2, 53100 Siena, Italy
* Correspondence: g.spizzirri@unical.it
† These authors contributed equally to this work.

Abstract: An ultrasound-assisted extraction method, employing ethanol and water as solvents at low temperature (30 °C) and reduced time (15 min), was proposed to extract bioactive molecules from different cultivars (*Magliocco Canino*, *Magliocco Rosato*, *Gaglioppo*, and *Nocera Rosso*) of wine lees. All the extract yields were evaluated and their contents of phenolic acids, flavonoids, and total polyphenols were determined by means of colorimetric assays and high-performance liquid chromatography coupled with diode-array detection (HPLC-DAD) and Fourier transform infrared (FTIR) techniques. Radical scavenging assays were performed and the *Magliocco Canino* extracted with a hydroalcoholic mixture returned the best results both against ABTS (0.451 mg mL^{-1}) and DPPH (0.395 mg mL^{-1}) radicals. The chemometric algorithms principal component analysis (PCA) and partial least square regression (PLS) were used to process the data obtained from all qualitative–quantitative sample determinations with the aim of highlighting data patterns and finding possible correlations between composition and antioxidant features of the different wine lees cultivars and the extraction procedures. Wine lees from *Magliocco Canino* and *Magliocco Rosato* were found to be the best vegetable matrices in terms of metabolite content and antioxidant properties. The components extracted with alcoholic or hydroalcoholic solvents, specifically (−)-epigallocatechin gallate, chlorogenic acid, and *trans*-caftaric acid, were found to be correlated with the antioxidant capacity of the extracts. Multivariate data processing was able to identify the compounds related to the antioxidant features. Two PLS models were optimized by using their concentration levels to predict the IC_{50} values of the extracts in terms of DPPH and ABTS with high values of correlation coefficient R^2, 0.932 and 0.824, respectively, and a prediction error lower than 0.07. Finally, cellular (SH-SY5Y cells) antioxidant assays were performed on the best extract (the hydroalcoholic extract of *Magliocco Canino cv*) to confirm its biological performance against radical species. All these recorded data strongly outline the aptness of valorizing wine lees as a valuable source of antioxidants.

Keywords: wine lees; green extraction procedure; principal component analysis; partial least square regression; antioxidant properties

1. Introduction

Wine is produced in all parts of the world, but France, Italy, Spain, and some emerging countries such as Australia, Chile, South Africa, and the United States represent the main world producers [1]. The market data highlight the extreme complexity of the wine sector, often based on thousands of small farms that produce small quantities of wine, together with other large companies with high wine production [2]. Italy, together with France, ranks at the top of the classification of wine-producing countries. Italy is still the leading wine-producing country with 44,500 hectoliters, while European Union countries reached 145,000 hectoliters in 2021, with a substantial decrease of 13% (−21,000 hectoliters) compared to 2020, almost achieving 60% of world wine production [3].

However, the wine industry generates enormous quantities of waste every year, among which are pomace, grape seeds, stems, leaves, lees, and cellar waste. The literature data report that for each produced hectoliter of wine, 20 kg of pomace, 3.85 kg of stalks, and 6.36 kg of lees and clarification solids are produced [4]. Their disposal, even in the face of the considerable quantities and their molecular composition, has an environmental impact that should not be underestimated. For this reason, it is important to adopt strategies for the recovery and valorization of wine wastes. The reduction in by-products and waste produced during the winemaking process plays a crucial role in providing a green and clean vision of this agri-food sector. The aim can be easily realized by providing new and innovative strategies able to transform the winemaking waste into high-added value products. Winemaking wastes represent a valuable supply of active molecules, mainly polyphenols, that can be largely reused as supplements in pharmaceutical and biomedical fields, as well as in the food industry. Recently, mixtures of grape seeds and skins were used to produce extracts useful as food supplements [5,6]. Nevertheless, wine lees generated in post-fermentation are poorly investigated, even though the lees represent about 14% of the total organic waste produced during winemaking [7].

The lees are the residue accumulated after the fermentation of the wine consisting predominantly of yeasts and impurities originating from grapes. Two main fractions comprise lees by-products [8]: a combination of proteins, insoluble carbohydrates, organic acids, yeasts, inorganic salts, and phenolic molecules provides the solid fraction [9], while ethanol, acetic acid, and lactic acid are the main compounds of the liquid fraction [10]. Environmental conditions, grape variety, and regions of origin are agronomic parameters that deeply influence the chemical composition of lees [11]. Lees have usually been a key raw material to produce ethanol and tartaric acid for application in the food industry [12] and represent a resource of high-added-value substances with remarkable antioxidant capacity and the ability to prevent cardiovascular diseases, as well as a remarkable mix of anti-inflammatory and anticancer molecules [13].

Starting from lees produced by winemaking with different grape cultivars, the challenge of this research was to propose an innovative and eco-friendly extraction protocol able to provide a mix of chemical molecules with notable antioxidant features. In this regard, different solvents were tested, while ultrasound-assisted extraction was employed to reduce the time and temperature of the process, preserving the chemical and biological integrity of the active compounds. The extracts were deeply characterized by chromatographic and spectroscopic methodologies and antioxidant performance and the collected data were analyzed by chemometric tools in order to highlight data patterns and the relationship between the chemical composition of the samples and their antioxidant capacities.

2. Materials and Methods

2.1. Chemicals

Gallic acid, (+)-hydrated catechin, (−)-epigallocatechin, procyanidin B_2, epigallocatechin gallate, (−)-epicatechin, chlorogenic acid, caffeic acid, p-coumaric acid, ferulic acid, Folin–Ciocalteu reagent, sodium carbonate (Na_2CO_3) radical 2,2′-diphenyl-1-picrylyhydrazyl (DPPH), radical 2,2′-azino-bis(3-ethylbenzothiazolin-6-sulfonic) (ABTS), sodium nitrite ($NaNO_2$), sodium phosphate (Na_3PO_4), aluminum chloride ($AlCl_3$), hydrochloric acid (HCl), sodium hydroxide (NaOH), absolute ethanol, Dulbecco's modified Eagle's medium (DMEM), DMEM without phenol red, phosphate buffer solution (PBS), 2′,7′-dichlorofluorescein diacetate (DCF-DA), hydrogen peroxide (H_2O_2), *L*-glutamine, penicillin, streptomycin, and Whatman No. 3 filter paper were purchased from Sigma Aldrich (Sigma Chemical Co., St. Louis, MO, USA). Delphinidin-3-*O*-glucoside (DG), cyanidin-3*O*-glucoside (CG), petunidin-3*O*-glucoside (PTG), peonidin-3*O*-glucoside (POG), and malvidin-3*O*-glucoside (MG) were purchased from Extrasynthese (Genay, France).

HPLC-grade water and acetonitrile were purchased from VWR (Chromasolv, VWR International Srl, Milano, Italy).

2.2. Sample Collection and Preparation

A total of four lees samples of autochthonous Calabria *Vitis vinifera* red grape varieties (*Nocera Rosso* (1), *Magliocco Rosato* (2), *Magliocco Canino* (3), and *Gaglioppo* (4)) were collected in September 2021 from a local producer (Azienda Agricola Donna Fidelia, Belvedere Marittimo, Italy). The grapes were harvested at technological maturation, and the agronomic practices as well as the winemaking process were the same for all analyzed samples. The removal of the ethanol from the lees samples was accomplished by rotary evaporation (ALC Multispeed Centrifuge Thermo Electron Corporation, Waltham, MA, USA) for 15 min at 35 °C and the concentrated solution was frozen at −18 °C and then freeze-dried at a pressure of 0.45 mbar (Micro Modulyo, Edwards). Freeze-dried lees samples were crushed and kept in hermetically sealed containers at −18 °C until further analysis.

2.3. Wine Lees Extraction

Lees samples were extracted as described by Carullo et al. [13]. Two hundred mL of ethanol (E), HCl solution at pH = 2.0 (W), or hydroalcoholic solution (50% v/v) acidified at pH 2.0 with HCl (WE) were added to 1.0 g of a freeze-dried sample of each cultivar, and the samples were extracted using an ultrasound-bath Branson model 3800-CPXH (Milan, Italy) at 30 °C (10 cycles/sec) for 15 min at an ultrasonic frequency of 40 kHz. The supernatants were decanted and the solid was removed, while the solution was evaporated, frozen, and freeze-dried to provide a vaporized solid. Wine lees and sample preparation were performed in triplicate.

2.4. Chemical Characterization of Lyophilized Wine Lees

2.4.1. HPLC-DAD Analysis of Lyophilized Wine Lees

High-performance liquid chromatography coupled to diode array detection (HPLC-DAD) analysis of polyphenols was performed by an HPLC 1260 system equipped with a degasser, quaternary pump solvent delivery, thermostatic column compartment, autosampler, and diode array detector (DAD) in a series configuration (Agilent Technologies, Palo Alto, CA, USA). The wine lees extracts were resuspended in 1.5 mL ethanol/water (70:30, v/v), filtered through 0.45 µm pore size regenerated cellulose filters (VWR International Srl, Milano, Italy), and injected onto a reversed stationary phase column, ZORBAX Eclipse Plus C_{18} (250 × 4.6 mm i.d., particle size 5 µm, Agilent Technologies, Palo Alto, CA, USA) protected by a C_{18} Guard Cartridge (4.0 × 2.0 mm i.d., Phenomenex, Torrance, CA, USA). HPLC separation was accomplished by using a binary mobile phase composed of (solvent A) H_2O/formic acid 10% (v/v) and (solvent B) acetonitrile. The following gradient was employed: 0 min, 5% B; 10 min, 13% B; 20 min, 15% B; 30 min, 22% B; 50 min, 22% B; 51 min, 100% B; 61 min, 100% B; and 62 min, 5% B. This was followed by washing and re-equilibrating the column. The column temperature was controlled at 25 °C, and the flow was maintained at 0.7 mL min^{-1}. DAD wavelengths were set at 280, 320, 360, and 520 nm corresponding to the maximum absorptions of flavan-3-ols and benzoic acids, hydroxycinnamic acids, flavonols, and anthocyanins, respectively.

The tentative identification of the compounds in the extracts was achieved by matching the positions of absorption maxima (λ_{max}), absorption spectra profiles, and retention times (RT) with those from commercially available pure standards and studies already reported in the literature for comparable matrices [14,15]. Moreover, the quantification was performed using the calibration curves in the concentration range of 100–0.2 µg mL^{-1} of malvidin-3O-glucoside (R^2 = 0.9983), caffeic acid (R^2 = 0.9988), epicatechin (R^2 = 0.9944), and gallic acid (R^2 = 0.9991).

2.4.2. Fourier Transform Infrared Analysis of Lyophilized Wine Lees

The infrared fingerprints of the lyophilized wine lees samples were acquired by using the Spectrum Two infrared spectrometer (Perkin Elmer Italia Spa, Milan, Italy) supplied with an attenuated total reflection (ATR) accessory with a ZnSe crystal on the sampling flat plate. The ATR detector was cleaned with ethanol after each spectral collection and then dried. The infrared spectrum of the laboratory air was considered as background to check the instrumental status and H_2O/CO_2 interferences. The FTIR spectra of the samples (3 samples for each extraction procedure), placed on the ATR detector, were recorded in triplicate in the range 4000–450 cm^{-1}, with 32 scans and a resolution of 4 cm^{-1}. The fingerprint analysis of samples was focused on a specific wavenumber range, the variables selection was carried out by taking out the spectral window 4000–1850 cm^{-1} [16,17]. The interval 4000–2500 cm^{-1} contained mainly signals of the stretching vibrations due to -OH functions and aromatic bonds (C-H), and information about phenolic compounds was relatively poor. The 2500–1850 cm^{-1} interval also contained no relevant spectral information besides the band corresponding to CO_2. The remaining 1800–450 cm^{-1} interval was set in matrix form and subjected to chemometric modeling after opportune pre-treatment and signal transformation from reflectance to absorbance data.

2.4.3. Polyphenols Total Content

The total phenol content (TPC) of wine lees extracts was determined as described by Spizzirri et al. [18]. In a volumetric flask, 6.0 mL of an aqueous solution of each lees extract, 1.0 mL of Folin–Ciocalteu reagent, and 2.0 mL of Na_2CO_3 solution (2% *w/v*) were added. After two hours at room temperature, the absorbance was spectrophotometrically measured at 720 nm by a Jasco V-530 UV/Vis spectrometer (Jasco, Tokyo, Japan) against a control. This analysis was performed in triplicate and the TPC value was determined by a standard curve constructed using gallic acid (GA) in the range of 8–40 μM (R^2 = 0.9988). The TPC for each extract was expressed as mg GA equivalents per gram of dry matrix (mg GA/g).

2.4.4. Phenolic Acid Content

The phenolic acid content (PAC) of each dry matrix sample was evaluated by a literature procedure with some changes [19]. In a volumetric flask (10.0 mL) 1.0 mL of an aqueous solution of each extract, 1.0 mL of HCl (0.5 mol L^{-1}), 1.0 mL of Arnov's reagent (Na_2MoO_4 and $NaNO_3$ 0.1 mg mL^{-1}), 1.0 mL of NaOH (1.0 mol L^{-1}), and distilled water were added. The absorbance of the solutions was spectrophotometrically determined at 490 nm. This analysis was performed in triplicate and the PAC value was determined by a standard curve constructed using GA in the range of 10–80 μM (R^2 = 0.9973). The PAC for each extract was expressed as mg GA equivalents per gram of dry matrix (mg GA/g).

2.4.5. Flavonoid Content

Flavonoid content (FC) in the lees extracts was spectrophotometrically determined by a literature procedure with some changes and expressing the results as the mass of catechin (CT) per gram of dry sample (mg CT g^{-1}) [20]. Briefly, in a 5.0 mL volumetric flask, 0.5 mL of an aqueous solution of each extract was added to 0.15 mL of $NaNO_2$ (5% *w/v*). After 6 min, 0.3 mL of $AlCl_3$ (6% *w/v*), and after 5 min, 1.0 mL of NaOH 1.0 M were added to the mixture by measuring the absorbance at 510 nm against a control. A calibration curve of CT was built in the concentration range of 10.0–100.0 μM (R^2 = 0.9975).

2.5. Antioxidant Properties

The antioxidant features of the lees extracts were evaluated by specific measurements able to quantify their scavenger activities in organic and aqueous media against hydrophilic and lipophilic radical species, respectively.

The scavenger capacity of the extracts in an organic environment was evaluated by analyzing the concentration decrease in DPPH radical, slightly modifying a literature procedure [21]. Briefly, in a volumetric flask (10 mL) 1.0 mL of hydroalcoholic solutions (50:50 v/v) of each extract, 4.0 mL of a hydroalcoholic mixture (50:50 v/v), and 5.0 mL of a 200 μM ethanolic solution of DPPH were mixed. The mixture was kept at room temperature for 30 min and the residual concentration of the radical species was spectrophotometrically measured at 517 nm. The scavenging capacity of each lees extract against DPPH was expressed in terms of IC_{50}. Ascorbic acid was used as a positive control.

The scavenging activity of the extracts in the aqueous medium was evaluated in terms of the decrease in ABTS radical following a literature procedure with some changes [22]. Briefly, 2.0 mL of the aqueous solution 1.23×10^{-4} mol L^{-1} of the ABTS radical was added to 500 μL of aqueous solutions of each extract, and the mixture was kept in the dark for 6 min. The remaining ABTS concentration was spectrophotometrically evaluated at 734 nm, expressing the scavenging capacity in terms of IC_{50}. Ascorbic acid was used as a positive control.

2.6. *Effect of LWE3 on H_2O_2-Induced Reactive Oxygen Species Production in SH-SY5Y Cells*

2.6.1. Cell Cultures

Human SH-SY5Y neuroblastoma cells (ECACC Cat# 94030304, passages 7–20) were cultured in Dulbecco's modified Eagle's medium (DMEM), supplemented with 10% heat-inactivated fetal bovine serum (FBS), 100 U mL^{-1} penicillin, and 100 μg mL^{-1} streptomycin. Cell cultures were maintained in a humidified atmosphere at 37 °C and 5% CO_2.

2.6.2. Reactive Oxygen Species Detection

Intracellular reactive oxygen species (ROS) formation was investigated by using 2′,7′-dichlorofluorescein diacetate (DCF-DA). SH-SY5Y cells were seeded (2×10^4 cells/well) into a 96-well plate, grown for 24 h under standard conditions, treated with LWE3 (10 and 25 mg mL^{-1}) for 5 h at 37 °C, washed with PBS, and loaded with 10 μM DCF-DA for 30 min at 37 °C. The cells, rinsed twice with PBS, were treated with 2 mM H_2O_2 in DMEM without phenol red and the intracellular fluorescence was read immediately for 60 min with the Thermo Labsystems Synergy HTX reader (BioTek, Winooski, VT, USA) (485 nm excitation, 528 nm emission). The Area Under $Curve_{(0\text{–}60min)}$ of the curve describing changes in fluorescence monitored every 5 min was calculated.

2.7. *Statistical and Chemometric Analysis*

HPLC-DAD analyses and antioxidant tests of the samples were performed in triplicate. Data were expressed as means ± SD and analyzed using the Wilcoxon test. A value of $p < 0.05$ was considered statistically significant. Biological experiment data are shown as the mean ± S.E.M. and analyzed by using ANOVA followed by the Tukey post-test with GraphPad Prism version 5.04 (GraphPad Software Inc., San Diego, CA, USA). In all comparisons, $p < 0.05$ was considered significant.

Principal component analysis (PCA) is an exploratory technique to extract the information contained in complex data systems, such as the spectral fingerprint of samples subjected to instrumental analysis. Samples and spectral variables are projected into the multidimensional space of the new principal components (PCs). PCA was performed to assess the composition differences in terms of the phenolic and flavonoid compounds of the wine lees extracts that can be detected by infrared spectral fingerprinting. The original data consisting of the extracts' analysis were organized into a matrix, in which 108 samples were described by their FTIR-ATR spectra. PCA analysis was elaborated by the Singular Value Decomposition (SVD) algorithm and the full cross-validation (FCV) procedure allowed for the determination of the appropriate number of PCs [23].

Partial least square regression (PLS) is a factor analysis method for the elaboration of the multivariate model with predictive ability, where descriptor variables X and vector y containing the response variables are decomposed in orthogonal factors. Consecutive factors are evaluated until the covariance between descriptors and responses is maximized. PLS modeling is achieved when the factors that explain most of the covariation between both data sets are found. The number of factors is chosen by calculating the figures of the merit root mean square error of validation (RMSEV) and correlation coefficient R^2 [24].

The multivariate analysis of the experimental data was carried out using the software Unscrambler X version 10.5 (CAMO, Trondheim, Norway).

3. Results and Discussion

An eco-friendly procedure was proposed to isolate antioxidant compounds from four different autochthones cultivars (*Magliocco Canino*, *Magliocco Rosato*, *Gaglioppo*, and *Nocera Rosso*) wine lees (Table 1).

Table 1. Ultrasound-assisted extractions of wine lees from different cultivars.

Sample		Extraction Conditions				Yield	
Code	*Mass Dry Extract* (g)	*Solvent*	*Volume* (mL)	*T* (°C)	*t* (min)	*Mass* (g)	%
LE1	1.0	Ethanol	200	30	15	0.063 ± 0.005 [c]	6.3 ± 0.5 [ca]
LEW1	1.0	Water (pH = 2.0)/Ethanol 50:50 *v*/*v*	200	30	15	0.202 ± 0.014 [f]	20.2 ± 1.5 [f]
LW1	1.0	Water (pH = 2.0)	200	30	15	0.358 ± 0.007 [i]	35.8 ± 0.6 [i]
LE2	1.0	Ethanol	200	30	15	0.025 ± 0.001 [a]	2.5 ± 0.1 [a]
LEW2	1.0	Water (pH = 2.0)/Ethanol 50:50 *v*/*v*	200	30	15	0.132 ± 0.006 [d]	13.2 ± 0.5 [d]
LW2	1.0	Water (pH = 2.0)	200	30	15	0.277 ± 0.008 [g]	27.7 ± 0.7 [g]
LE3	1.0	Ethanol	200	30	15	0.040 ± 0.003 [b]	4.0 ± 0.3 [b]
LEW3	1.0	Water (pH = 2.0)/Ethanol 50:50 *v*/*v*	200	30	15	0.137 ± 0.014 [d]	13.7 ± 1.5 [d]
LW3	1.0	Water (pH = 2.0)	200	30	15	0.313 ± 0.007 [h]	31.3 ± 0.6 [h]
LE4	1.0	Ethanol	200	30	15	0.024 ± 0.001 [a]	2.4 ± 0.1 [a]
LEW4	1.0	Water (pH = 2.0)/Ethanol 50:50 *v*/*v*	200	30	15	0.169 ± 0.006 [e]	16.9 ± 0.5 [e]
LW4	1.0	Water (pH = 2.0)	200	30	15	0.278 ± 0.008 [g]	27.8 ± 0.7 [g]

LE1 = lees of *Nocera Rosso* in ethanol; LWE1 = lees of *Nocera Rosso* in water (pH = 2)/ethanol; LW1 = l lees of *Nocera Rosso* in water (pH = 2); LE2 = lees of *Magliocco Rosato* in ethanol; LWE2 = lees of *Magliocco Rosato* in water (pH = 2)/ethanol; LW2 = lees of *Magliocco Rosato* in water (pH = 2); LE3 = lees of *Magliocco Canino* in ethanol; LWE3 = lees of *Magliocco Canino* in water (pH = 2)/ethanol; LW3 = lees of *Magliocco Canino* in water (pH = 2); LE4 = lees of *Gaglioppo* in ethanol; LWE4 = lees of *Gaglioppo* in water (pH = 2)/ethanol; LW4 = lees of *Gaglioppo* in water (pH = 2). Different letters in the same column express significant differences ($p < 0.05$).

Specifically, water (pH = 2.0), ethanol, and a water (pH = 2.0)/ethanol (50/50 *v*/*v*) mixture were employed, while the extractions were performed at low temperature (30 °C) and reduced time (15 min) to preserve the structural integrity of the bioactive compounds. For all the analyzed cultivars, the extraction procedure performed by employing acidic water returned the best results in terms of yield (range 27.7–35.8%), while the hydroalcoholic mixture performance displayed values statistically ($p < 0.05$) reduced (13.2–20.2%). Finally, pure ethanol represented the worst extraction solvent for all the analyzed cultivars (2.4–6.3%). The recorded analytical results clearly highlight that winery by-products are rich in highly hydrophilic compounds, poorly interacting with the organic solvents. In all cases, the cultivar *Nocera Rosso* guarantees the highest yields. Focusing our attention on the phenolic molecules, the wine lees represent a vegetable matrix rich in high-added-value compounds, such as flavonoids, tannins, and phenolic acids [25]. The literature has established that the chemical integrity and biological characteristics of the active molecules can be successfully preserved by employing eco-friendly procedures, considering low temperatures, reduced extraction times, and green solvents [26]. Specifically, bioactive molecules were effectively extracted from the vegetal raw material by employing an ultrasound-assisted methodology, able to decrease both extraction time and temperature, avoiding the loss of the biological properties of the active compounds [27]. The chemical compositions and yields of the extracts are strictly related to the hydrophilicity of the solvent and the solid–solvent ratio. Usually, an increase in the solvent volume ensures a better swelling of the vegetal raw material, making easy the transfer of the polyphenols and enhancing the yield of the extraction procedure [28]. Additionally, the employment of a binary solvent system based on water and eco-friendly organic solvents was suggested by the literature and can guarantee high performance for the extraction of polyphenols from the vegetal matrix [29]. Specifically, the effect of ethanol concentration on the extraction yield was reported in the literature and the highest extraction yields of phenolic molecules were obtained when hydroalcoholic mixtures were used [30] due to the presence of a more polar medium increasing the polyphenol extraction efficiency [31]. In this regard, Kalia et al. found a 50% (v/v) ethanol solution in water to be the most effective for the extraction of phenolics from *Potentilla atrosanguinea* [32].

A detailed characterization of the extracts was performed by HPLC-DAD and FTIR spectroscopy.

3.1. HPLC-DAD Characterization of Polyphenols in Wine Lees Extracts

Free phenolics are among the main constituents of wine lees [14]; therefore, HPLC-DAD analyses were performed to identify and quantify the main polyphenols in the different lees extracts (Figure 1), taking into consideration four wavelengths (280, 320, 360, and 520 nm) at which the absorption of flavan-3-ols and benzoic acids, hydroxycinnamic acids, flavonols, and anthocyanins, respectively, is maximum [33].

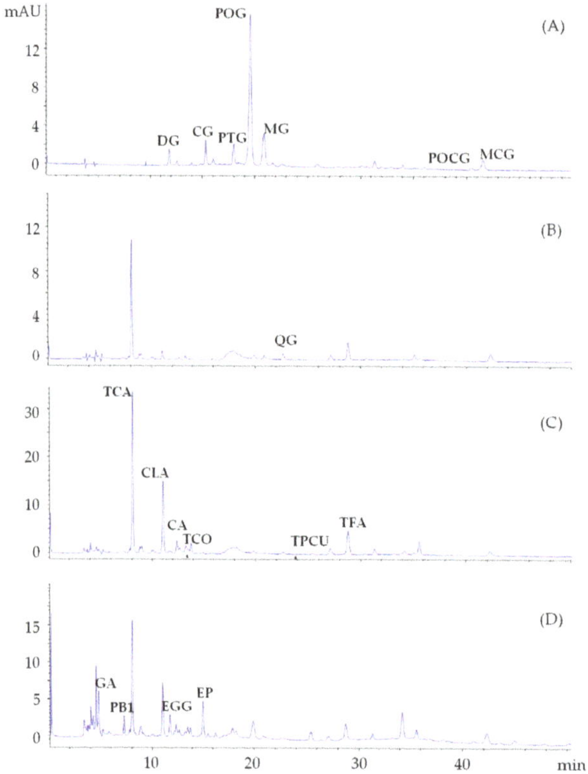

Figure 1. HPLC chromatograms registered at (**A**) 520 nm (DG = delphinidin-3*O*-glucoside; CG = cyanidin-3*O*-glucoside; PTG = petunidin-3*O*-glucoside; POG = peonidin-3*O*-glucoside; MG = malvidin-3*O*-glucoside; POCG = peonidin-3*O*-t-coumaroylglucoside; MCG = malvidin-3*O*-t-coumaroylglucoside), (**B**) 360 nm (QG = quercetin-3*O*-glucoside), (**C**) 320 nm (TCA = *trans*-caftaric acid; CLA = chlorogenic acid; CA = caffeic acid; TCOA = *trans*-coutaric acid; TPCUA = *trans*-p-coumaric acid; TFA = *trans*-ferulic acid), and (**D**) 280 nm (GA = gallic acid; PB1 = procyanidin B1; EG = (−)-epigallocatechin; PB2 = procyanidin B2; (−)-EGG = epigallocatechin gallate; EP = (−)-epicatechin).

Starting from anthocyanins, seven compounds were unequivocally identified—delphinidin-3*O*-glucoside, cyanidin-3*O*-glucoside, petunidin-3*O*-glucoside, peonidin-3*O*-glucoside, and malvidin-3*O*-glucoside—because of the matching with commercial standards, while peonidin-3*O*-*trans*-coumaroylglucoside (POCG) and malvidin-3*O*-*trans*-coumaroylglucoside (MCG) were identified due to their characteristic chromatographic and spectrophotometric behavior many times reported in the literature [14,15]. Conversely, insufficient information was available to correctly identify the other anthocyanin conjugates in the extracts (Figure 1A).

Regarding their content, as expected [14], anthocyanins were more concentrated in lees from red wines (*Nocera Rosso* cv) and particularly in the water extracts due to the high polarity of these compounds; indeed, either the mono-glucoside anthocyanins or the two coumaroyl conjugates (POCG and MCG) were significantly more concentrated in LW1 than LWE1 and LE1 (Table 2).

Chlorogenic acid (CLA), caffeic acid (CA), *trans*-p-coumaric acid (TPCUA), and *trans*-ferulic acid (TFA) were revealed with the help of reference standards (Figure 1C). Generally, they were more concentrated in the hydroalcoholic extracts (LWE); in particular, the highest amounts of CLA (830 mg g^{-1}), CA (180 mg g^{-1}), TPCUA (46 mg g^{-1}), and TFA (150 mg g^{-1}) were quantified in *Magliocco Canino* (LWE3) and *Nocera Rosso* (LWE1), respectively (Table 2). It is worth noting that lower values of CLA, CA, and TPCUA were reported by Landeka et al. in methanolic (pH = 2) extracts of wine lees [34]. However, according to a previous report [14], the main hydroxycinnamic acid present in the extracts was *trans*-caftaric acid (TCA), reaching values of 2100 mg g^{-1} in LWE3 samples; this compound was tentatively identified together with *trans*-coutaric acid (TCOA) based on their typical UV spectra and chromatographic elution [14].

Gallic acid (GA) and five flavan-3-ols, namely procyanidin B_1 (PB_1), (−)-epigallocatechin (EG), procyanidin B_2 (PB_2), (−)-epigallocatechin gallate (EGG), and (−)-epicatechin (EP), showing variegated presence in the extracts, were also recognized (Figure 1D). In agreement with their polarity, the greater amounts of less hydrophilic PB1 (up to 700 mg g^{-1}), PB2 (110 mg g^{-1}), and EP (160 mg g^{-1}) were found in the LWE extracts of *Nocera Rosso* and *Magliocco Canino*, whereas the more hydrophilic GA and EG were more concentrated in water extracts, specifically in LW1 (650 mg g^{-1}) and LW2 (220 mg g^{-1}), respectively. It is worth pointing out that the behavior of EGG was an exception because its values were prevalent in all LE extracts ranging from 820 to 2900 mg g^{-1} (Table 2). Finally, just quercetin-3*O*-glucoside (QG) was identified as a flavonol compound (Figure 1B) at higher levels in LWE1 and LWE3.

Table 2. Content (expressed in mg g^{-1}) of the identified polyphenols into the wine lees extracts.

Compound	RT (min)	LE1	LWE1	LW1	LE2	LWE2	LW2	LE3	LWE3	LW3	LE4	LWE4	LW4
						λ = 280 nm							
Gallic acid	4.733	n.d.	390 ± 60 [b]	650 ± 90 [a]	n.d.	0.39 ± 0.04 [d]	19 ± 3 [c]	n.d.	n.d.	tr	n.d.	34 ± 6 [c]	15 ± 3 [c]
Procyanidin B_1	7.124	tr	180 ± 40 [b]	44 ± 8 [c]	n.d.	n.d.	n.d.	n.d.	700 ± 140 [a]	n.d.	tr	tr	n.d.
Unknown	7.745	n.d.	n.d.	n.d.	n.d.	n.d.	460 ± 90 [ab]	340 ± 60 [b]	620 ± 120 [a]	tr	140 ± 20 [c]	180 ± 40 [c]	400 ± 60 [ab]
(−)-epigallocatechin	8.643	n.d.	n.d.	n.d.	n.d.	n.d.	220 ± 50 [a]	n.d.	n.d.	n.d.	n.d.	160 ± 30 [b]	110 ± 20 [b]
Procyanidin B_2	10.699	n.d.	n.d.	n.d.	n.d.	n.d.	21 ± 3 [b]	n.d.	110 ± 20 [a]	n.d.	tr	tr	12.8 ± 1.9 [b]
Epigallocatechin gallate	11.736	820 ± 160 [c]	250 ± 50 [d]	n.d.	1800 ± 400 [b]	190 ± 40 [d]	n.d.	2900 ± 700 [a]	1200 ± 300 [b]	n.d.	880 ± 190 [c]	260 ± 50 [d]	n.d.
(−)-Epicatechin	13.544	n.d.	120 ± 20 [a]	34 ± 5 [b]	n.d.	n.d.	n.d.	n.d.	n.d.	n.d.	tr	tr	5.5 ± 0.8 [c]
Unknown	14.795	210 ± 40 [b]	370 ± 80 [ab]	110 ± 20 [c]	n.d.	n.d.	n.d.	n.d.	410 ± 90 [a]	n.d.	n.d.	n.d.	n.d.
Unknown	16.224	n.d.	40 ± 7	n.d.	n.d.	n.d.	n.d.	n.d.	n.d.	n.d.	n.d.	n.d.	n.d.
Unknown	25.406	n.d.	160 ± 30	n.d.	n.d.	n.d.	n.d.	n.d.	n.d.	n.d.	n.d.	n.d.	n.d.
						λ = 320 nm							
Unknown	6.363	n.d.	n.d.	n.d.	n.d.	n.d.	n.d.	n.d.	170 ± 40 [a]	n.d.	20 ± 3 [b]	5.8 ± 0.4 [c]	1.37 ± 0.14 [c]
Unknown	7.081	n.d.	n.d.	n.d.	56 ± 12 [a]	42 ± 8 [ab]	26 ± 5 [b]	n.d.	51 ± 10 [a]	n.d.	n.d.	7.2 ± 0.8 [c]	12 ± 2 [bc]
trans-caftaric acid	7.899	710 ± 140 [c]	570 ± 120 [cd]	330 ± 70 [d]	1200 ± 300 [b]	500 ± 100 [cd]	220 ± 40 [b]	170 ± 30 [e]	2100 ± 400 [a]	48 ± 8 [b]	520 ± 90 [cd]	230 ± 40 [de]	250 ± 50 [d]
Unknown	8.380	n.d.	n.d.	87 ± 19 [a]	n.d.	7.8 ± 0.9 [b]	1.9 ± 0.4 [b]	n.d.	n.d.	n.d.	n.d.	tr	n.d.
Unknown	8.625	27 ± 6 [b]	20 ± 4 [b]	20 ± 3 [b]	tr	13 ± 3 [c]	n.d.	n.d.	66 ± 9 [a]	tr	n.d.	tr	3.2 ± 0.7 [d]
Unknown	8.774	29 ± 6 [b]	31 ± 8 [b]	41 ± 7 [ab]	n.d.	21 ± 5 [b]	5.2 ± 1.1 [c]	n.d.	72 ± 14 [a]	tr	n.d.	3.2 ± 0.7 [c]	1.5 ± 0.3 [c]
Chlorogenic acid	10.871	370 ± 70 [b]	290 ± 60 [b]	170 ± 30 [bc]	230 ± 50 [b]	102 ± 14 [c]	60 ± 12 [d]	66 ± 13 [d]	830 ± 140 [a]	27 ± 5 [e]	130 ± 30 [c]	55 ± 10 [d]	51 ± 10 [d]
Unknown	11.41	11 ± 3 [b]	9 ± 2 [b]	11 ± 3 [b]	n.d.	n.d.	n.d.	n.d.	25 ± 6 [a]	n.d.	n.d.	n.d.	n.d.
Unknown	12.403	16 ± 3 [bc]	50 ± 9 [b]	n.d.	tr	4.8 ± 0.9 [c]	8.4 ± 1.5 [c]	n.d.	160 ± 40 [a]	n.d.	n.d.	2.6 ± 0.5 [c]	3.4 ± 0.6 [c]
Unknown	12.691	16 ± 4 [a]	21 ± 5 [a]	n.d.	n.d.	n.d.	n.d.	n.d.	n.d.	n.d.	12 ± 4 [a]	n.d.	n.d.
Caffeic acid	13.097	n.d.	35 ± 8 [b]	25 ± 5 [b]	tr	12 ± 3 [b]	5.6 ± 1.2 [c]	n.d.	180 ± 50 [a]	5.0 ± 1.1 [c]	20 ± 4 [b]	7.5 ± 1.8 [c]	7.5 ± 1.4 [c]
trans-coutaric acid	13.794	10 ± 2 [b]	37 ± 10 [a]	n.d.	n.d.	n.d.	n.d.	n.d.	16 ± 4 [b]	n.d.	n.d.	n.d.	n.d.
trans-p-coumaric acid	27.072	n.d.	46 ± 9	n.d.	n.d.	n.d.	n.d.	n.d.	n.d.	n.d.	n.d.	n.d.	n.d.
trans-ferulic acid	28.728	n.d.	150 ± 30 [a]	n.d.	n.d.	33 ± 9 [b]	n.d.	n.d.	n.d.	n.d.	n.d.	n.d.	n.d.
Unknown	31.306	n.d.	31 ± 7	n.d.	n.d.	n.d.	n.d.	n.d.	n.d.	n.d.	n.d.	n.d.	n.d.
Unknown	34.182	n.d.	18 ± 3	n.d.	n.d.	n.d.	n.d.	n.d.	n.d.	n.d.	n.d.	n.d.	n.d.
Unknown	35.586	n.d.	69 ± 15	n.d.	n.d.	n.d.	n.d.	n.d.	n.d.	n.d.	n.d.	n.d.	n.d.
						λ = 360 nm							
Quercetin-3O-glucoside	22.627	tr	26 ± 6 [b]	n.d.	n.d.	8.3 ± 1.8 [bc]	n.d.	n.d.	90 ± 20 [a]	n.d.	25 ± 5 [b]	4.5 ± 1.0 [c]	4.70 ± 0.8 [c]

Table 2. *Cont.*

Compound	RT (min)	LE1	LWE1	LW1	LE2	LWE2	LW2	LE3	LWE3	LW3	LE4	LWE4	LW4
						λ = 520 nm							
Delphinidin-3*O*-glucoside	11.782	16 ± 4 [b]	n.d.	86 ± 18 [a]	n.d.	n.d.	n.d.	n.d.	n.d.	n.d.	n.d.	n.d.	n.d.
Cyanidin -3*O*-glucoside	15.303	30 ± 7 [b]	12 ± 3 [b]	135 ± 30 [a]	n.d.	n.d.	n.d.	n.d.	n.d.	n.d.	n.d.	n.d.	n.d.
Petunidin -3*O*-glucoside	17.959	52 ± 11 [ab]	20 ± 4 [b]	87 ± 16 [a]	n.d.	n.d.	n.d.	n.d.	n.d.	n.d.	n.d.	n.d.	n.d.
Peonidin-3*O*-glucoside	19.531	400 ± 90 [b]	190 ± 40 [b]	1400 ± 300 [a]	n.d.	16 ± 3 [c]	n.d.	n.d.	n.d.	n.d.	n.d.	n.d.	n.d.
Malvidin-3 *O*-glucoside	20.843	n.d.	9.0 ± 1.9 [b]	330 ± 70 [a]	n.d.	5.3 ± 1.3 [b]	n.d.	n.d.	n.d.	n.d.	n.d.	n.d.	n.d.
Unknown	21.744	n.d.	n.d.	24 ± 7	n.d.	n.d.	n.d.	n.d.	n.d.	n.d.	n.d.	n.d.	n.d.
Unknown	22.549	n.d.	n.d.	33 ± 8	n.d.	n.d.	n.d.	n.d.	n.d.	n.d.	n.d.	n.d.	n.d.
Unknown	25.853	n.d.	n.d.	21 ± 4	n.d.	n.d.	n.d.	n.d.	n.d.	n.d.	n.d.	n.d.	n.d.
Unknown	31.293	n.d.	n.d.	52 ± 12	n.d.	n.d.	n.d.	n.d.	n.d.	n.d.	n.d.	n.d.	n.d.
Unknown	33.991	n.d.	n.d.	22 ± 5	n.d.	n.d.	n.d.	n.d.	n.d.	n.d.	n.d.	n.d.	n.d.
Peonidin-3*O*-*trans*-coumaroylglucoside	40.364	31 ± 7 [a]	11 ± 3 [b]	24 ± 5 [a]	n.d.	n.d.	n.d.	n.d.	n.d.	n.d.	n.d.	n.d.	n.d.
Malvidin-3 *O*-*trans*-coumaroylglucoside	41.482	72 ± 13 [b]	79 ± 15 [b]	110 ± 20 [a]	n.d.	n.d.	n.d.	n.d.	n.d.	n.d.	n.d.	n.d.	n.d.
Total		2820 ± 623	3045 ± 642	3802 ± 749 [b]	3286 ± 741	929 ± 180	1026 ± 196	3476 ± 685 [b]	6800 ± 1445 [a]	75 ± 14	1747 ± 358	919 ± 167	838 ± 145

n.d. = not detected; tr = trace. RT = retention time. LE1 = lees of *Nocera Rosso* in ethanol; LWE1 = lees of *Nocera Rosso* in water/ethanol; LW1 = lees of *Nocera Rosso* in water; LE2 = lees of *Magliocco Rosato* in ethanol; LWE2 = lees of *Magliocco Rosato* in water/ethanol; LW2 = lees of *Magliocco Rosato* in water; LE3 = lees of *Magliocco Canino* in ethanol; LWE3 = lees of *Magliocco Canino* in water/ethanol; LW3 = lees of *Magliocco Canino* in water; LE4 = lees of *Gaglioppo* in ethanol; LWE4 = lees of *Gaglioppo* in water/ethanol; LW4 = lees of *Gaglioppo* in water. Different letters in the same row express significant differences ($p < 0.05$) (Duncan test).

3.2. Characterization of Wine Lees Extracts Via FTIR and PCA

The FTIR fingerprints of the wine lees are shown in Figure 2, where the variation in sample composition due to different cultivars and extraction strategies can be seen. The wavenumber window 1850–450 cm^{-1} presented the characteristic bands of phenolic compounds for all samples. The bands between 1470 and 950 cm^{-1} were due to the methoxy group of some phenolic acids. In the range of 1755–1630 cm^{-1}, phenolic acids can be distinguished from flavonoids by the typical bands of the carboxyl groups, while flavonoid moieties are mainly distinguished by bands associated with benzo-γ-pyrone and benzopyrylium signals in the regions 1650–1400 and 1200–450 cm^{-1} [16].

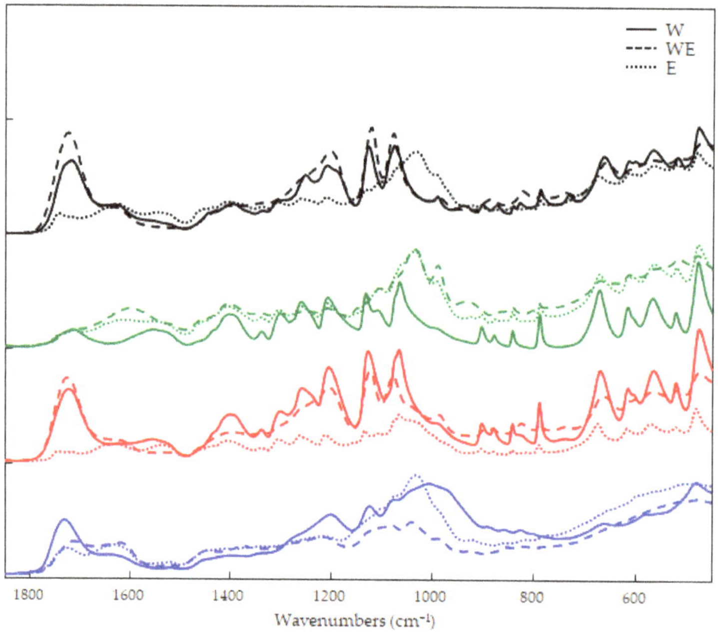

Figure 2. FTIR spectra for the different wine lees extractions: *Nocera Rosso* L1 (blue line), *Magliocco Rosato* L2 (red line), *Magliocco Canino* L3 (green line), and *Gaglioppo* L4 (black line), extracted by water (W, solid line), ethanol (E, dotted line), and hydroalcoholic (WE, dashed line) solutions.

Considering the intense overlapping of the signals from different compound families, a PCA was performed to investigate more specific differences in spectral fingerprints. Figure 3 describes the 3D plot scores by considering the principal components **1**, **2**, and **3** with a total explained variance of 93%. The clustering of the samples was immediately evident, and it was possible to distinguish the samples according to the type of solvent used to extract the phenolic compounds. The only exception was the sample LWE3, which stood out from the others by forming a distinct group. Analyzing the x-loading values, calculated for the processed wave variables with respect to the first three PCs, some characteristic peaks for each extraction technique or cultivar were highlighted.

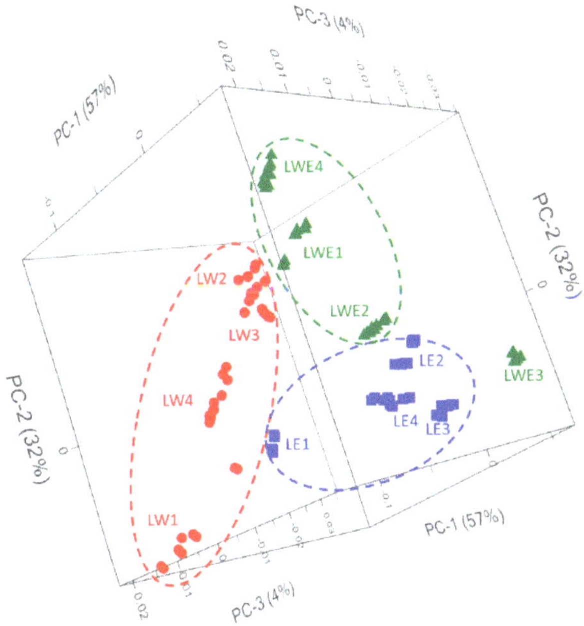

Figure 3. Three-dimensional score plot PC1-3 obtained by the PCA modeling of FTIR data from *Nocera Rosso* L1, *Magliocco Rosato* L2, *Magliocco Canino* L3, and *Gaglioppo* L4 extracts in the range 1850–450 cm^{-1} with a total explained variance of 93%.

PCA processing was able to handle and highlight a relative abundance of useful information in four spectral regions: 1736, 1720, 1390, and 1075 cm^{-1}. The first band at 1736 cm^{-1} was apparently not responsible for the clustering of samples in the 3D-scores space; however, these characteristic bands could be attributed to the anthocyanins such as POCG and MCG, which have been detected for samples belonging to *Nocera Rosso* cultivar (L1) (Table 2 and Figure 2). Signals at 1720, 1120, and 1075 cm^{-1} were able to give enough information to allow the grouping of the samples and especially the clusters consisting of wine lees extracted by ethanol (LE) and hydroalcoholic (LWE) solvents. Chlorogenic acid and esters of caffeic acid showed bands around 1720 cm^{-1}, which could be associated with the vibration of unsaturated aliphatic ester or the carbonyl stretching of protonated carboxylic acid; epigallocatechin gallate (EGG) is characterized by bands in the range 1120–1050 cm^{-1} and showed a band around 800 cm^{-1} [16]. Chromatographic analysis showed a relative abundance in the content of metabolites TCA, CA, CLA, and EGG for samples extracted in ethanol (LE) or hydroalcoholic (LWE) solvents, which was confirmed by evaluating the infrared fingerprint of the sample. The higher levels of these metabolites in the LWE3 sample were also evident in the infrared signals and were able to push the samples out of the LWE cluster by forming a distinct cluster.

3.3. Antioxidant Characterization of the Wine Lees Extracts

The total polyphenol content of wine lees extracts was accomplished according to the Folin–Ciocalteu methodology and the obtained results are reported in Table 3. The literature data reported that the phenolic profile in lees is strictly related to the type of crushed grapes and other factors that are present during vinification [8].

Table 3. Total phenolic content, phenolic acid content, flavonoid content, and antioxidant activity of the extracts from wine lees.

Sample	TPC (mg *GA* g^{-1} *extract*)	PAC (mg *GA* g^{-1} *extract*)	FC (mg *CT* g^{-1} *extract*)	IC_{50} (mg mL^{-1})	
				DPPH	*ABTS*
LE1	18.94 ± 0.37 [e]	5.89 ± 0.15 [f]	9.54 ± 0.17 [f]	0.470 ± 0.017 [c]	0.770 ± 0.027 [d]
LWE1	20.01 ± 0.46 [f]	6.58 ± 0.16 [g]	10.89 ± 0.26 [g]	0.490 ± 0.022 [c]	0.690 ± 0.025 [c]
LW1	27.23 ± 0.49 [h]	10.25 ± 0.49 [l]	18.15 ± 0.38 [l]	0.608 ± 0.019 [e]	0.500 ± 0.019 [b]
LE2	24.25 ± 0.47 [g]	9.14 ± 0.17 [h]	13.23 ± 0.17 [h]	0.457 ± 0.022 [c]	0.790 ± 0.027 [d]
LWE2	11.02 ± 0.36 [c]	3.12 ± 0.08 [c]	7.59 ± 0.16 [d]	0.643 ± 0.025 [e]	0.710 ± 0.030 [c]
LW2	10.89 ± 0.29 [c]	3.26 ± 0.10 [c]	8.25 ± 0.19 [e]	0.803 ± 0.038 [f]	0.680 ± 0.032 [c]
LE3	23.72 ± 0.27 [g]	8.89 ± 0.17 [h]	16.24 ± 0.26 [i]	0.419 ± 0.013 [a]	0.700 ± 0.027 [c]
LWE3	49.56 ± 0.56 [i]	22.67 ± 0.56 [i]	20.15 ± 0.32 [m]	0.395 ± 0.016 [a]	0.451 ± 0.015 [a]
LW3	4.61 ± 0.09 [a]	1.58 ± 0.07 [a]	1.54 ± 0.07 [a]	1.360 ± 0.067 [h]	1.480 ± 0.049 [g]
LE4	12.24 ± 0.22 [d]	5.54 ± 0.12 [e]	6.25 ± 0.22 [c]	0.560 ± 0.028 [d]	0.850 ± 0.032 [ef]
LWE4	11.35 ± 0.26 [c]	2.54 ± 0.08 [b]	8.01 ± 0.16 [e]	0.630 ± 0.026 [e]	0.800 ± 0.026 [de]
LW4	10.29 ± 0.23 [b]	2.65 ± 0.07 [b]	5.23 ± 0.13 [b]	1.080 ± 0.050 [g]	0.912 ± 0.035 [f]
Positive control					
Ascorbic acid				0.017 ± 0.002	0.050 ± 0.002

TPC = total phenolic content; PAC = phenolic acid content; FC = flavonoid content; GA = gallic acid; CT = catechin; DPPH = (2.2-diphenyl-1-picrylhydrazyl); ABTS = (2.2′-azinobis (3-ethylbenzothiazoline-6-sulphonic acid)); LE1 = lees of *Nocera Rosso* in ethanol; LWE1 = lees of *Nocera Rosso* in water (pH = 2)/ethanol; LW1 = l lees of *Nocera Rosso* in water (pH = 2); LE2 = lees of *Magliocco Rosato* in ethanol; LWE2 = lees of *Magliocco Rosato* in water (pH = 2)/ethanol; LW2 = lees of *Magliocco Rosato* in water (pH = 2); LE3 = lees of *Magliocco Canino* in ethanol; LWE3 = lees of *Magliocco Canino* in water (pH = 2)/ethanol; LW3 = lees of *Magliocco Canino* in water (pH = 2); LE4 = lees of *Gaglioppo* in ethanol; LWE4 = lees of *Gaglioppo* in water (pH = 2)/ethanol; LW4 = lees of *Gaglioppo* in water (pH = 2). Each measurement was carried out in triplicate and data are expressed as means (±SD). Different letters express significant differences ($p < 0.05$).

The recorded data displayed as the cultivar is an important parameter to be considered and deeply influences the performance of the extraction mixture. Ethanolic extracts returned the highest TPC values for *Magliocco Rosato* and *Magliocco Canino* cultivars, while the acidic water extraction of *Nocera Rosso* significantly guaranteed the best performance. Finally, the hydroalcoholic extract of *Magliocco Canino* displayed the highest TPC value (49.56 mg GA per g of extract) according to the data recovered by HPLC-DAD analysis. Recorded TPC value is in the same order of magnitude reported in the literature and related to wine lees deriving from different grape varieties and performing the extraction by several analytical methodologies. In particular, solvents with different polarities were also evaluated in the analyses of *Tempranillo* wines lees, returning TPC values in the range of 26 (acetone)-254 (ethanol/water 25:75 v/v) mg GA per gram of dry matter [35], according to another study performed a conventional extraction procedure and reporting a phenolic concentration equal to 547 mg GA per gram of dry matter [7]. Additionally, the TPC values of different extracts deriving from various red wines (*Cabernet Sauvignon*, *Cabernet Franc*, *Merlot*) by ultrasound were in the range of 44.02–58.71 mg GA per gram of dry extract [30], while other studies displayed decreased values of 23.2–30.9 mg GA per gram of dry extract [34,36]. On the other hand, these partial discrepancies can be largely due to the wine lees types, strictly related to the vinification process and grape variety as well as the extraction procedure.

LWE3 also showed the greatest concentration of flavonoid (20.15 mg GA per g of extract) and phenolic acid (22.67 mg CT per g of extract) compounds. Concerning the phenolic acids, *p*-coumaric and caffeic acids as well as their derivatives such as *trans*-coutaric acid and *trans*-caftaric acid, respectively, have been found in wine lees samples, according to the literature data reporting *trans*-caftaric acid as the predominant compounds in both *Vitis vinifera* and *non-vinifera* types [36].

Polyphenol moieties display numerous beneficial effects such as a remarkable scavenger ability against various radical species [37]. As antioxidant bio-compounds explain their action through different mechanisms, usually, various tests should be explored to fully estimate the antioxidant capacity of a compound mixture [38]. For this reason, the antioxidant profile of the extracts was evaluated in terms of scavenger activity both in aqueous and organic environments against DPPH and ABTS radicals, respectively. The capacity of the extracts to inhibit the lipophilic DPPH radical, expressed in terms of IC_{50} (mg mL^{-1}), is reported in Table 3. The recorded results are in the range of 0.395–1.360 mg mL^{-1} and LWE3 appears as the more active extract. This trend was also established in the hydrophilic environment against the ABTS radical (IC_{50} for LWE3 equal to 0.451 mg mL^{-1}), highlighting a greater scavenger effect of the extract in the organic environment with respect to the aqueous one. In general, scavenger activity measurements confirmed the TPC, PAC, and FC values. Specifically, a direct correlation between the antioxidant capacity of the extracts was carried out, verifying the existence of a direct dependence between TPC value and the scavenger activity, considering the sum of the contributions of the various antioxidant compounds in the sample and their possible synergistic effects.

3.4. *Effect of LWE3 on H_2O_2-Induced ROS Production in SH-SY5Y Cells*

In SH-SY5Y cells, treatment with H_2O_2 markedly increased the intracellular level of ROS (Figure 4). However, pre-treatment with LWE3 significantly prevented ROS production in a concentration-dependent manner, suggesting that the extract protected neuroblastoma cells against oxidative stress damage.

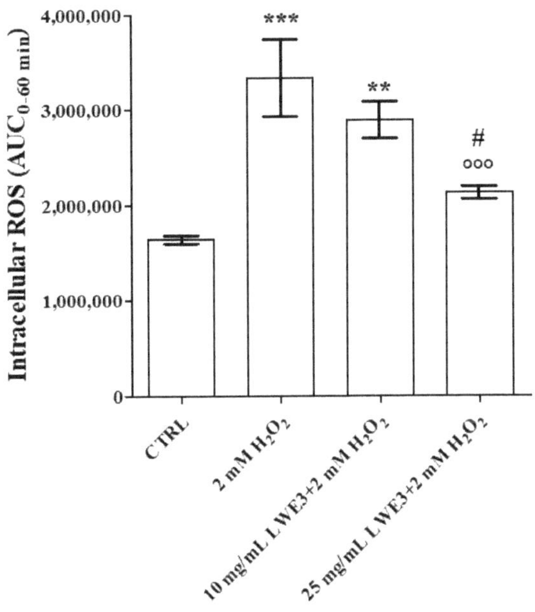

Figure 4. Total amount of intracellular reactive oxygen species in the control condition (CTRL) in presence of 2 mM H_2O_2, of 10 mg mL^{-1} LWE3 plus 2 mM H_2O_2 and of 25 mg mL^{-1} LWE3 plus 2 mM H_2O_2 during 60 min, expressed as Area Under $Curve_{(0–60\ min)}$. Data are reported as the mean ± S.E.M. of at least 3 independent experiments. LWE3 = lees of *Magliocco Canino* in water (pH = 2)/ethanol. *** $p < 0.001$ vs. CTRL, ** $p < 0.01$ vs. CTRL, °°° $p < 0.001$ vs. H_2O_2, # $p < 0.05$ vs. 10 mg mL^{-1} LWE3 + 2 mM H_2O_2, ANOVA followed by Tukey post-test.

3.5. *Relationship between Antioxidant Properties and Metabolite Composition*

In the present study, the PLS algorithm was applied to study the relationship between antioxidant properties and the metabolite composition of the extracts. The root mean square error of validation (RMSEV) and the correlation coefficient R^2 were used to evaluate the fitting of the multivariate models with the experimental results. Usually, an R^2 value higher than 0.5 is indicative of an acceptable model and a value over 0.8 proves an excellent correlation [39].

The chemical composition detected by HPLC analysis was used as a descriptor variable (matrix X) for each sample, and two different response vectors, y_{DPPH} and y_{ABTS}, consisting of the respective IC_{50} values evaluated for each sample, were selected. All variables used in the building of the model were re-scaled and standardized prior to elaboration; they were normalized by dividing by the standard deviation value in the original scale and in logarithmic form.

First, multivariate calibration built two PLS models with very low predictive performance with R^2 below 0.6 for both y_{DPPH} and y_{ABTS}. These models were used as an initial screening of the correlation between the compound concentrations and the antioxidant power of the extracts. After evaluating the regression coefficients of each variable, it was possible to determine which of them provided the most information in the calibration of the models. Figure 5 shows the weighted regression coefficients (Bw) plot. Regression coefficients describe the relationship between all the descriptors (x-variables) and a given response (y-variable). Bw coefficients provide information about the importance of the x-variables: a high Bw value means an important role in the building of the models, while x-variables with small coefficients may be negligible; a positive coefficient shows a direct proportionality with the response, and a negative coefficient shows an indirect proportionality. The most important variables were TCA, CLA, and EGG for the prediction of y_{DPPH} and TCA and CLA for the prediction of y_{ABTS}.

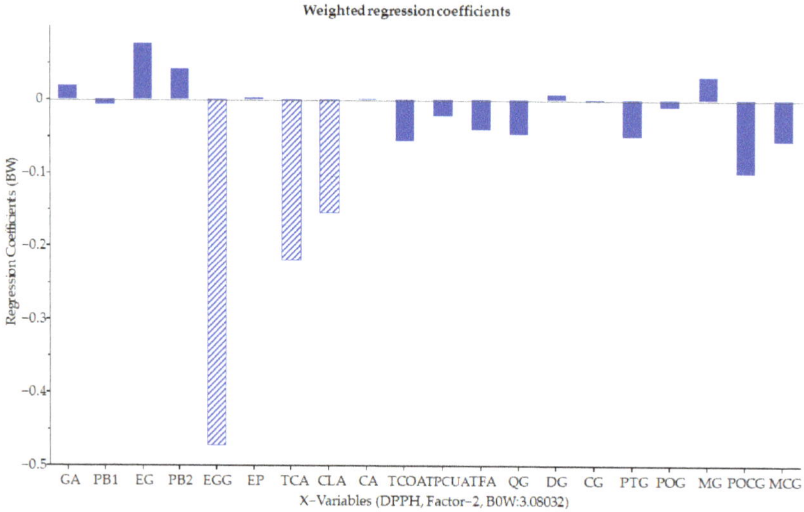

Figure 5. The weighted regression coefficients (Bw) were calculated for all the x-variables used in PLS calibration for the prediction of DPPH IC_{50} (y_{DPPH}).

A new calibration procedure was thus optimized by considering just the variables TCA, CLA, and EGG. A significant improvement in the statistical parameters was observed when the concentration levels of phenolic acids and flavonoids were considered on the logarithmic scale. The PLS model built to predict the DPPH IC_{50} gave good statistical parameters with a correlation coefficient R^2 value of 0.932 and a prediction error RMSEV of 0.023 by using three factors, while ABTS IC_{50} was correlated with R^2 of 0.824 an RMSEV of 0.064 by using two factors.

4. Conclusions

In this study, wine lees from different cultivars (*Magliocco Canino*, *Magliocco Rosato*, *Gaglioppo*, and *Nocera Rosso*) were extracted with an ultrasound-assisted method using an *eco*-friendly procedure employing low temperature and reduced time and ethanol and water as solvents to obtain polyphenolic fractions deeply analyzed by HPLC-DAD and FTIR techniques. Specifically, anthocyanins were more concentrated in lees from red winemaking (*Nocera Rosso cv*) and particularly in the water extracts due to the high polarity of these compounds, while the main hydroxycinnamic acid present in the extracts was *trans*-caftaric acid, reaching values of 2100 mg g^{-1} in LWE3 samples. Additionally, colorimetric tests allowed for the evaluation of total polyphenol, phenolic acid, and flavonoid contents, while radical scavenging assays were performed to quantify the antioxidant performances of the extracts, both in organic and aqueous media, against DPPH and ABTS radicals, respectively. The combined use of multivariate tools and FTIR spectral analysis proved very effective in characterizing samples from different cultivars and extraction procedures, grouping samples with respect to their spectral fingerprint, and highlighting the correspondence between spectral bands and metabolite abundance in extracts. The collected data confirmed the spectroscopic recovery, highlighting LWE3 as representing the higher-performing extract. Cellular (SH-SY5Y cells) antioxidant assays were performed on the best extract (LWE3) to confirm its biological performance against radical species.

The chemometric processing of the qualitative–quantitative experimental data allowed the correlations between chemical composition and antioxidant features of the different wine lees extracts to be found. PLS optimization identified the metabolites responsible for the detected antioxidant effects, and two PLS models were built to predict the IC_{50} values of DPPH and ABTS radicals with good predictive ability by using the concentration values of the compounds TCA, CLA, and EGG.

Further studies will employ the best extract to prepare innovative high-value functional foods. Alternative antioxidant extracts will be involved in a radical conjugation process to synthesize more stable macromolecular systems able to be used as an additive in the food industry.

Author Contributions: Conceptualization and design: U.G.S.; methodology: U.G.S., M.D.L., S.S. and P.C.; validation: U.G.S., D.R. and P.C.; formal analysis, U.G.S., M.D.L., G.I., B.G. and P.C.; investigation: U.G.S., S.S., M.D.L. and P.C.; resources: D.R., M.L.C., M.D.L. and F.A.; data curation: U.G.S., S.S., P.C. and M.D.L.; writing—original draft preparation: U.G.S., M.D.L., G.I., P.C. and S.S.; writing—review and editing: U.G.S., D.R., F.A., G.I., M.L.C. and M.D.L.; visualization: M.D.L. and P.C.; supervision: D.R. and F.A.; funding acquisition: M.D.L., P.C., D.R., S.S. and F.A. All authors contributed experimental assistance and intellectual input to this study. All authors have read and agreed to the published version of the manuscript.

Funding: Pasquale Crupi is funded by Research for Innovation REFIN-POR Puglia FESR-FSE 2014/2020.

Institutional Review Board Statement: Not applicable.

Informed Consent Statement: Not applicable.

Data Availability Statement: The data presented in this study are available on request from the corresponding author. The data are not publicly available as they contain information that could compromise the privacy of research participants.

Conflicts of Interest: The authors declare no conflict of interest.

References

1. Moscovici, D.; Gow, J.; Alonso Ugaglia, A.; Rezwanul, R.; Valenzuela, L.; Mihailescu, R. Consumer Preferences for Organic Wine-Global Analysis of People and Place. *J. Clean Prod.* **2022**, *368*, 133215. [CrossRef]
2. Sellers, R.; Alampi-Sottini, V. The Influence of Size on Winery Performance: Evidence from Italy. *Wine Econ. Policy* **2016**, *5*, 33–41. [CrossRef]
3. Lavelli, V.; Sri Harsha, P.S.C.; Ferranti, P.; Scarafoni, A.; Iametti, S. Grape Skin Phenolics as Inhibitors of Mammalian α-Glucosidase and α-Amylase-Effect of Food Matrix and Processing on Efficacy. *Food Funct.* **2016**, *7*, 1655–1663. [CrossRef] [PubMed]

4. González-Paramás, A.M.; Esteban-Ruano, S.; Santos-Buelga, C.; de Pascual-Teresa, S.; Rivas-Gonzalo, J.C. Flavanol Content and Antioxidant Activity in Winery Byproducts. *J. Agric. Food Chem.* **2004**, *52*, 234–238. [CrossRef] [PubMed]
5. Restuccia, D.; Giorgi, G.; Gianfranco Spizzirri, U.; Sciubba, F.; Capuani, G.; Rago, V.; Carullo, G.; Aiello, F. Autochthonous White Grape Pomaces as Bioactive Source for Functional Jams. *Int. J. Food Sci. Technol.* **2019**, *54*, 1313–1320. [CrossRef]
6. Ruggieri, L.; Cadena, E.; Martínez-Blanco, J.; Gasol, C.M.; Rieradevall, J.; Gabarrell, X.; Gea, T.; Sort, X.; Sánchez, A. Recovery of Organic Wastes in the Spanish Wine Industry. Technical, Economic and Environmental Analyses of the Composting Process. *J. Clean Prod.* **2009**, *17*, 830–838. [CrossRef]
7. Pérez-Serradilla, J.A.; Luque de Castro, M.D. Microwave-Assisted Extraction of Phenolic Compounds from Wine Lees and Spray-Drying of the Extract. *Food Chem.* **2011**, *124*, 1652–1659. [CrossRef]
8. Jara-Palacios, M.J. Wine Lees as a Source of Antioxidant Compounds. *Antioxidants* **2019**, *8*, 45. [CrossRef]
9. Barcia, M.T.; Pertuzatti, P.B.; Gómez-Alonso, S.; Godoy, H.T.; Hermosín-Gutiérrez, I. Phenolic Composition of Grape and Winemaking By-Products of Brazilian Hybrid Cultivars BRS Violeta and BRS Lorena. *Food Chem.* **2014**, *159*, 95–105. [CrossRef]
10. Irimia, L.M.; Patriche, C.V.; Murariu, O.C. The Impact of Climate Change on Viticultural Potential and Wine Grape Varieties of a Temperate Wine Growing Region. *Appl. Ecol. Environ. Res.* **2018**, *16*, 2663–2680. [CrossRef]
11. Versari, A.; Castellari, M.; Spinabelli, U.; Galassi, S. Recovery of Tartaric Acid from Industrial Enological Wastes. *J. Chem. Technol. Biotechnol.* **2001**, *76*, 485–488. [CrossRef]
12. Alarcón, M.; López-Viñas, M.; Pérez-Coello, M.S.; Díaz-Maroto, M.C.; Alañón, M.E.; Soriano, A. Effect of Wine Lees as Alternative Antioxidants on Physicochemical and Sensorial Composition of Deer Burgers Stored during Chilled Storage. *Antioxidants* **2020**, *9*, 687. [CrossRef] [PubMed]
13. Carullo, G.; Durante, M.; Sciubba, F.; Restuccia, D.; Spizzirri, U.G.; Ahmed, A.; di Cocco, M.E.; Saponara, S.; Aiello, F.; Fusi, F. Vasoactivity of Mantonico and Pecorello Grape Pomaces on Rat Aorta Rings: An Insight into Nutraceutical Development. *J. Funct. Foods* **2019**, *57*, 328–334. [CrossRef]
14. Matos, M.S.; Romero-Díez, R.; Álvarez, A.; Bronze, M.R.; Rodríguez-Rojo, S.; Mato, R.B.; Cocero, M.J.; Matias, A.A. Polyphenol-Rich Extracts Obtained from Winemakingwaste Streams as Natural Ingredients with Cosmeceutical Potential. *Antioxidants* **2019**, *8*, 355. [CrossRef]
15. Alba, V.; Natrella, G.; Gambacorta, G.; Crupi, P.; Coletta, A. Effect of over Crop and Reduced Yield by Cluster Thinning on Phenolic and Volatile Compounds of Grapes and Wines of 'Sangiovese' Trained to Tendone. *J. Sci. Food Agric.* **2022**, *102*, 7155–7163. [CrossRef]
16. Abbas, O.; Compère, G.; Larondelle, Y.; Pompeu, D.; Rogez, H.; Baeten, V. Phenolic Compound Explorer: A Mid-Infrared Spectroscopy Database. *Vib. Spectrosc.* **2017**, *92*, 111–118. [CrossRef]
17. Ceramella, J.; la Torre, C.; De Luca, M.; Iacopetta, D.; Fazio, A.; Catalano, A.; Ragno, G.; Longo, P.; Sinicropi, M.S.; Rosano, C. Exploring the Anticancer and Antioxidant Properties of *Vicia faba* L. Pods Extracts, a Promising Source of Nutraceuticals. *PeerJ* **2022**, *10*, e13683. [CrossRef]
18. Spizzirri, U.G.; Carullo, G.; de Cicco, L.; Crispini, A.; Scarpelli, F.; Restuccia, D.; Aiello, F. Synthesis and Characterization of a (+)-Catechin and L-(+)-Ascorbic Acid Cocrystal as a New Functional Ingredient for Tea Drinks. *Heliyon* **2019**, *5*, e02291. [CrossRef] [PubMed]
19. Spizzirri, U.G.; Caputo, P.; Oliviero Rossi, C.; Crupi, P.; Muraglia, M.; Rago, V.; Malivindi, R.; Clodoveo, M.L.; Restuccia, D.; Aiello, F. A Tara Gum/Olive Mill Wastewaters Phytochemicals Conjugate as a New Ingredient for the Formulation of an Antioxidant-Enriched Pudding. *Foods* **2022**, *11*, 158. [CrossRef] [PubMed]
20. Spizzirri, U.G.; Carullo, G.; Aiello, F.; Paolino, D.; Restuccia, D. Valorisation of Olive Oil Pomace Extracts for a Functional Pear Beverage Formulation. *Int. J. Food Sci. Technol.* **2021**, *56*, 5497–5505. [CrossRef]
21. Spizzirri, U.G.; Abduvakhidov, A.; Caputo, P.; Crupi, P.; Muraglia, M.; Rossi, C.O.; Clodoveo, M.L.; Aiello, F.; Restuccia, D. Kefir Enriched with Carob (*Ceratonia siliqua* L.) Leaves Extract as a New Ingredient during a Gluten-Free Bread-Making Process. *Fermentation* **2022**, *8*, 305. [CrossRef]
22. Carullo, G.; Spizzirri, U.G.; Montopoli, M.; Cocetta, V.; Armentano, B.; Tinazzi, M.; Sciubba, F.; Giorgi, G.; Enrica Di Cocco, M.; Bohn, T.; et al. Milk Kefir Enriched with Inulin-Grafted Seed Extract from White Wine Pomace: Chemical Characterisation, Antioxidant Profile and in Vitro Gastrointestinal Digestion. *Int. J. Food Sci. Technol.* **2022**, *57*, 4086–4095. [CrossRef]
23. Spatari, C.; De Luca, M.; Ioele, G.; Ragno, G. A Critical Evaluation of the Analytical Techniques in the Photodegradation Monitoring of Edible Oils. *LWT* **2017**, *76*, 147–155. [CrossRef]
24. De Luca, M.; Ioele, G.; Spatari, C.; Caruso, L.; Galasso, M.P.; Ragno, G. Evaluation of Human Breastmilk Adulteration by Combining Fourier Transform Infrared Spectroscopy and Partial Least Square Modeling. *Food Sci. Nutr.* **2019**, *7*, 2194–2201. [CrossRef]
25. Chang, Y.; Shi, X.; He, F.; Wu, T.; Jiang, L.; Normakhamatov, N.; Sharipov, A.; Wang, T.; Wen, M.; Aisa, H.A. Valorization of Food Processing Waste to Produce Valuable Polyphenolics. *J. Agric. Food Chem.* **2022**, *70*, 8855–8870. [CrossRef]
26. Cañadas, R.; González-Miquel, M.; González, E.J.; Díaz, I.; Rodríguez, M. Overview of Neoteric Solvents as Extractants in Food Industry: A Focus on Phenolic Compounds Separation from Liquid Streams. *Food Res.* **2020**, *136*, 109558. [CrossRef] [PubMed]
27. Montenegro-Landívar, M.F.; Tapia-Quirós, P.; Vecino, X.; Reig, M.; Valderrama, C.; Granados, M.; Cortina, J.L.; Saurina, J. Fruit and Vegetable Processing Wastes as Natural Sources of Antioxidant-Rich Extracts: Evaluation of Advanced Extraction Technologies by Surface Response Methodology. *J. Environ. Chem. Eng.* **2021**, *9*, 105330. [CrossRef]

28. Clodoveo, M.L.; Crupi, P.; Muraglia, M.; Corbo, F. Ultrasound Assisted Extraction of Polyphenols from Ripe Carob Pods (*Ceratonia siliqua* L.): Combined Designs for Screening and Optimizing the Processing Parameters. *Foods* **2022**, *11*, 284. [CrossRef] [PubMed]
29. Rached, I.; Barros, L.; Fernandes, I.P.; Santos-Buelga, C.; Rodrigues, A.E.; Ferchichi, A.; Barreiro, M.F.; Ferreira, I.C.F.R. *Ceratonia siliqua* L. Hydroethanolic Extract Obtained by Ultrasonication: Antioxidant Activity, Phenolic Compounds Profile and Effects in Yogurts Functionalized with Their Free and Microencapsulated Forms. *Food Funct.* **2016**, *7*, 1319–1328. [CrossRef] [PubMed]
30. Tao, Y.; Wu, D.; Zhang, Q.A.; Sun, D.W. Ultrasound-Assisted Extraction of Phenolics from Wine Lees: Modeling, Optimization and Stability of Extracts during Storage. *Ultrason. Sonochem.* **2014**, *21*, 706–715. [CrossRef]
31. de Bruno, A.; Romeo, R.; Fedele, F.L.; Sicari, A.; Piscopo, A.; Poiana, M. Antioxidant Activity Shown by Olive Pomace Extracts. *J. Environ. Sci. Health B* **2018**, *53*, 526–533. [CrossRef] [PubMed]
32. Kalia, K.; Sharma, K.; Singh, H.P.; Singh, B. Effects of Extraction Methods on Phenolic Contents and Antioxidant Activity in Aerial Parts of Potentilla Atrosanguinea Lodd. and Quantification of Its Phenolic Constituents by RP-HPLC. *J. Agric. Food Chem.* **2008**, *56*, 10129–10134. [CrossRef]
33. Crupi, P.; Antonacci, D.; Savino, M.; Genghi, R.; Perniola, R.; Coletta, A. Girdling and Gibberellic Acid Effects on Yield and Quality of a Seedless Red Table Grape for Saving Irrigation Water Supply. *Eur. J. Agron.* **2016**, *80*, 21–31. [CrossRef]
34. Jurcevic, I.L.; Dora, M.; Guberovic, I.; Petras, M.; Brncic, S.R.; Dikic, D. Polyphenols from Wine Lees as a Novel Functional Bioactive Compound in the Protection against Oxidative Stress and Hyperlipidaemia. *Food Technol. Biotechnol.* **2017**, *55*, 109–116. [CrossRef]
35. Romero-Díez, R.; Rodríguez-Rojo, S.; Cocero, M.J.; Duarte, C.M.M.; Matias, A.A.; Bronze, M.R. Phenolic Characterization of Aging Wine Lees: Correlation with Antioxidant Activities. *Food Chem.* **2018**, *259*, 188–195. [CrossRef] [PubMed]
36. Reis, G.M.; Faccin, H.; Viana, C.; da Rosa, M.B.; de Carvalho, L.M. *Vitis vinifera* L. Cv Pinot Noir Pomace and Lees as Potential Sources of Bioactive Compounds. *Int. J. Food Sci. Nutr.* **2016**, *67*, 789–796. [CrossRef]
37. Ruskovska, T.; Maksimova, V.; Milenkovic, D. Polyphenols in Human Nutrition: From the in Vitro Antioxidant Capacity to the Beneficial Effects on Cardiometabolic Health and Related Inter-Individual Variability-An Overview and Perspective. *Br. J. Nutr.* **2020**, *123*, 241–254. [CrossRef]
38. Pellegrini, N.; Serafini, M.; Colombi, B.; del Rio, D.; Salvatore, S.; Bianchi, M.; Brighenti, F. Total Antioxidant Capacity of Plant Foods, Beverages and Oils Consumed in Italy Assessed by Three Different in Vitro Assays. *J. Nutr.* **2003**, *133*, 2812–2819. [CrossRef]
39. Ioele, G.; De Luca, M.; Oliverio, F.; Ragno, G. Prediction of Photosensitivity of 1,4-Dihydropyridine Antihypertensives by Quantitative Structure-Property Relationship. *Talanta* **2009**, *79*, 1418–1424. [CrossRef]

antioxidants

MDPI

Article

The Utilization of an Aloe Vera Rind By-Product: Deep Eutectic Solvents as Eco-Friendly and Recyclable Extraction Media of Polyphenolic Compounds

Georgia D. Ioannou [1], Katerina A. Ioannou [1], Atalanti Christou [1], Ioannis J. Stavrou [2] and Constantina P. Kapnissi-Christodoulou [1,*]

1 Department of Chemistry, University of Cyprus, 1678 Nicosia, Cyprus; gioann02@ucy.ac.cy (G.D.I.); ioannou.katerina@ucy.ac.cy (K.A.I.); achris54@ucy.ac.cy (A.C.)
2 Department of Life Sciences, European University Cyprus, 2404 Nicosia, Cyprus; io.stavrou@euc.ac.cy
* Correspondence: ckapni1@ucy.ac.cy

Abstract: In this study, an optimized environmentally friendly procedure was employed to enhance the sustainable utilization of phenolic antioxidants derived from aloe vera rind by-products. The procedure involved the application of ultrasound-assisted extraction (UAE) in combination with deep eutectic solvents (DESs). Eleven different DESs and three conventional solvents were employed as extraction media for polyphenolic compounds. Choline chloride–citric acid (ChCl-CA) was selected as the most suitable extractant, considering its extraction efficiency in relation to the total phenolic content. The operating conditions of UAE were optimized and modeled by the use of response surface methodology in order to maximize the yield of total phenolics and antioxidant capacity. The optimal operational parameters for the UAE procedure were determined to be 16.5 min, 74% (*v*/*v*) DES in water, and a solvent-to-solid ratio equal to 192. HPLC analysis, which was performed on the optimum extract, revealed significant levels of phenolics present in the aloe rind. Efficient recovery of the extracted antioxidants was obtained by the use of solid-phase extraction (SPE) and polyamide cartridges. The ChCl-CA DES exhibited excellent recycling capability with a yield of over 90% through SPE. Finally, the greenness of the method was evaluated using the green AGREE and AGREEprep metrics. The results highlighted the sustainability and the greenness of the proposed extraction procedure for the aloe by-product.

Keywords: *Aloe barbadensis* Miller; aloe vera rind; ultrasound-assisted extraction; response surface methodology (RSM); deep eutectic solvents (DESs); green metrics; by-product; agrowaste; polyphenols; antioxidants

1. Introduction

The aloe vera plant, scientifically known as *Aloe barbadensis* Miller, is widely known for its remarkable pharmacological and therapeutic properties. Some of its beneficial properties include wound healing, anti-inflammatory and antibacterial effects, and laxative and antioxidant activities [1–4]. All these have led to the widespread utilization of the aloe plant and particularly its gel, in various industries, such as pharmaceuticals, food, and cosmetics [5]. Statistical analysis of economic data reveals a consistent upward trend in the revenue generated by the aloe industry [5].

Aloe vera belongs to the Liliacceae family, particularly the Aloe genus, which contains more than 400 species [6]. The aloe plant is a perennial succulent xerophyte with turgid pointed green leaves joined at the stem in a rosette pattern [7]. The leaf of aloe consists of three different layers: the inner gel, the latex, and the outer green rind. Aloe gel is the most extensively studied part of the plant due to its therapeutic properties, which are attributed to bioactive compounds. Aloe latex, a yellow liquid, is rich in anthrones, which are responsible for the laxative effect of the plant. The outer protective layer of the plant is a green thick rind, which is considered agrowaste and a by-product in aloe-related industries. The aloe rind corresponds to a significant percentage of the aloe leaves' total weight, ranging from 20 to 30% [8].

In recent decades, the scientific community has aimed to increase the valorization of agricultural by-products and minimize waste generation in productive processes due to environmental issues [9,10]. A number of studies have recently reported the recovery of valuable bioactive compounds from agrowastes as renewable plant materials [11–13]. A significant example involves the aloe rind, which was found to contain significant amounts of polyphenolic compounds [14,15].

Polyphenols are a widespread class of compounds, formed through the secondary metabolism of plants. They are divided into subcategories, based on the number of phenol rings they contain and the structural differences in the binding between these rings [16,17]. The main classes of polyphenols are phenolic acids, flavonoids, stilbenes, and tannins. Phenolics, which are acknowledged for their role as natural antioxidants, have been extensively associated with a wide range of valuable effects on human health. In particular, polyphenols can protect important cellular components from oxidative damage through their effective scavenging of free radicals. As a consequence, the risk of degenerative diseases associated with oxidative stress is significantly reduced [18,19].

The extraction optimization of antioxidant compounds from aloe rind by-products has received limited attention, with only a small number of studies published on the subject. The antioxidant capacity of various parts of the plant (gel, rind, flower, and root) has been studied and compared, but the optimization of phenolic extraction has not yet been addressed [14,20,21]. Some studies have employed spectrophotometric assays to evaluate the antioxidant activity of aloe rinds, and their findings have indicated the high content of polyphenols [22,23]. Añibarro-Ortega et al. optimized the extraction procedure of a specific chromone, aloesin, from aloe rinds using alternative green solvents (glycerol and propylene glycol) along with a thermostatic magnetic stirring bath [24]. In another study, Solaberrieta et al. reported the optimization of the extraction procedure of polyphenols using non-conventional microwave-assisted extraction (MAE) [15].

The utilization of alternative extraction techniques results in an environmentally friendly sample preparation process due to reduced processing time and solvent consumption. Different non-conventional approaches are employed to extract phenolic components from plant matrices, including supercritical fluid extraction (SFE), pressurized liquid extraction (PLE), MAE, and ultrasound-assisted extraction (UAE) [25,26]. The application of UAE has acquired significant attention due to its numerous advantages. It is considered a simple, cost-effective, environmentally friendly, and highly efficient approach for phenolic extraction [12]. The enhancement of process efficiency by sonication is mainly attributed to the phenomenon of acoustic cavitation, leading to the breakdown of the cellular structure of plant material and the release of valuable polyphenolic compounds [27]. Additionally, this technique enables an efficient and selective extraction in short processing times, without the requirement of a high temperature. Consequently, it is considered to be more suitable for the recovery of thermally sensitive antioxidant compounds [28]. To the best of our knowledge, no prior research has, so far, been conducted to optimize the phenolics extraction procedure using UAE from aloe rinds.

The selection of the appropriate solvent is a critical step in sample preparation. In recent decades, there has been a shift toward sustainable and eco-friendly neoteric solvents as extraction media [29]. Among these solvents, ionic liquids (ILs) and deep eutectic solvents (DESs), classified as neoteric, have gained significant attention, with DESs exhibiting several advantages, including lower cost and an easier preparation process compared to ILs [30]. DESs consist of a hydrogen bond donor (HBD) and a hydrogen bond acceptor (HBA) in solid or liquid form [31,32]. The initial components can be varied, depending on the desired properties of the DES. Among them, the main categories include organic acids, monosaccharides, polyols, and amino acids.

DESs possess a range of notable properties, including low melting points, negligible vapor pressure, thermal stability, non-flammability, non-toxicity, and biodegradability [33,34]. These characteristics make DESs highly versatile and applicable in a wide range of fields, including catalysis and electrochemistry, and they can be used as additives in liquid chromatography and capillary electrophoresis and for extraction solvents [29,35–37]. In the existing literature, DESs have been reported to be employed as extraction media by the use of different extraction methods, mainly UAE and MAE, for the recovery of valuable components from plant matrices. According to these studies, DESs are more selective and efficient extractants of phytochemicals than conventional solvents [38–40]. However, to date, DESs have not been utilized for the recovery of high-value-added compounds from aloe vera.

Within this framework, different DESs were prepared and evaluated to determine the most suitable for the recovery of antioxidants from aloe rind by-products. The operational parameters from the UAE of aloe rind phenolics were optimized by spectrophotometric assays and modeled by response surface methodology (RSM). Phytochemical analysis of the extract under optimal conditions was performed by HPLC-PDA. Solid-phase extraction was applied on the aloe rind extract in order to recover the phenolics and the DES in different fractions. In addition, the greenness of the proposed extraction approach was evaluated using green metrics.

2. Materials and Methods

2.1. Chemicals and Reagents

The starting materials of DESs, choline chloride (≥98%), urea, ethylene glycol, 1,3-butanedion (99.5%), glycerol, citric acid monohydrate, D-fructose (≥99%), and D-sorbitol (≥98%) were purchased from Sigma-Aldrich (St. Louis, MO, USA). D-glucose anhydrous and citric acid monohydrate were acquired from CARLO ERBA Reagents SAS (Val de Reuil Cedex, France) and Merck (Darmstadt, Germany), respectively.

For HPLC analysis, acetonitrile (ACN) and methanol (MeOH) were provided by Sigma Aldrich (St. Louis, MO, USA), while trifluoroacetic acid (TFA) was purchased from Merck (Darmstadt, Germany). The analytical standards of catechin, quercitrin, and myricetin were obtained from HWI ANALYTIK GMBH (Rülzheim, Germany), while apigenin, epicatechin, quercetin, sinapic acid, caffeic acid, and gallic acid were purchased from Sigma Aldrich (St. Louis, MO, USA). Rutin was obtained from PhytoLab GmbH & Co (Vestenbergsgreuth, Germany).

The reagents for spectrophotometric assays, Folin–Ciocalteu reagent, sodium carbonate (Na_2CO_3), 2,4,6-tris(2-pyridyl)-s-triazine) (TPTZ), iron(III) chloride hexahydrate ($FeCl_3{\cdot}6H_2O$), and sodium acetate were purchased from Sigma Aldrich (St. Louis, MO, USA), and DPPH was purchased from TCI (Tokyo, Japan).

2.2. Preparation of Deep Eutectic Solvents

In this study, the eleven DESs were prepared by the heating method. HBAs (choline chloride, glycerol, citric acid) and HBDs (organic acids, sugars, alcohols) were mixed, according to the appropriate molar ratio, as demonstrated in Table 1. The mixtures were then heated on a rotary evaporator at 80 °C until a clear liquid was formed. All DESs were stored in a desiccator at room temperature until the extraction procedure. The obtained DESs and their starting materials were analyzed by FTIR in order to confirm the formation of DESs (Figures S1–S11 in the Supplementary Material).

2.3. Plant Material

Aloe barbadensis Miller plants were generously provided by Puro Aloe Vera Care (Ormideia, Cyprus). Aloe vera leaves were cut from three-year-old plants during the summer and winter periods. Subsequently, aloe leaves were washed thoroughly with distilled water to remove any contaminants and soil particles, and with a knife, the green aloe skin was cautiously separated from the inner gel. The aloe rind was washed once again with distilled water in order to remove any residual gel. Then, the aloe skin was cut into small pieces and lyophilized (LyoDry Compact Benchtop Freeze Dryer, MECHATECH SYSTEMS LTD, Bristol, UK). The freeze-dried rind was ground to a fine powder using a Thermomix TM5 (VORWERK, Wuppertal, Germany) and was passed through a 250 μm sieve (Endecotts, London, UK) to obtain uniformly sized particles. Samples of different plants were homogenized, vacuum-packed, and stored at −20 °C until further extraction and analysis.

Table 1. Composition and abbreviation of the prepared DESs.

HBA	HBD	Abbreviation	Molar Ratio
Choline Chloride	Ethylene Glycol	ChCl-EG	1:2
	Glycerol	ChCl-Gly	1:1
	Urea	ChCl-Ur	1:2
	1,3-Butylene Glycol	ChCl-BG	1:2
	Citric Acid	ChCl-CA	1:1
	D-Glucose	ChCl-D-Glu	2:1
	D-Fructose	ChCl-D-Fru	2:1
	D-Sorbitol	ChCl-D-Sor	1:1
Citric Acid	Glycerol	CA-Gly	1:2
Glycerol	Urea	Gly-Ur	1:1
	D-Fructose	Gly-D-Fru	3:1

2.4. *Ultrasound-Assisted Extraction of Polyphenols from Aloe Vera Rinds*

The UAE of polyphenols was carried out by the use of a 500 W power and a 20 kHz frequency ultrasonic probe system (CY-500, Optic Ivymen System®, Barcelona, Spain). For the extraction, an appropriate amount of aloe rind powder was mixed with 10 mL of the extraction solvent, and the obtained mixture was exposed to ultrasound, following the experimental design conditions. In particular, the extraction procedure was performed using various extraction times, solvent-to-solid ratios, and concentrations of DESs. The ultrasound-treated solution was centrifuged in duplicate at 4400 rpm for 10 min, filtered, and stored at 4 °C until further analysis. All extracts were prepared in triplicate.

2.5. *Determination of Total Phenolic Content*

The TPC of aloe rind extracts was determined by the Folin–Ciocalteu spectrophotometric method, as described by Ozturk et al. [11], with minor modifications. Briefly, 80 μL of filtrated extract was diluted and mixed with 3.12 mL of distilled water. Then, a volume of 200 μL of Folin–Ciocalteu reagent 10% (*v*/*v*) in distilled water was added, and a vortex mixer was used for one minute. After 1–5 min, a 600 μL freshly prepared saturated solution of Na_2CO_3, 20% *w*/*v* was added into the reaction mixture and vigorously shaken. A UV-Vis spectrophotometer (UV-1900, Shimadzu, Tokyo, Japan) was used to measure the absorbance of the extracts (i) after 1 h of reaction in the dark and (ii) at room temperature at 750 nm. Gallic acid was employed as a reference standard, and the quantification of total phenolic content was expressed as the mg of gallic acid equivalents (GAE) per g of dried aloe rind. All analytical procedures were conducted in triplicate, and the outcomes were presented as the mean value along with its associated standard deviation.

2.6. *Determination of Radical Scavenging Activity by DPPH*

To evaluate the antioxidant capacity of the phenolic extracts by scavenging of free radicals of 2,2-diphenyl-1-picrylhydrazyl (DPPH), the method followed in this study was previously described by Xu and Chang [41]. An ethanolic solution of DPPH (0.1 mM) was freshly prepared. A volume of 3.8 mL DPPH solution was mixed with 0.2 mL of aloe rind extract and vigorously shaken. The mixtures were kept under light-obscured conditions at room temperature for a duration of 30 min, and the decrease in absorption was measured at 517 nm by use of a UV-Vis spectrophotometer (UV-1900, Shimadzu, Tokyo, Japan). The same amount of DPPH solution and a volume of 0.2 mL of the extraction solvent, without the sample, were added for the preparation of a blank sample, and its absorption was measured (t = 0 min). Radical scavenging activity (%) was calculated as $[((1 - Abs_{ext})/Abs_{bl}) \times 100]$, where Abs_{ext} is the absorption of extract solution and Abs_{bl} is the absorption of a blank sample. Trolox was employed as a reference standard, and the outcomes of antioxidant activity based on DPPH were expressed as the mM of Trolox equivalents (TE) per g of dried aloe rind.

2.7. Determination of Ferric Reducing Antioxidant Power (FRAP)

The antioxidant activities of aloe rind extracts were evaluated through a reduction in ferric ion (Fe^{3+}) to ferrous ion (Fe^{2+}), according to the FRAP assay method, as outlined by Benzie and Strain [42]. Firstly, the working solution was prepared by adding 300 mM acetate buffer (pH 3.6), 10 mM TPTZ in 40 mM HCl, and 20 mM $FeCl_3$. $6H_2O$ solutions at a ratio of 10:1:1 were incubated at 37 °C for 30 min. Then, a 150 µL aliquot of the sample extract underwent a reaction with 2850 µL FRAP working solution in the dark at room temperature for a duration of 30 min. The absorbance of the blue-colored solution was measured at a wavelength of 593 nm by use of a UV-Vis spectrophotometer (UV-1900, Shimadzu, Tokyo, Japan). Results were expressed as µM TE per g of dried aloe rind using a Trolox as the standard compound.

2.8. Experimental Design and Statistical Analysis

The Box–Behnken design is one of the designs used to provide maximum information about a procedure using a minimum number of experimental data. Box–Behnken design was used to determine optimal conditions and evaluate the impact of three independent variables: extraction time (A), solvent-to-solid ratio (B), and percent content of the DES (C). The ranges of independent variables were evaluated in preliminary experiments, and Table S1 summarizes the three levels of independent factors that were investigated in the experimental design. The responses (dependent variables) were the TPC, DPPH, and FRAP in the dried aloe rind. A summary of the effect of extraction parameters on the responses of aloe rind extract is presented in Table 2. Design Expert version 13.0.5 software (Stat-Ease Inc., Minneapolis, MN, USA) was used for the analysis of variance (ANOVA) test in order to investigate the correlation between independent factors and responses.

2.9. Quantification of Polyphenolic Compounds through HPLC

For the identification and quantification of individual phenolic compounds in the aloe rind extracts, chromatographic analysis was performed by use of an HPLC system (Shimadzu, Tokyo, Japan) equipped with a photodiode array detector (PDA) (SPD-M20A). The chromatographic determination was conducted using the external standard method, employing ten analytical standards of phenolics (gallic acid, catechin, epicatechin, caffeic acid, rutin, sinapic acid, quercitrin, myricetin, quercetin, and apigenin). The chromatographic conditions employed in this study were similar to the ones used in the methodology described by Kumar et al. [43]. The PDA detector was set at 280 nm for the determination of all analytes under study. The analytical column (Venusil XSP C18—150 mm × 4.6 mm, 5 µm) was equipped with a pre-column composed of the same material, and the temperature was maintained constant at 25 °C. The mobile phase consisted of Milli Q water (mobile phase A) and 0.02% (*v*/*v*) TFA in ACN (mobile phase B), and the flow rate was 1 mL/min. A gradient elution program was implemented starting at 80% for the first five min. Mobile phase A was then decreased linearly to 60% at 8 min and subsequently to 50% at 12 min. Finally, mobile phase A increased gradually to 60% until 17 min and then was reset to its initial composition at 21 min, where it remained constant until the 25th min. The injection volume was 20 μL of extract for each analysis, and all experimental procedures were conducted in triplicate.

Table 2. Box–Behnken design of the UAE of independent factors and experimental results for the TPC (mg GAE/g of dried aloe rinds), DPPH (mM TE/g of dried aloe rinds), and FRAP (μM TE/g of dried aloe rinds).

Run	Independent Factors			Responses		
	Time (min)	Solvent/Solid (mL/g)	% DES	TPC	DPPH	FRAP
1	15	100	60	42.1	7.4	799
2	10	150	60	45.8	11.9	1570
3	20	150	60	52.1	11.0	1423
4	15	200	60	64.6	14.3	1132
5	20	100	70	40.5	8.3	1338
6	10	100	70	49.7	8.4	1655
7	15	150	70	53.8	11.8	1889
8	15	150	70	53.9	11.8	1889
9	15	150	70	53.8	11.7	1889
10	15	150	70	53.8	11.8	1889
11	20	200	70	65.4	16.8	2234
12	10	200	70	69.5	17.1	2339
13	15	100	80	36.6	8.3	1846
14	10	150	80	45.9	12.6	2234
15	20	150	80	52.0	12.6	1907
16	15	200	80	69.7	16.0	2535

2.10. *Recovery of Polyphenols and DESs through Solid-Phase Extraction*

2.10.1. Optimization of Polyphenol Recovery—Selection of SPE Cartridges

A solid-phase extraction (SPE) was performed in order to separate the polyphenols from the DES extracts. Three commercially available SPE cartridges were employed in this study, namely Maxi-Clean™ C18 (900 mg, GRACE, Tyrone, PA, USA), Oasis® HLB (400 mg, Waters, Milford, MA, USA), and Discovery® DPA-6S (500 mg, SUPELCO, Bellefonte, PA, USA). The evaluation criteria involved the recovery of polyphenols and the yield of the obtained DES. All SPE experiments were conducted using a vacuum manifold system with a 12-position rack (Visiprep™ SPE Vacuum Manifold, SUPELCO). The sorbent materials of the cartridges were first preconditioned with 5 mL of methanol and equilibrated with 5 mL of an acidified methanolic solution, 20:80 (*v*/*v*) MeOH:H_2O acidified to pH 2.0 with HCl. Subsequently, 5 mL of an acidified standard mixture solution containing 30 μg/mL of each analyte and the appropriate amount of DESs in 20:80 (*v*/*v*) MeOH:H_2O acidified to pH 2.0 with HCl were passed through each type of cartridge. The DES fractions were collected during this process. The acidification of the standard mixture solution was a necessary step to prevent the ionization of polyphenols and minimize their loss during the SPE procedure. The cartridges were washed with 5 mL of acidified water (pH 2.0, HCl). Finally, the fractions of analytes were obtained by eluting the bound phenolics from the cartridges. For C18 and HLB sorbent materials, elution was performed using 80:20 *v*/*v* MeOH:H_2O (2 × 5 mL), while for polyamide DPA-6S cartridges, elution was carried out using a recommended mixture of acetone:H_2O (80:20 *v*/*v*, 2 × 5 mL). The elution fractions were evaporated to dryness using a rotary evaporator and a lyophilizer. The collected DES fraction was weighed to determine its yield, and its FT-IR spectrum was acquired for comparison with the initial spectrum of the DES. The polyphenolic fraction was redissolved in 1 mL of MeOH, filtered through a 0.45 μm pore size membrane filter, and then injected into the HPLC system for further analysis.

2.10.2. Recovery of Polyphenols and DESs from the Rind Extract

According to preliminary findings, the Discovery® DPA-6S cartridge was employed for the recovery of polyphenols and DESs from aloe rind extracts. As mentioned, the polyamide cartridges were conditioned and equilibrated using 5 mL MeOH and 5 mL acidified methanolic solutions, respectively. The 15 mL sample mixture was prepared by three-fold dilution of the obtained DES extract in an acidified methanolic solution. It was then loaded into the sorbents, and the DES fraction was collected. The cartridges underwent a washing step that involved 5 mL of acidified water to eliminate any co-extracted compounds. Finally, the retained phenolics were eluted using a mixture of aqueous acetone (2 × 5 mL). The resulting fractions were subjected to evaporation until dryness was achieved. The FT-IR spectrum of the DES fraction was obtained and compared with the spectrum of the initial DES. The phenolics fraction was redissolved in 1 mL of MeOH, followed by filtration through a membrane filter with a pore size of 0.45 μm, and the resulting solution was introduced into the HPLC system for analysis.

3. Results and Discussion

3.1. Selection of a Suitable Green Solvent for Phenolic Extraction

The selection of an optimal solvent is a critical step in the extraction procedure since it affects the recovery of the targeted bioactive compounds from a given matrix. Different eco-friendly solvents, including three conventional (water, ethanol, and 50% ethanol) and eleven non-conventional (DESs) solvents, were examined through single-factor experiments in the medium level of independent variables (extraction time: 15 min, solvent-to-solid ratio: 150, and percent content of the DES: 70%). The selection of the appropriate solvent was based on the TPC of their extracts, as demonstrated in Figure 1.

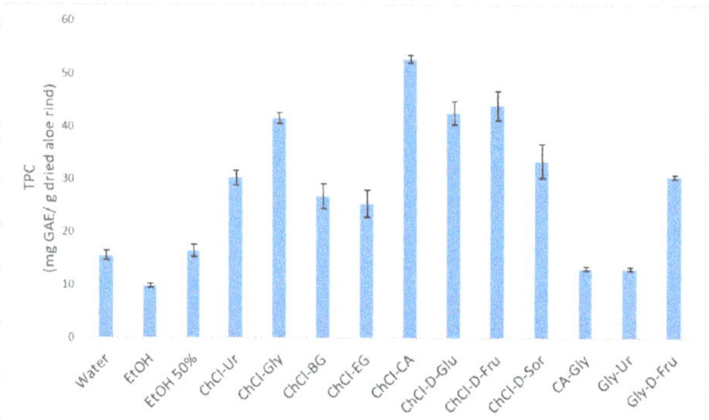

Figure 1. The TPC of aloe rind extracts using different green solvents. Extraction conditions: extraction time, 15 min; solvent-to-solid ratio, 150; DES percentage, 70%. Error bars indicate SD (n = 3).

The TPC values of the extracts of different types of solvents ranged between 9.89 and 52.75 mg GAE/g of dried rind. DESs demonstrated a greater TPC than conventional solvents, except for CA-Gly and Gly-Ur, whose values were at the same level as water and 50% ethanol. Higher TPC values were obtained when DESs that consisted of glycerol and citric acid, as well as the monosaccharides glucose and fructose as an HBD and choline chloride as an HBA were used. Although the two starting materials of CA-Gly combined with choline chloride demonstrated significant amounts of the TPC, the obtained value was considerably less than expected. Thus, it appears that HBDs and HBAs have a significant impact on the physicochemical properties of DESs. Consequently, these characteristics directly affect the ability of the DES to extract polyphenolic compounds from a plant matrix. The ChCl-CA demonstrated the highest TPC when it was utilized for the extraction of bioactive compounds from aloe vera rinds. Therefore, it was selected as the optimal solvent to conduct subsequent experiments.

3.2. Optimization of the Antioxidant Extraction Procedure from Aloe Rinds

RSM was applied through Box–Behnken design in order to determine the optimal operating parameters for the UAE of polyphenols from aloe vera rind by-products. It was employed to estimate the effect of multiple variables and their interactions on the responses with a minimum number of experiments. In particular, three independent variables, namely extraction time (A), solvent-to-solid ratio (B), and percent content of the DES (C) were investigated at three equally spaced levels (−1, 0, +1), which were selected based on preliminary experiments. The complete design included a total of sixteen experiments consisting of twelve combinations of the variables and four replicates performed at the central point. To mitigate the systematic error, the 16 experiments were performed in triplicate and random order. The derived extracts were subjected to analysis to determine the TPC and antioxidant capacity through DPPH and FRAP, which were defined as the dependent variables of the experimental design. The mean values of the responses obtained from three replicates are presented in Table 2. Under the established operating parameters, the experimental values varied between 36.6 and 69.7 mg GAE/g of dried aloe rinds, 7.4 to 17.1 mM TE/g of dried aloe rinds, and 799–2535 μM TE/g of dried aloe rinds for the TPC, DPPH, and FRAP, respectively.

3.2.1. Statistical Analysis and Model Fitting

Individual statistical analyses were conducted for each dependent variable (TPC, DPPH, FRAP) within the experimental design. This approach was employed to determine the factors that exhibit a significant effect on the extraction process for each respective response. The outcomes from the statistical examination of variance (ANOVA) depicted in Table 3 indicate a strong level of significance for the extracted models ($p < 0.0001$) for all dependent variables. The R^2 values serve as valuable metrics for evaluating the fitting of the model. The closer the R^2 adjust value is to 1, the stronger the correlation of the experimental data to the mathematical equation [44]. The obtained R^2 adjust values were 0.797, 0.984, and 0.775 for the TPC, DPPH, and FRAP, respectively, indicating good adequacy of the model to the response variables. The polynomial mathematical equations of response variables, which were obtained by fitting the experimental data, are presented below.

$$\mathrm{YTPC} = 53.05 - 0.12\,\mathrm{A} + 12.53\,\mathrm{B} - 0.05\,\mathrm{C} \quad (1)$$

$$Y_{DPPH} = 11.75 - 0.15\,\mathrm{A} + 3.97\,\mathrm{B} + 0.62\,\mathrm{C} - 0.04\,\mathrm{AB} + 0.25\,\mathrm{AC} + 0.17\,\mathrm{BC} + 0.71\,\mathrm{A}^2 + 0.19\,\mathrm{B}^2 - 0.46\,\mathrm{C}^2 \quad (2)$$

$$Y_{FRAP} = 1785.51 \quad 112.00\,\mathrm{A} + 325.14\,\mathrm{B} + 449.65\,\mathrm{C} \quad (3)$$

According to the regression analysis outcomes obtained using Design-Expert software, the best-fit model for the TPC and FRAP was the linear model, while the quadratic model was suggested for DPPH. The superior performance of the linear model for the TPC and FRAP can be attributed to the non-significant effect of quadratic and interaction terms on the respective responses. The statistical analysis performed confirmed the statistical significance of the coefficients derived from the polynomial models obtained. In the case of the TPC, only the linear term of the solvent-to-solid ratio (B) exhibited a significant effect. However, for FRAP, both the linear terms of the solvent-to-solid ratio (B) and the percentage of the DES (C) showed statistical significance. Notably, the percentage of the DES (C) made the most substantial contribution to the model, as indicated by its *p*-value, which was less than 0.0001. The variables with the largest impact on DPPH response were the linear coefficient of the solvent-to-solid ratio (B) and the percent content of the DES (C), along with the quadratic coefficient of extraction time (A^2) and the percent content of the DES (C^2). Conversely, the linear coefficient of extraction time (A) did not exhibit any notable effects on the TPC, DPPH, and FRAP values ($p > 0.05$). Based on all response variables, it can be concluded that the solvent-to-solid ratio is the most critical factor that affects the recovery of polyphenols from aloe by-products.

Table 3. ANOVA results for the TPC, DPPH, and FRAP models of aloe rind extracts.

Source	Sum of Squares (SS)	Degree of Freedom (DF)	Mean Square (MS)	F-Value	*p*-Value
TPC model				20.59	<0.0001 ***
A	0.1	1	0.1	0.01	0.9437
B	1256.5	1	1256.5	61.77	<0.0001 ***
C	0.1	1	0.1	0.01	0.9780
Residuals	244.1	12	20.34		
		R^2 = 0.8373, R^2_{adj} = 0.797, R^2_{pred} = 0.757			
DPPH model				103.69	<0.0001 ***
A	0.2	1	0.2	1.25	0.3070
B	125.9	1	125.9	886.43	<0.0001 ***
C	3.1	1	3.1	21.76	0.0034 **
AB	0.0	1	0.0	0.03	0.8588
AC	0.2	1	0.2	1.73	0.2370
BC	0.1	1	0.1	0.86	0.3908
A^2	2.1	1	2.1	14.33	0.0091 **
B^2	0.1	1	0.1	0.98	0.3602
C^2	0.8	1	0.8	5.85	0.0497 *
Residuals	0.9	6	0.1		
		R^2 = 0.994, R^2_{adj} = 0.984, R^2_{pred} = 0.899			
FRAP model				18.26	<0.0001 ***
A	1.0×10^5	1	1.0×10^5	2.14	0.1688
B	8.5×10^5	1	8.5×10^5	18.07	0.0011 **
C	1.6×10^5	1	1.6×10^5	34.56	<0.0001 ***
Residuals	5.6×10^5	12	46,798.8		
		R^2 = 0.8203, R^2_{adj} = 0.775, R^2_{pred} = 0.733			

* Significant at $p \leq 0.05$. ** Significant at $p \leq 0.01$.*** Significant at $p \leq 0.001$.

3.2.2. Effect of Process Variables

As previously indicated, the solvent-to-solid ratio has been identified as the most important parameter in the extraction of these valuable bioactive compounds. Based on the experimental outcomes, an increase in the solvent-to-solid ratio leads to an elevation in the TPC and antioxidant activity (DPPH, FRAP) values. These findings confirmed that an increase in the amount of solvent promotes the interactions between the plant matrix and solvent, thereby enhancing the mass transfer of polyphenolic compounds and, subsequently, the extraction efficiency [11,45]. A lower ratio leads to the rapid saturation of the solvent, which, in turn, limits the quantity of extractable polyphenols [39].

The addition of water into the DES results in a reduction in the viscosity and an increase in the polarity of the extraction solvent. The presence of water in the DES affects the physicochemical properties of the DES, facilitating a more effective penetration of the solvent into the ruptured plant cell, enhancing the mass transfer and, consequently, improving the recovery of polyphenols [46]. On the other hand, excessive amounts of water (>50%) may negatively impact extraction efficiency by weakening or disrupting the intermolecular hydrogen bond interactions within the DES starting materials [38,46]. A water composition ranging from 20 to 40% was selected in order to avoid any interference with the DES. The composition of the DES and water in the extraction solvent significantly affects the antioxidant capacity of the extracts. In particular, an increase in the percentage of the DES leads to higher values of FRAP and DPPH.

The extraction time of bioactive compounds from a plant matrix plays a crucial role in the optimization of sample preparation. A prolonged extraction time may cause a degradation of sensitive polyphenolic compounds, while a reduction in the time may not result in the expected release and extraction of polyphenols from the plant cell [47–49]. Surprisingly, based on statistical analysis, the extraction time was found to have a non-significant effect on the recovery of valuable polyphenols from aloe rinds. This finding was unexpected, considering that similar studies performed on other plant matrices, such as ginger, pomegranate by-products, and cranberry, where UAE was performed with the DES as an extraction solvent, demonstrated a significant impact on extraction time [50–52]. Solaberrieta et al., who optimized the MAE of polyphenols from aloe rinds, reported that the extraction time and temperature were not important factors affecting antioxidant recovery and, therefore, the TPC, DPPH, and FRAP [15]. Given the consistency of our results with the above-mentioned finding, it is concluded that aloe vera rind is a unique plant matrix, and the sample processing time does not influence the release of phenolics.

3.2.3. Optimal Conditions and Model Validation

Based on the acquired polynomial equations of antioxidant activity and the TPC, three-dimensional response surface plots were constructed to visually depict the correlation between the operating parameters and the response variables. Figure 2 exhibits these response surface plots, illustrating the association between the independent variables, namely the percent content of the DES and the solvent-to-solid ratio with the TPC, DPPH, and FRAP of aloe vera rinds.

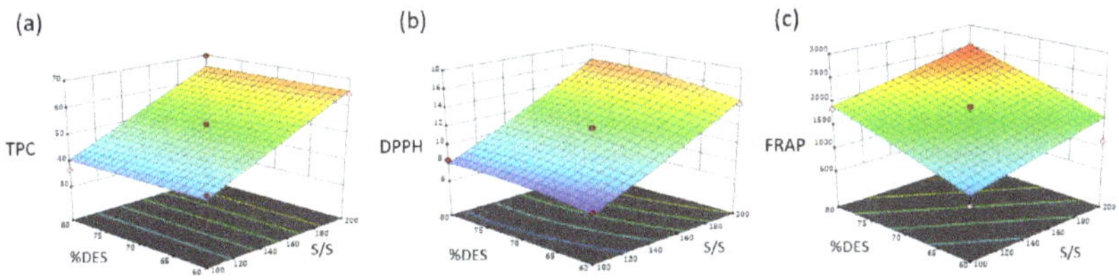

Figure 2. Three-dimensional response surface plots demonstrating the effect of the solvent-to-solid ratio and percentage content of the DES on (**a**) the TPC, (**b**) DPPH, and (**c**) FRAP.

In order to determine the optimum level of each operating parameter, a multiple response optimization was performed, with the objective of maximizing the TPC and the antioxidant activity of the extract. The results obtained indicated that the optimum conditions were as follows: an extraction time of 16.5 min, a solvent-to-solid ratio equal to 192, and an extraction solvent consisting of 74% (v/v) of the DES in water. The predictive ability of the response surface models was evaluated by conducting extractions under the estimated optimal conditions. The experimental results were in agreement with the predicted values, with a percentage of error ranging from 0.62 to 2.20% (Table 4). The strong correlation between the experimental and predicted values confirms the reliability and effectiveness of the models to correlate the independent and dependent variables and, consequently, to determine the optimal extraction conditions of phenolic components from aloe vera rinds.

Table 4. Experimental and predicted values in the optimum extraction conditions.

Dependent Variables	Predicted Value	Experimental Value	Percentage Error (%)
TPC (mg GAE/g)	63.56	64.96 ± 3.04	2.20
DPPH (mM TE/g)	15.51	15.69 ± 0.35	1.19
FRAP (μM TE/g)	2203	2217 ± 39	0.62

The quantitative comparison of the results obtained from the analysis of aloe vera rinds, in terms of total phenolics and antioxidant activity, with the literature proved to be a challenging task. The main difficulty encountered was the variation in units of measurement used to express the results. In particular, FRAP values can be expressed in terms of either Fe^{3+} or gallic acid equivalents, while DPPH values can be described as % inhibition or IC_{50} [14,53,54]. For comparison purposes, the optimum DPPH value was expressed as 78.7 ± 0.62% inhibition. The DPPH results obtained in this study demonstrated a comparable antioxidant potential to that reported by Bushra et al. (77.6% inhibition), who employed conventional extraction techniques using 80% methanol as the extraction solvent [55]. However, the % inhibition of DPPH of aloe rind extracts obtained in the present work was higher than the values reported by Lopez et al. (58.8 ± 0.4%) and Hu et al. (39.7 ± 0.07%) [14,54]. In terms of the TPC, our findings are higher than those reported by Hossen et al. (3.52 mg GAE/g sample) [53]. Therefore, based on these comparisons, it can be concluded that the optimized operating conditions of the aloe rind extraction procedure employed in this study yielded higher levels of total phenolics and antioxidant capacity compared to the literature. Consequently, this optimization led to a greater recovery of valuable bioactive compounds.

3.3. Phenolic Profile of Aloe Rind Extracts—HPLC Analysis

Despite the fact that spectrophotometric assays enable rapid screening for the determination of polyphenolic compounds, they are susceptible to the potential overestimation of both phenolic content and antioxidant capacity due to cross-reactions with other reducing components [12,56]. Consequently, it became imperative to employ a chromatographic analysis for the identification and quantification of individual phenolics present in aloe rind extracts.

A rapid and accurate HPLC method was employed to determine the phenolic antioxidants. The method was validated prior to analysis in terms of precision, limit of detection, and limit of quantitation, as listed in Table S2 (Supplementary Material). All analytes exhibited excellent linearity, with the coefficients of determination varied above 0.997. The precision of the analytical method was evaluated by relative standard deviations (RSDs) of peak areas. The RSD values for repeatability (intraday precision) and reproducibility (interday precision) were lower than 1.04% and 2.68%, respectively. The limit of detection (LOD) and quantification (LOQ) of the method ranged from 0.1 to 0.9 μg/mL and 0.3 to 2.8 μg/mL, correspondingly.

The qualitative and quantitative results obtained from the chromatographic determination of aloe rind extracts, under the optimum extraction parameters, are presented in Table 5. The aloe rind was found to consist of a wide range of polyphenolic components. As demonstrated in Figure S12, the aloe rind extract is a complex plant matrix, with a variety of phytochemicals. Therefore, the detection of phenolics was performed by spiking the sample with pure individual standards. Among the ten phenolic compounds examined, the chromatographic method successfully detected eight. Myricetin exhibited the highest abundance among the antioxidants present in the aloe rind, surpassing catechin by approximately 70% in terms of concentration. Catechin, gallic acid, rutin, apigenin, quercetin, and epicatechin exhibited significant contributions to the overall phenolic content of the aloe rind, while caffeic acid was found to be present in relatively minor quantities compared to the aforementioned analytes.

Table 5. Quantitative data for the HPLC analysis of the optimum aloe rind extract.

Compound	Concentration (mg/g Dried Aloe Rind)	% Content
Gallic acid	1.37 ± 0.14	14.2
Catechin	1.44 ± 0.09	14.9
Epicatechin	0.91 ± 0.04	9.4
Caffeic acid	0.21 ± 0.02	2.2
Rutin	1.20 ± 0.04	12.4
Sinapic acid	ND	0
Quercitrin	ND	0
Myricetin	2.45 ± 0.04	25.4
Quercetin	0.98 ± 0.03	10.1
Apigenin	1.11 ± 0.04	11.4
Total	9.67	100

ND: non-detected.

In comparison with other studies, significant variations were noted in regard to the type and composition of phenolic compounds [14,15,57]. The variances observed in the phenolic profile are indicative of the impact of several factors, including geographical origin, plant variety, harvest season, soil characteristics, the extraction process, and the analytical method employed. For example, according to Lopez et al., catechin was found to be the most prevalent phenolic compound, followed by sinapic acid, while, according to our findings, sinapic acid could not be detected by HPLC in the optimum extract [14].

3.4. Recovery of Polyphenols and DESs from Aloe Rind Extracts

The isolation and recovery of extracted compounds from extracts is challenging due to the negligible vapor pressure of DESs [58–60]. In recent years, several approaches have been proposed to facilitate the recovery of valuable extracted compounds, including the applications of anti-solvents, macro-porous resins, and supercritical carbon dioxide [61–66]. The SPE procedure has proven to be a simple and efficient method for the isolation of phytochemicals from DES extracts [58,59,67]. Therefore, preliminary studies were performed to select the most suitable cartridge for recovering the extracted phenolics and the ChCl-CA, in different fractions, from the optimal aloe rind extracts. Three commercially available SPE sorbents (Maxi-Clean™ C18, Oasis® HLB, Discovery® DPA-6S), known for their favorable retention properties toward polyphenols, were evaluated for their ability to recover and isolate polyphenols and DESs. The recoveries of the polyphenolic compounds under study on different SPE cartridges, along with the standard deviations (SDs), are presented in Figure 3. Discovery® DPA-6S sorbents demonstrated superior recovery ability of the target compounds and were consequently selected as the most suitable cartridges. A polyamide resin cartridge (DPA-6S) is typically employed for the absorption of polar compounds, particularly polyphenols, through hydrogen bonding between the hydroxyl groups of the compounds and the amide groups of the resin [12].

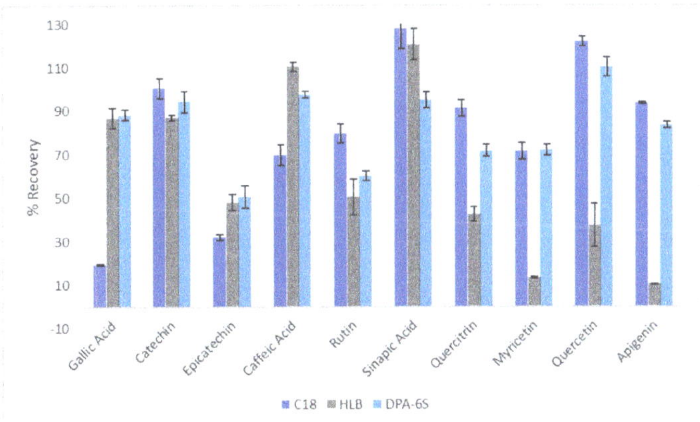

Figure 3. Recovery of the polyphenolic compounds on different SPE cartridges.

Following the optimization of the SPE method, the procedure was performed utilizing the aloe rind extracts under optimum conditions. The recovery of phenolics was determined to be at satisfactory levels, ranging from 54.3 to 96.1%. The lowest recovery values were observed for epicatechin and myricetin. The obtained DES fraction exhibited a yield of 95.98% ± 2.86. For confirmation purposes, FTIR experiments were conducted. The spectroscopic analysis confirmed a high degree of similarity between the findings and the initial DES (Figure S13, Supplementary Materials). These findings highlight the ability of the DES to be recycled and employed in subsequent extraction cycles.

3.5. Green Evaluation Using Green Metrics

The green metrics have emerged as innovative tools in order to assess the greenness of analytical methods. The AGREE® (version 0.5) [68] and AGREEprep® (version 0.91) [69] tools are gaining attention nowadays due to their easy, user-friendly, and open-access software. Both metric tools employ a scoring system ranging from 0 to 1, along with a red-yellow-green scale, indicating the strengths and weaknesses of the analytical method. An overall score greater than 0.6 is considered indicative of a green method. The AGREE® Calculator metric provides information about the entire analytical methodology. It consists of 12 criteria that align with the 12 categories defined by the Principles of Green Analytical Chemistry. Various parameters of the method, such as the nature and volume of reagents, energy consumption, generated waste, and the number of procedural steps, are taken into consideration. In contrast, the AGREEprep® Calculator metric tool focuses on sample preparation and depends on 10 environmental impact criteria, including the type of solvents, sample size, waste generation, and energy consumption.

The present extraction procedure was compared with other methodologies described in the literature for the recovery of bioactive compounds in aloe vera rind samples, as illustrated in Table 6. Pictograms representing the chosen studies were generated using AGREE and AGREEprep software. The current sample preparation approach, which employs UAE combined with the DES, accomplished the greenest methodology, with an overall score greater than 0.7 in both metrics. The main drawback of the proposed procedure is the requirement to conduct sampling of the plant material (criteria 1). The substitution of organic and hazardous solvents with the DES contributes to the development of a more sustainable and green analytical method. In addition, the selection of UAE and the reduced process time contribute to low energy consumption. The HPLC-PDA system proved to be suitable for the chromatographic analysis of the DES extracts. However, the use of a mass spectrometer, as a detector in HPLC, may lead to potential damage due to the low volatility of the DES, the increased energy consumption, and equipment cost [70]. Despite these challenges, it is important to note that identifying complex mixtures with overlapping peaks in their chromatogram is still not possible without a mass spectrometer detector.

Table 6. Comparison of the extraction procedure from aloe rinds with the developed method.

Extraction Method	Extraction Time	Extraction Solvent	Mass of Aloe Rind	Solvent Volume	Detection System	AGREE	AGREEprep	Ref.
Soxhlet	12 h (4 × 3 h)	Hex, Ace, EtOH, MeOH	10 g	700 mL (4 × 175 mL)	HPLC-DAD	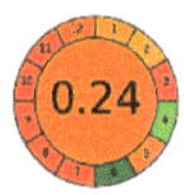	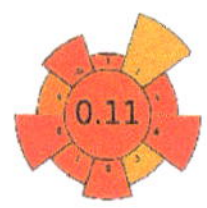	[14]
MAE	36.6 min	80% EtOH	1.5 g	50 mL	HPLC-ESI-MS/MS	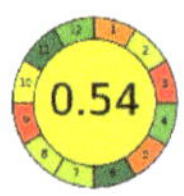	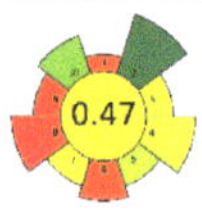	[15]
Stirring	3 days	Acidic MeOH	100 g	500 mL	UV	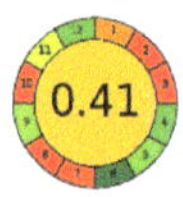	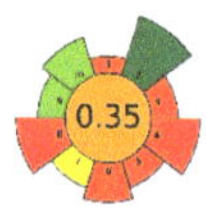	[53]
UAE	16.5 min	74% DES (ChCl-CA)	0.052 g	10 mL	HPLC-PDA	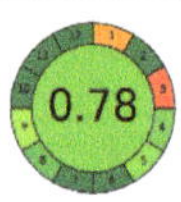	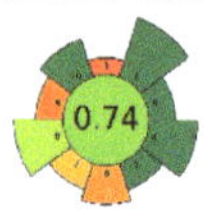	This work

4. Conclusions

In the present study, the ultrasound-assisted extraction of phenolic antioxidants from aloe rind agrowaste, using ChCl-CA DES as the suitable green solvent, was optimized by RSM. Under the optimum operating conditions (16.5 min, solvent to solid 192, and 74% DES), high values of the TPC and antioxidant activity (DPPH and FRAP) were obtained. The aloe rind extract was subjected to chromatographic analysis, which revealed a notable presence of polyphenolic compounds, with myricetin identified as the most abundant compound. Furthermore, in order to recover the bioactive components and DESs from the extract, SPE utilizing DPA-6S cartridges was employed. This method exhibited excellent recovery of valuable phenolics, thereby demonstrating the recyclability of the DES. The greenness of the method was evaluated by employing green metrics. The extraction procedure achieved a score greater than 0.7, indicating that it is aligned with the concept of green chemistry. In summary, the combination of UAE and the DES provides a sustainable, efficient, and alternative methodology for the recovery of polyphenols from aloe vera rinds. This integrated approach is promising for the widespread application and utilization of aloe vera by-products on an industrial scale.

Supplementary Materials: The following supporting information can be downloaded at https://www.mdpi.com/article/10.3390/antiox13020162/s1, Figure S1: The FTIR spectra of ChCl, Ur, and ChCl-Ur; Figure S2: The FTIR spectra of ChCl, Gly, and ChCl-Gly; Figure S3: The FTIR spectra of ChCl, BG, and ChCl-BG; Figure S4: The FTIR spectra of ChCl, EG, and ChCl-EG; Figure S5: The FTIR spectra of ChCl, CA, and ChCl-CA; Figure S6: The FTIR spectra of ChCl, D-Glu, and ChCl-D-Glu; Figure S7: The FTIR spectra of ChCl, D-Fru, and ChCl-D-Fru; Figure S8: The FTIR spectra of ChCl, D-Sor, and ChCl-D-Sor; Figure S9: The FTIR spectra of CA, Gly, and CA-Gly; Figure S10: The FTIR spectra of Gly, Ur, and Gly-Ur; Figure S11: The FTIR spectra of Gly, D-Fru, and Gly-D-Fru; Figure S12: HPLC chromatograph of optimum aloe rind extracts. (1) Gallic acid, (2) catechin, (3) epicatechin, (4) caffeic acid, (5) rutin, (8) myricetin, (9) quercetin, and (10) apigenin; Figure S13: The FTIR spectra of (A) ChCl-CA and (B) obtained ChCl-CA by SPE; Table S1: The three levels of independent variables of experimental design; Table S2: Validation of the HPLC method.

Author Contributions: Methodology, G.D.I.; Investigation, G.D.I., K.A.I. and A.C.; Data curation, K.A.I.; Writing—original draft, G.D.I.; Writing—review & editing, A.C., I.J.S. and C.P.K.-C.; Supervision, I.J.S. and C.P.K.-C.; Project administration, C.P.K.-C.; Funding acquisition, C.P.K.-C. All authors have read and agreed to the published version of the manuscript.

Funding: This research received no external funding.

Data Availability Statement: Data are contained within the article and Supplementary Materials.

Conflicts of Interest: The authors declare no conflict of interest.

References

1. Kumar, S.; Yadav, J.P. Ethnobotanical and Pharmacological Properties of Aloe Vera: A Review. *J. Med. Plant Res.* **2014**, *8*, 1387–1398. [CrossRef]
2. Kumar, R.; Singh, A.K.; Gupta, A.; Bishayee, A.; Pandey, A.K. Therapeutic Potential of Aloe Vera—A Miracle Gift of Nature. *Phytomedicine* **2019**, *60*, 152996. [CrossRef] [PubMed]
3. Sahu, P.K.; Giri, D.D.; Singh, R.; Pandey, P.; Gupta, S. Therapeutic and Medicinal Uses of Aloe Vera: A Review. *Pharmacol. Pharm.* **2013**, *4*, 599–610. [CrossRef]
4. Radha, M.H.; Laxmipriya, N.P. Evaluation of Biological Properties and Clinical Effectiveness of Aloe Vera: A Systematic Review. *J. Tradit. Complement. Med.* **2015**, *5*, 21–26. [CrossRef] [PubMed]
5. Javed, S.; Atta-Ur, R. *Aloe Vera Gel in Food, Health Products, and Cosmetics Industry*, 1st ed.; Elsevier B.V.: Amsterdam, The Netherlands, 2014; Volume 41, ISBN 9780444632944.
6. Bozzi, A.; Perrin, C.; Austin, S.; Vera, F.A. Quality and Authenticity of Commercial Aloe Vera Gel Powders. *Food Chem.* **2007**, *103*, 22–30. [CrossRef]
7. Ramachandra, C.T.; Srinivasa Rao, P. Processing of Aloe Vera Leaf Gel: A Review. *Am. J. Agric. Biol. Sci.* **2008**, *3*, 502–510. [CrossRef]
8. Guo, X.; Mei, N. Aloe Vera: A Review of Toxicity and Adverse Clinical Effects. *J. Environ. Sci. Health* **2016**, *34*, 77–96. [CrossRef] [PubMed]

9. Esposito, B.; Sessa, M.R.; Sica, D.; Malandrino, O. Towards Circular Economy in the Agri-Food Sector. A Systematic Literature Review. *Sustainability* **2020**, *12*, 7401. [CrossRef]
10. Gullón, P.; Gullón, B.; Romaní, A.; Rocchetti, G.; Manuel, J. Trends in Food Science & Technology Smart Advanced Solvents for Bioactive Compounds Recovery from Agri-Food by-Products: A Review. *Trends Food Sci. Technol.* **2020**, *101*, 182–197. [CrossRef]
11. Ozturk, B.; Parkinson, C.; Gonzalez-Miquel, M. Extraction of Polyphenolic Antioxidants from Orange Peel Waste Using Deep Eutectic Solvents. *Sep. Purif. Technol.* **2018**, *206*, 1–13. [CrossRef]
12. Christou, A.; Stavrou, I.J.; Kapnissi-Christodoulou, C.P. Continuous and Pulsed Ultrasound-Assisted Extraction of Carob's Antioxidants: Processing Parameters Optimization and Identification of Polyphenolic Composition. *Ultrason. Sonochem.* **2021**, *76*, 105630. [CrossRef]
13. Pal, C.B.T.; Jadeja, G.C. Microwave-Assisted Deep Eutectic Solvent Extraction of Phenolic Antioxidants from Onion (*Allium Cepa* L.) Peel: A Box–Behnken Design Approach for Optimization. *J. Food Sci. Technol.* **2019**, *56*, 4211–4223. [CrossRef] [PubMed]
14. López, A.; De Tangil, M.S.; Vega-orellana, O.; Ramírez, A.S.; Rico, M. Phenolic Constituents, Antioxidant and Preliminary Antimycoplasmic Activities of Leaf Skin and Flowers of *Aloe Vera* (L.) Burm. f. (Syn. A. Barbadensis Mill.) from the Canary Islands (Spain). *Molecules* **2013**, *18*, 4942–4954. [CrossRef]
15. Solaberrieta, I.; Jimenez, A.; Garrigos, M.C. Valorization of Aloe Vera Skin By-Products to Obtain Bioactive Compounds by Microwave-Assisted Extraction: Antioxidant Activity and Chemical Composition. *Antioxidants* **2022**, *11*, 1058. [CrossRef] [PubMed]
16. Stavrou, I.J.; Christou, A.; Kapnissi-Christodoulou, C.P. Polyphenols in Carobs: A Review on Their Composition, Antioxidant Capacity and Cytotoxic Effects, and Health Impact. *Food Chem.* **2018**, *269*, 355–374. [CrossRef] [PubMed]
17. Khurana, S.; Venkataraman, K.; Hollingsworth, A.; Piche, M.; Tai, T.C. Polyphenols: Benefits to the Cardiovascular System in Health and in Aging. *Nutrients* **2013**, *5*, 3779–3827. [CrossRef]
18. Scalbert, A.; Manach, C.; Morand, C.; Rémésy, C.; Jiménez, L. Dietary Polyphenols and the Prevention of Diseases. *Crit. Rev. Food Sci. Nutr.* **2005**, *45*, 287–306. [CrossRef] [PubMed]
19. Ningappa, M.B.; Dinesha, R.; Srinivas, L. Antioxidant and Free Radical Scavenging Activities of Polyphenol-Enriched Curry Leaf (*Murraya Koenigii* L.) Extracts. *Food Chem.* **2008**, *106*, 720–728. [CrossRef]
20. Quispe, C.; Villalobos, M.; Bórquez, J.; Simirgiotis, M. Chemical Composition and Antioxidant Activity of Aloe Vera from the Pica Oasis (Tarapacá, Chile) by UHPLC-Q/Orbitrap/MS/MS. *J. Chem.* **2018**, *2018*, 1–12. [CrossRef]
21. Añibarro-Ortega, M.; Pinela, J.; Barros, L.; Ciric, A.; Silva, S.P.; Coelho, E.; Mocan, A.; Calhelha, R.C.; Sokovic, M.; Coimbra, M.A.; et al. Compositional Features and Bioactive Properties of Aloe Vera Leaf (Fillet, Mucilage and Rind) and Flower. *Antioxidants* **2019**, *8*, 444. [CrossRef]
22. Miladi, S.; Mohamed, D. In Vitro Antioxidant Activities of Aloe Vera Leaf Skin Extracts. *J. La Société Chim. Tunis.* **2008**, *10*, 101–109.
23. Kammoun, M.; Miladi, S.; Ali, Y.B.; Damak, M.; Gargouri, Y.; Bezzine, S. In Vitro Study of the PLA2 Inhibition and Antioxidant Activities of Aloe Vera Leaf Skin Extracts. *Lipids Health Dis.* **2011**, *10*, 30. [CrossRef]
24. Añibarro-Ortega, M.; Pinela, J.; Ćirić, A.; Lopes, E.; Molina, A.K.; Calhelha, R.C.; Soković, M.; Ferreira, O.; Ferreira, I.C.F.R.; Barros, L. Extraction of Aloesin from Aloe Vera Rind Using Alternative Green Solvents: Process Optimization and Biological Activity Assessment. *Biology* **2021**, *10*, 951. [CrossRef] [PubMed]
25. Ameer, K.; Shahbaz, H.M.; Kwon, J.H. Green Extraction Methods for Polyphenols from Plant Matrices and Their Byproducts: A Review. *Compr. Rev. Food Sci. Food Saf.* **2017**, *16*, 295–315. [CrossRef] [PubMed]
26. Talmaciu, A.I.; Volf, I.; Popa, V.I. A Comparative Analysis of the "Green" Techniques Applied for Polyphenols Extraction from Bioresources. *Chem. Biodiv.* **2015**, *12*, 1635–1651. [CrossRef]
27. Ramić, M.; Vidović, S.; Zeković, Z.; Vladić, J.; Cvejin, A.; Pavlić, B. Modeling and Optimization of Ultrasound-Assisted Extraction of Polyphenolic Compounds from Aronia Melanocarpa by-Products from Filter-Tea Factory. *Ultrason. Sonochem.* **2015**, *23*, 360–368. [CrossRef]
28. Ajila, C.M.; Brar, S.K.; Verma, M.; Tyagi, R.D.; Godbout, S.; Valéro, J.R. Extraction and Analysis of Polyphenols: Recent Trends. *Crit. Rev. Biotechnol.* **2011**, *31*, 227–249. [CrossRef] [PubMed]
29. Torres-Valenzuela, L.S.; Ballesteros-Gómez, A.; Rubio, S. Green Solvents for the Extraction of High Added-Value Compounds from Agri-Food Waste. *Food Eng. Rev.* **2020**, *12*, 83–100. [CrossRef]
30. Choi, Y.H.; Verpoorte, R. Green Solvents for the Extraction of Bioactive Compounds from Natural Products Using Ionic Liquids and Deep Eutectic Solvents. *Curr. Opin. Food Sci.* **2019**, *26*, 87–93. [CrossRef]
31. Liu, Y.; Friesen, J.B.; McAlpine, J.B.; Lankin, D.C.; Chen, S.N.; Pauli, G.F. Natural Deep Eutectic Solvents: Properties, Applications, and Perspectives. *J. Nat. Prod.* **2018**, *81*, 679–690. [CrossRef]
32. El Achkar, T.; Greige-Gerges, H.; Fourmentin, S. Basics and Properties of Deep Eutectic Solvents: A Review. *Environ. Chem. Lett.* **2021**, *19*, 3397–3408. [CrossRef]
33. Pena-Pereira, F.; Namieśnik, J. Ionic Liquids and Deep Eutectic Mixtures: Sustainable Solvents for Extraction Processes. *ChemSusChem* **2014**, *7*, 1784–1800. [CrossRef] [PubMed]
34. Hansen, B.B.; Spittle, S.; Chen, B.; Poe, D.; Zhang, Y.; Klein, J.M.; Horton, A.; Adhikari, L.; Zelovich, T.; Doherty, B.W.; et al. Deep Eutectic Solvents: A Review of Fundamentals and Applications. *Chem. Rev.* **2021**, *121*, 1232–1285. [CrossRef] [PubMed]
35. Shishov, A.; Bulatov, A.; Locatelli, M.; Carradori, S.; Andruch, V. Application of Deep Eutectic Solvents in Analytical Chemistry. A Review. *Microchem. J.* **2017**, *135*, 33–38. [CrossRef]

36. Bajkacz, S.; Adamek, J.; Sobska, A. Application of Deep Eutectic Solvents and Ionic Liquids in the Extraction of Catechins from Tea. *Molecules* **2020**, *25*, 3216. [CrossRef]
37. Tan, T.; Zhang, M.; Wan, Y.; Qiu, H. Utilization of Deep Eutectic Solvents as Novel Mobile Phase Additives for Improving the Separation of Bioactive Quaternary Alkaloids. *Talanta* **2016**, *149*, 85–90. [CrossRef]
38. Bener, M.; Sen, F.B.; Onem, A.N.; Bekdeser, B.; Celik, S.E.; Lalikoglu, M.; Asci, Y.S.; Capanoglu, E.; Apak, R. Microwave-Assisted Extraction of Antioxidant Compounds from by-Products of Turkish Hazelnut (*Corylus Avellana* L.) Using Natural Deep Eutectic Solvents: Modeling, Optimization and Phenolic Characterization. *Food Chem.* **2022**, *385*, 132633. [CrossRef]
39. Cai, C.; Li, F.; Liu, L.; Tan, Z. Deep Eutectic Solvents Used as the Green Media for the Efficient Extraction of Caffeine from Chinese Dark Tea. *Sep. Purif. Technol.* **2019**, *227*, 115723. [CrossRef]
40. Mouratoglou, E.; Malliou, V.; Makris, D.P. Novel Glycerol-Based Natural Eutectic Mixtures and Their Efficiency in the Ultrasound-Assisted Extraction of Antioxidant Polyphenols from Agri-Food Waste Biomass. *Waste Biomass Valorization* **2016**, *7*, 1377–1387. [CrossRef]
41. Xu, B.J.; Chang, S.K.C. A Comparative Study on Phenolic Profiles and Antioxidant Activities of Legumes as Affected by Extraction Solvents. *J. Food Sci.* **2007**, *72*, S159–S166. [CrossRef]
42. Benzie, I.F.F.; Strain, J.J. The Ferric Reducing Ability of Plasma (FRAP) as a Measure of 'Antioxidant Power': The FRAP Assay. *Anal. Biochem.* **1996**, *239*, 70–76. [CrossRef]
43. Kumar, N.; Bhandari, P.; Singh, B.; Gupta, A.P.; Kaul, V.K. Reversed Phase-HPLC for Rapid Determination of Polyphenols in Flowers of Rose Species. *J. Sep. Sci.* **2008**, *31*, 262–267. [CrossRef] [PubMed]
44. Pinto, D.; Vieira, E.F.; Peixoto, A.F.; Freire, C.; Freitas, V.; Costa, P.; Delerue-Matos, C.; Rodrigues, F. Optimizing the Extraction of Phenolic Antioxidants from Chestnut Shells by Subcritical Water Extraction Using Response Surface Methodology. *Food Chem.* **2021**, *334*, 127521. [CrossRef]
45. Xia, B.; Yan, D.; Bai, Y.; Xie, J.; Cao, Y.; Liao, D.; Lin, L. Determination of Phenolic Acids in *Prunella Vulgaris* L.: A Safe and Green Extraction Method Using Alcohol-Based Deep Eutectic Solvents. *Anal. Methods* **2015**, *7*, 9354–9364. [CrossRef]
46. Vilková, M.; Justyna, P.; Andruch, V. The Role of Water in Deep Eutectic Solvent-Base Extraction. *J. Mol. Liq.* **2020**, *304*, 112747. [CrossRef]
47. Garcia-salas, P.; Morales-soto, A.; Segura-carretero, A.; Fernández-gutiérrez, A. Phenolic-Compound-Extraction Systems for Fruit and Vegetable Samples. *Molecules* **2010**, *15*, 8813–8826. [CrossRef]
48. Dai, J.; Mumper, R.J. Plant Phenolics: Extraction, Analysis and Their Antioxidant and Anticancer Properties. *Molecules* **2010**, *15*, 7313–7352. [CrossRef]
49. Vural, N.; Cavuldak, Ö.A.; Anlı, R.E. Multi Response Optimisation of Polyphenol Extraction Conditions from Grape Seeds by Using Ultrasound Assisted Extraction (UAE). *Sep. Sci. Technol.* **2018**, *53*, 1540–1551. [CrossRef]
50. Hsieh, Y.; Li, Y.; Pan, Z.; Chen, Z.; Lu, J.; Yuan, J. Ultrasonication-Assisted Synthesis of Alcohol-Based Deep Eutectic Solvents for Extraction of Active Compounds from Ginger. *Ultrason. Sonochem.* **2020**, *63*, 104915. [CrossRef] [PubMed]
51. Alrugaibah, M.; Yagiz, Y.; Gu, L. Use Natural Deep Eutectic Solvents as Efficient Green Reagents to Extract Procyanidins and Anthocyanins from Cranberry Pomace and Predictive Modeling by RSM and Artificial Neural Networking. *Sep. Purif. Technol.* **2021**, *255*, 117720. [CrossRef]
52. Bertolo, M.R.V.; Martins, V.C.A.; Plepis, A.M.G.; Junior, S.B. Utilization of Pomegranate Peel Waste: Natural Deep Eutectic Solvents as a Green Strategy to Recover Valuable Phenolic Compounds. *J. Clean. Prod.* **2021**, *327*, 129471. [CrossRef]
53. Hossen, M.; Lokman, M.; Mitra, K.; Hossain, B. Phytochemicals and In-Vitro Antioxidant Activity Analysis of Aloe Vera by-Products (Skin) in Different Solvent Extract. *J. Agric. Food Res.* **2022**, *10*, 100460. [CrossRef]
54. Hu, Q.; Hu, Y.; Xu, J. Free Radical-Scavenging Activity of Aloe Vera (*Aloe barbadensis* Miller) Extracts by Supercritical Carbon Dioxide Extraction. *Food Chem.* **2005**, *91*, 85–90. [CrossRef]
55. Bushra, S.; Farooq, A.; Muhammad, A. Effect of Extraction Solvent/Technique on the Antioxidant Activity of Selected Medicinal Plant Extracts. *Molecules* **2009**, *14*, 2167–2180. [CrossRef]
56. Papagiannopoulos, M.; Wollseifen, H.R.; Mellenthin, A.; Haber, B.; Galensa, R. Identification and Quantification of Polyphenols in Carob Fruits (*Ceratonia Siliqua* L.) and Derived Products by HPLC-UV-ESI/MSn. *J. Agric. Food Chem.* **2004**, *52*, 3784–3791. [CrossRef] [PubMed]
57. Lucini, L.; Pellizzoni, M.; Pellegrino, R.; Pietro, G.; Colla, G. Phytochemical Constituents and in Vitro Radical Scavenging Activity of Different Aloe Species. *Food Bioprod. Process. Chem.* **2015**, *170*, 501–507. [CrossRef] [PubMed]
58. Min, K.; Sang, M.; Woo, M.; Zhao, J.; Jin, Y.; Lee, D.; Won, S.; Hoon, J.; Lee, J. Tailoring and Recycling of Deep Eutectic Solvents as Sustainable and Efficient Extraction Media. *J. Chromatogr. A* **2015**, *1424*, 10–17. [CrossRef]
59. Nam, M.W.; Zhao, J.; Lee, M.S.; Jeong, J.H.; Lee, J. Enhanced Extraction of Bioactive Natural Products Using Tailor-Made Deep Eutectic Solvents: Application to Flavonoid Extraction from Flos Sophorae. *Green Chem.* **2015**, *17*, 1718–1727. [CrossRef]
60. Dai, Y.; Van Spronsen, J.; Witkamp, G.J.; Verpoorte, R.; Choi, Y.H. Ionic Liquids and Deep Eutectic Solvents in Natural Products Research: Mixtures of Solids as Extraction Solvents. *J. Nat. Prod.* **2013**, *76*, 2162–2173. [CrossRef]
61. Zhou, P.; Wang, X.; Liu, P.; Huang, J.; Wang, C.; Pan, M. Enhanced Phenolic Compounds Extraction from *Morus Alba* L. Leaves by Deep Eutectic Solvents Combined with Ultrasonic-Assisted Extraction. *Ind. Crop. Prod.* **2018**, *120*, 147–154. [CrossRef]
62. Huang, Y.; Feng, F.; Jiang, J.; Qiao, Y.; Wu, T.; Voglmeir, J.; Chen, Z. Green and Efficient Extraction of Rutin from Tartary Buckwheat Hull by Using Natural Deep Eutectic Solvents. *Food Chem.* **2017**, *221*, 1400–1405. [CrossRef] [PubMed]

63. Cao, J.; Yang, M.; Cao, F.; Wang, J.; Su, E. Tailor-Made Hydrophobic Deep Eutectic Solvents for Cleaner Extraction of Polyprenyl Acetates from Ginkgo Biloba Leaves. *J. Clean. Prod.* **2017**, *152*, 399–405. [CrossRef]
64. Cui, Q.; Liu, J.; Wang, L.; Kang, Y.; Meng, Y.; Jiao, J.; Fu, Y. Sustainable Deep Eutectic Solvents Preparation and Their Ef Fi Ciency in Extraction and Enrichment of Main Bioactive Fl Avonoids from Sea Buckthorn Leaves. *J. Clean. Prod.* **2018**, *184*, 826–835. [CrossRef]
65. Plaza, A.; Tapia, X.; Yañez, C.; Vilches, F.; Candia, O.; Cabezas, R. Obtaining Hydroxytyrosol from Olive Mill Waste Using Deep Eutectic Solvents and Then Supercritical—CO_2. *Waste Biomass Valorization* **2020**, *11*, 6273–6284. [CrossRef]
66. Della Posta, S.; Gallo, V.; Gentili, A.; Fanali, C. Strategies for the Recovery of Bioactive Molecules from Deep Eutectic Solvents Extracts. *Trends Anal. Chem.* **2022**, *157*, 116798. [CrossRef]
67. Fu, N.; Lv, R.; Guo, Z.; Guo, Y.; You, X.; Tang, B.; Han, D.; Yan, H.; Ho, K. Environmentally Friendly and Non-Polluting Solvent Pretreatment of Palm Samples for Polyphenol Analysis Using Choline Chloride Deep Eutectic Solvents. *J. Chromatogr. A* **2017**, *1492*, 1–11. [CrossRef]
68. Pena-Pereira, F.; Wojnowski, W.; Tobiszewski, M. AGREE—Analytical GREEnness Metric Approach and Software. *Anal. Chem.* **2020**, *92*, 10076–10082. [CrossRef]
69. Wojnowski, W.; Tobiszewski, M.; Pena-Pereira, F.; Psillakis, E. AGREEprep—Analytical Greenness Metric for Sample Preparation. *TrAC Trends Anal. Chem.* **2022**, *149*, 116553. [CrossRef]
70. Mammana, S.B.; Gagliardi, L.G.; Silva, M.F. Sustainable Sample Preparation Method Based on Hydrophobic Natural Deep Eutectic Solvents. Chemometric Tools and Green Metrics for Ibuprofen in Groundwater. *Sep. Purif. Technol.* **2022**, *303*, 122240. [CrossRef]

antioxidants

MDPI

Article

Microwave-Assisted Extraction of Bioactive Compounds from Mandarin Peel: A Comprehensive Biorefinery Strategy

Marina Jurić [1], Nikolina Golub [1,*], Emerik Galić [1], Kristina Radić [1], Luna Maslov Bandić [2] and Dubravka Vitali Čepo [1,*]

1 Department of Nutrition and Dietetics, University of Zagreb Faculty of Pharmacy and Biochemistry, Ante Kovačića 1, 10000 Zagreb, Croatia; marina.juric@pharma.unizg.hr (M.J.); emerik.galic@pharma.unizg.hr (E.G.); kristina.radic@pharma.unizg.hr (K.R.)

2 Department of Chemistry, University of Zagreb Faculty of Agriculture, Svetošimunska 25, 10000 Zagreb, Croatia; lmaslov@agr.hr

* Correspondence: nikolina.golub@pharma.unizg.hr (N.G.); dubravka.vitali@pharma.unizg.hr (D.V.Č.)

Abstract: Mandarin peel is a valuable but underutilized source of numerous bioactive compounds. The main focus of this work was to develop an integrated two-step process for the subsequent extraction of polyphenols and carotenoids (step 1) and pectin (step 2) from mandarin peel by microwave-assisted extraction (MAE), using only green solvents. This represents a novel, scale-up-suitable approach that might contribute to the improved revalorization of mandarin peel. Response surface methodology was used to maximize the yields of polyphenols, flavonoids, and carotenoids, as well as antioxidative activity (DPPH- and ABTS-radical scavenging capacity). The sample-to-solvent ratio and solvent type significantly influenced extractability of polyphenols and carotenoids, while extraction time and power were the key variables influencing pectin yield. Optimal extracts contained 21.76 ± 0.46 mg GAE/g of polyphenols (with 139.7 ± 2.28 mg/g and 703.62 ± 51.72 µg/g of tangeretin and nobiletin, respectively); 352.3 ± 17.4 µg/g of β-carotene and 273 ± 23 mg/g of pectin. MAE resulted in either higher yields, reduced extraction times or both, compared to conventional solvent extraction (CSE), depending on the target compound. The energy consumption of MAE was considerably lower, compared to CSE, in four out of five developed extraction procedures. Pectin obtained in the integrated two-step process had higher purity compared to pectin extracted from intact mandarin peel.

Keywords: mandarin peel; response surface methodology; carotenoids; polyphenols; pectin; biorefinery approach; microwave-assisted extraction

1. Introduction

More than 120 million tonnes of mandarins (*Citrus reticulata* Blanco) are produced worldwide [1], and during processing 50–60% of the whole fruit remains as a by-product (peels, pomace, and seeds). In Croatia, the average annual mandarin production between 2020 and 2024 was 38,981 tonnes [2]. Considering that Medved et al. obtained 72 g of mandarin peel powder from 1 kg of mandarin fruit, it can be estimated that Croatia produces around 2807 tonnes of mandarin peel annually [3].

Mandarin peel is rich in bioactive components such as polyphenols, flavonoids, carotenoids and pectin [4], with a huge market for application in the pharma and food industries. For example, in 2022, the global polyphenol market was estimated to be worth USD 1.68 billion. From 2023 to 2030, it is projected to expand at a compound annual growth rate of 7.4% [5]. Similar information has been provided by another report [6], which projected a market size of USD 2.5 billion by 2030 at a 7.5% annual growth rate. Pectin, on the other hand, is frequently employed as a gelling, stabilizing, emulsifying and thickening ingredient in food and pharmaceutical goods [7]. The pectin market was worth USD 1.31 billion in 2023 and is expected to grow at 6.9% up to 2032 [8]. The carotenoid market will be worth USD 9 billion by 2031, with an expected annual growth of 4.5% [9].

In view of attempts to enhance the sustainable recovery of valuable bioactive compounds from natural sources, the contemporary focus of scientific investigations is set on the development and application of innovative green extraction techniques. Among them, microwave-assisted extraction (MAE) offers significant advantages compared to conventional solvent extraction (CSE)—it is considered a reliable and safe method resulting in higher extraction yields, reduced solvent use and shorter time of extraction. Additionally, it leads to lower rates of oxidation and degradation of bioactive compounds of interest [10]. Importantly, MAE technology has matured to the point of industrial scale-up, with commercially available continuous-flow systems, thus supporting its economic feasibility and technological readiness for large-scale applications. This combination of sustainability, efficiency and scalability positions MAE as a promising alternative for the extraction of natural products in food, pharmaceutical and cosmetic industries.

Even though investigations focused on the valorisation of mandarin peel as the source of polyphenols are numerous, the application of MAE for this purpose has been investigated by only several researchers. Kaur et al. [11] applied methanol, ethanol, acetonitrile, ethyl acetate and hexane, obtaining the highest phenolic content and antioxidant activity with 80% ethanol. Similarly, Inoue et al. [12] and Nishad et al. [13] obtained the highest yields using 70% ethanol, while Hayat et al. [14] applied 80% methanol. It is important to emphasize that in the mentioned investigations, in-house fabricated microwave extraction systems were applied for extraction. Compared to this approach, the utilization of laboratory closed-vessel systems for MAE offers numerous advantages. It provides a wider range of microwave power and wider choice of solvents; prevents solvent evaporation and thus reduces solvent use; prevents overpressure incidents and enables uniform heating, which altogether might result in higher yields and lower environmental impact of the process [15]. It is also important to emphasize that, to our knowledge, there is no available research that specifically targeted MAE yields of the most abundant polyphenolic compounds in mandarin peel—flavonoids nobiletin and tangeretin [16]. They show protective effects against memory impairment in Alzheimer's disease, dementia and Parkinson's disease, so their content is particularly important in terms of obtaining functional mandarin-peel based polyphenol extracts [17,18].

The most abundant carotenoids in mandarin peel are β-cryptoxanthin, β-citraurin and violaxanthin, with β-cryptoxanthin often dominating (62.1% of total carotenoids in some varieties) [19]. Available research shows that the extraction of carotenoids from mandarin peel is usually conducted by utilizing organic solvents, such as hexane or acetone, and highlights ultrasound-assisted extraction (UAE) as more effective compared to CSE [20,21]. To our knowledge, there are no available investigations on the application of MAE for carotenoids from mandarin peel, and studies on the possibilities of green extraction solvents are limited. Anticona et al. [21] applied ethanol–water mixtures for UAE of antioxidants (including carotenoids) from mandarin peel while Maslov Bandić et al. [22] optimized solid–liquid extraction of carotenoids using limonene.

Both polyphenols and carotenoids are recognized as potential antioxidants; however, they act through distinct mechanisms. Polyphenols primarily neutralize free radicals via hydrogen atom transfer, while carotenoids quench singlet oxygen and scavenge peroxyl radicals. Additionally, due to different solubility, their physiological bioavailability and distribution to cell compartments differ significantly. Therefore, when combined, these compounds can exhibit synergistic effects, enhancing overall biological capacity beyond the sum of their individual actions. This is particularly relevant for obtaining functional extracts, as consumers increasingly seek multicomponent products that deliver broad-spectrum health benefits. In that context, extracts optimized for targeted functional characteristics are better positioned to meet both efficacy and market demand for multifunctional, natural health solutions. As such, the two following methods for the determination of antioxidant activity are frequently applied—antioxidant activity against the 2,2-azino-bis (3-ethylbenzothiazoline-6-sulfonic acid) (ABTS) radical, which reacts with both hydrophilic and lipophilic antioxidants, and activity against the 2,2-diphenyl-1-picrylhydrazyl (DPPH) radical, which predominantly reacts with lipophilic compounds [23].

While citrus peels supply approximately 85% of commercial pectin globally [24], mandarin remains understudied despite its potential. Emerging studies demonstrate mandarin peel pectin yields comparable to conventional sources: for example, Satsuma mandarin peel yields 15.34–18.99% pectin using high-hydrostatic-pressure-assisted methods [25]. The possibilities of the MAE of pectin from mandarin peel have not been thoroughly investigated. Karbuz and Tugrul [26] showed that MAE was superior to ultrasound-assisted extraction in terms of improved pectin yields and purity. Kumar and co-workers [27] applied MAE to compare grapefruit and mandarin peel as sources of pectin and investigated the impact of mandarin peel pretreatment on the yields and purity of the obtained pectin. Even though both investigations pointed out the advantages of MAE as an extraction technique and the applicability of mandarin peel as a source of high-quality pectin, again, as in the case of polyphenols, a kitchen microwave oven was applied for extraction. Consequently, the authors failed to conduct in-depth multiple-response optimization in order to investigate the significance of particular MAE conditions on the yields and characteristics of the obtained pectin.

Generally, current scientific research on the potential utilization of secondary raw materials, such as mandarin peel, primarily focuses on reducing the environmental footprint of developed procedures while improving the yields and quality of obtained products. Therefore, special emphasis is set on investigating solvent-free extraction or the utilization of green solvents and the application of contemporary extraction methods targeting those with a high level of technological readiness and potential for industrial application. Another innovative strategy is the development of a biorefinery approach that supports circular bioeconomy principles since it combines different biomass conversion processes to produce high-value-added products. It offers wide range of advantages in terms of a reduced environmental footprint (due to the focus on green processing technologies, improved resource efficiency and reduced waste generation), economic benefits (due to the consolidation of extraction steps, which reduces operational costs and infrastructure requirements, shorter extraction times or improved yields) and simplified scale-up (due to a reduced need for multiple separate processing lines) [28].

This research presents a comprehensive investigation into the application of MAE for isolating polyphenols, carotenoids and pectin from mandarin peel in the laboratory closed-vessel microwave extraction system that offers numerous benefits compared to a household microwave oven. In addition to aiming for maximal yields of major target compounds, it also investigates the possibility of obtaining the highest functionality (antioxidant activity) of the final product. Moreover, the focus is set on the application of green solvents—citric acid for pectin extraction and water–ethanol mixtures for the extraction of polyphenols and carotenoids. By utilizing multiple-response optimization, the study aims to elucidate the influence of specific MAE parameters on both the yield and quality of the extracted compounds. Furthermore, the work provides a comparative analysis of MAE versus CSE in terms of energy consumption, extraction efficiency and chemical composition of the products. Finally, the potential integration of optimized MAE processes into a continuous, two-step process is investigated. In this biorefinery approach, pectin is extracted from the residue remaining after the extraction of antioxidants, highlighting the numerous advantages in terms of enabling sustainable and efficient valorisation of mandarin peel.

2. Materials and Methods

2.1. Organization of Conducted Research

For antioxidant recovery, Satsuma mandarins (*Citrus unshiu* Marc.) were sourced from the local mandarin juice producer Novallis, located in Opuzen, Croatia. The fruits were manually peeled, and the peels were frozen at −50 °C and subsequently lyophilized for 36 h using an ALPHA freeze dryer (Christ, Osterode am Harz, Germany). Following lyophilization, the dried mandarin peels were milled to achieve a uniform particle size. The resulting material was then passed through a 0.45 mm stainless steel sieve to ensure homogeneity. The obtained powdered sample was stored at −20 °C until further experimentation. For pectin extraction, mandarin peel was dried in a laboratory oven at 60 °C until constant weight. After drying, the peel was ground, sieved through a 0.8 mm sieve and stored at 4 °C until extraction.

A schematic diagram of the research performed in this study is presented in Figure 1.

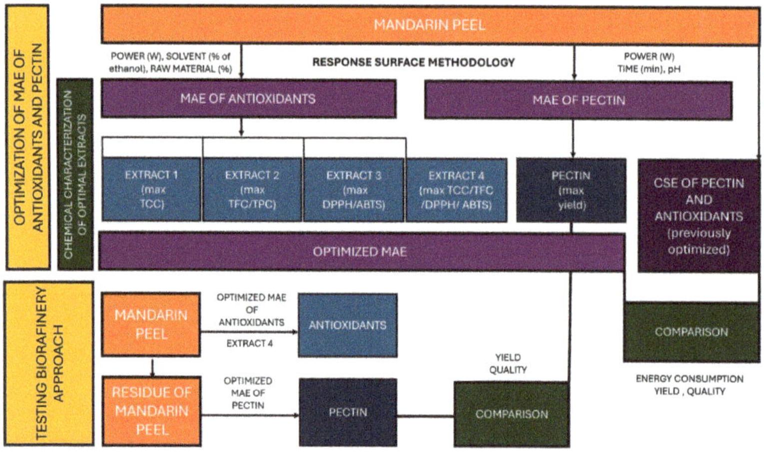

Figure 1. A schematic diagram of the experiments performed in this study. MAE—microwave-assisted extraction; TCC—total carotenoid content; TFC—total flavonoid content; TPC—total polyphenol content, ABTS—2,2-azino-bis (3-ethylbenzothiazoline-6-sulfonic acid) radical scavenging assay; DPPH—2,2-diphenyl-1-picrylhydrazyl radical scavenging assay.

Briefly, in the first phase of the investigation, response surface methodology (RSM) was used to optimize ethanol–water MAE of polyphenols and carotenoids form mandarin peel and determine major factors influencing yields. All together, 4 processes were optimized with the aim of obtaining extract 1 with maximal total carotenoid content; extract 2 with maximal content of polyphenols and flavonoids; extract 3 with maximal antioxidant activity and extract 4 where MAE conditions were optimized to yield maximal amounts of all targeted compounds. Parallelly, RSM was applied to optimize MAE for the extraction of pectin from mandarin peel. In order to investigate potential benefits of MAE, optimized MAE procedures were compared to optimal CSE procedures in terms of yields and energy consumption. For polyphenols, carotenoids and antioxidant potential, CSE procedures were optimized in the framework of preliminary investigations (unpublished data); for referent pectin, a CSE method available in the literature was used. In the second phase of the investigation, residues of mandarin peel remaining after obtaining extract 4 were used for the MAE of pectin. The characteristics of the obtained pectin were compared with those obtained from intact mandarin peel to investigate the applicability of the proposed biorefinery approach.

2.2. Experimental Design for Optimizing Extraction of Antioxidants

RSM coupled with the Box–Behnken design (three factors/three levels) (DesignExpert 7.0.0, Stat-Ease, Minneapolis, MN, USA) was used for the optimization of the MAE of antioxidants.

Prior to conducting a response surface analysis, initial factor screening using experimental designs such as Taguchi methods, Plackett–Burman designs, fractional factorial designs or single-factor-at-a-time experiments is critical to identify statistically significant parameters, thereby reducing experimental complexity and optimizing resource allocation by focusing subsequent surface exploration on influential variables [29–31]. In this case, preliminary research was conducted using a one-factor design, monitoring the influence of the solvent-to-raw material ratio; solvent type (ethanol, ethanol water mixtures or methanol) and temperature on the yields of polyphenols, flavonoids, carotenoids and antioxidative activity. Based on preliminary results, the following conditions were chosen for the RSM: ethanol–water mixtures as solvents (ranging from 30 to 90% v/v); microwave power (400–800 W) and the time of extraction adjusted to keep the maximal temperature of the reaction mixture below 75 °C to prevent the degradation of carotenoids.

Independent factors and their levels are shown in Table 1, with the following parameters—raw material (0.1–0.3%, w/v), power (400–800 W) and ethanol/water solvent ratio (30–90%, v/v)—while the temperature was monitored and adjusted to be below 75 °C. In that context, extraction was performed for 4 min (at a power of 400 W), for 2 min (600 W), and for 1 min (800 W) in a laboratory closed-vessel microwave system (Ethos Easy, Milestone, Sorisole, Italy). After extraction, the reaction mixtures were cooled down to room temperature and filtered. The obtained filtrates were used for the determination of antioxidant capacity, total carotenoid, total polyphenolic and total flavonoid content. A total of four optimal extracts were obtained, depending on the desired outcomes: 4 optimizations were performed by either maximizing selected responses (extracts 1–3: total carotenoids, total polyhenols/flavonoids, antioxidant activity) or by maximizing all responses (extract 4).

Table 1. Independent factors and their levels used in the design for the optimization of antioxidants.

Factor	Factor Level		
	−1	0	1
	Numeric Factors		
A: power (W)	400	600	800
B: solvent (%)	30	60	90
C: raw material (%)	0.1	0.2	0.3

CSE of antioxidants was optimized in the frameworks of preliminary investigations. The Box–Behnken design (three factors/three levels) was applied. Independent factors and their levels were as follows: raw material (0.1–0.3%, w/v), temperature (25–65 °C) and ethanol/water solvent ratio (30–90%, v/v). Optimization was equivalent to the optimization of MAE, and therefore, a total of 4 optimal extracts were obtained (extract 1–extract 4). Equations describing the relations between the CSE conditions and observed variables are presented in Table S1. Other data regarding CSE optimization are not shown in this study and are available on request.

2.3. Experimental Design for Determination of Pectin

RSM coupled with the Box–Behnken design (three factors/three levels) (Stat-Ease 360 22.0.8, Stat-Ease, Minneapolis, MN, USA) was used to optimize the MAE conditions for pectin. Independent factors and their levels are shown in Table 2.

Table 2. Independent factors and their levels used in the design for the optimization of pectin extraction.

Factor	Factor Level		
	−1	0	1
		Numeric Factors	
A: time (min)	1	3	5
B: power (W)	1000	1400	1800
C: pH	1	1.5	2

MAE was performed using a laboratory closed-vessel microwave system (Ethos Easy, Milestone, Sorisole, Italy). Each extraction began with a 10 s phase to reach the set microwave power, followed by a constant power phase for the designated extraction time, and ended with a cooling phase until the temperature reached 85 °C. The stirring speed was set to 10%. Time and power were chosen as independent factors based on extensive literature data pointing them out as the mostly influential in MAE [32]. Citric acid has been chosen as the solvent due to its good ecological acceptance and the literature pointing it out as particularly suitable for the extraction of pectin from similar matrices (citrus fruit) [33]. In addition to power and time, temperature can also have significant impact on pectin yields. It was not considered in the experimental design since the majority microwave digestion units (including ours) do not have an integrated cooling system installed that would enable the regulation of the temperature of the reaction mixture at the constant microwave power.

Temperature change was monitored during the process. A total of 1 g of mandarin peel was mixed in the vessel with 20 mL of 1% citric acid monohydrate (with the pH adjusted to 1, 1.5 or 2 using 6 M hydrochloric acid). The sample-to-solvent ratio was chosen based on available literature data and conducted preliminary research. Vessels were then closed and placed in the microwave rotor plate. Afterwards, the extract was passed through cotton gauze directly into a sinter funnel (grade 2) with FN3 filter paper and vacuum filtered, followed by a second filtration with filter paper. To precipitate pectin, an amount of 96% ethanol equal to twice the volume of the extraction solvent was added to the filtrate and the mixture was refrigerated at 4 °C. After 24 h, pectin was collected by filtration, dried at 45 °C until constant weight, ground in a mortar and stored at 4 °C.

The CSE of pectin was performed as described by Casas-Orozco et al. [34], with some modifications. Briefly, 5 g of mandarin peel was extracted in a water bath (2 h/85 °C) with 100 mL of 1% citric acid monohydrate (with the pH adjusted to the optimal MAE pH). All procedures following extraction were the same as described for MAE.

Once the optimal MAE conditions for polyphenol and pectin extraction were determined, polyphenols were extracted from lyophilized mandarin peel. After filtration, the residue was collected, dried and used for pectin extraction. The pectin's yield and characteristics were compared to pectin extracted from the sample where polyphenols were not extracted.

2.4. Determination and Chemical Characterization of Antioxidants

2.4.1. Spectrophotometric Determination of Antioxidants

Total carotenoid content (TCC) in mandarin peel extracts was determined according to the modified Barros et al. [35] method. Detection was performed by measuring absorbance at 453, 505 and 663 nm using a UV-Vis spectrophotometer (Model SpectraMax i3x Multi-Mode Detection Platform, Molecular Devices, San Jose, CA, USA). The content was calculated using Equation (1), and results are presented as μg of beta-carotene equivalent per g of dry peel.

$$\beta - \text{carotene}(\text{mg}/100\ \text{mL}) = (0.216 \times \text{A663}) - (0.304 \times \text{A505}) + (0.452 \times \text{A453}) \quad (1)$$

Total phenolic content (TPC) was determined by the modified Ainsworth & Gillespie et al. [36] method using the Folin–Ciocalteu (F-C) reagent (obtained from Merck, Darmstadt, Germany). A volume of 20 μL of extract and 50 μL of 10% (v/v) F-C reagent was added to the microplate, shaken and incubated for 5 min at 37 °C. Furthermore, 160 μL of 700 mM Na_2CO_3 (Lach-Ner, Tovarni, Czech Republic) was added and incubated for 30 min at the same temperature. Absorbance was measured at 750 nm, using a UV-VIS spectrophotometer (Model Victor x3, PerkinElmer, Waltham, MA, USA). The results are expressed as mg of gallic acid equivalents (GAE) per g of dry peel.

Total flavonoid content (TFC) in mandarin peel was detected using the spectrophotometric method of Ivanova et al. [37]. A volume of 4 mL of water and 1 mL of mandarin peel extract was mixed with 0.3 mL of $NaNO_2$ (0.5 g/L) in a volumetric flask. After 5 min, 0.3 mL of $AlCl_3$ (Sigma Aldrich, Steinheim, Germany) (1 g/L) was added. The reaction mixture was left for 6 min to react when 2 mL of NaOH (Sigma Aldrich, Steinheim, Germany) was added (1 mol/L). The volume was adjusted up to 10 mL with distilled water. Measurements were performed by measuring the absorbance at 360 nm using a UV-Vis spectrophotometer (Model SpectraMax i3x Multi-Mode Detection Platform, Molecular Devices, San Jose, CA, USA). The content of total flavonoids was quantified, and the results are expressed as mg quercetin equivalents (QE) per g of dry peel.

For the determination of antioxidant activity, DPPH and ABTS reagents were used (obtained from Sigma Aldrich, Steinheim, Germany). Antioxidant capacity determination using ABTS reagent was modified according to Re et al. [38]. A volume of 20 μL of extract was pipetted in the microplate with 200 μL of diluted $ABTS^{\cdot+}$ reagent. The absorbance was measured at 750 nm, using a UV-Vis spectrophotometer (Model SpectraMax i3x Multi-Mode Detection Platform, Molecular Devices, San Jose, CA, USA), and the results are expressed as the mmol Trolox equivalent (TE) per g of dry peel. The other method was modified according to Brand-Williams et al. [39]. In total, 150 μL of the DPPH methanol solution was mixed with 150 μL of extract. After 30 min of incubation, absorbance was measured at 530 nm, using a UV-VIS spectrophotometer (Model Victor x3, PerkinElmer, Waltham, MA, USA), and the results are expressed as mmol Trolox equivalent per g of dry peel.

2.4.2. HPLC Analysis of Polymethoxyflavones

In this research, optimal extracts were characterized by the determination of polymethoxyflavones (PMFs) using high-performance liquid chromatography, HPLC. All samples were evaporated to dryness and dissolved in 4 mL of water. A mixture was prepared by combining 0.6 mL of sample with 0.6 mL of a methanol/DMSO solution (1:1, v/v) in Eppendorf tubes. The mixture was then sonicated for 15 min at 50 °C, followed by centrifugation at 5000 rpm for 15 min at 4 °C. The resulting supernatant was transferred and filtered by 0.45 μm LLC-RC syringe filters prior to analysis to vials for HPLC analysis.

A modified method was used to determine the content of nobiletin and tangeretin by HPLC in the obtained extracts [17]. Nobiletin and tangeretin were obtained from Toronto Research Chemicals (Toronto, ON, Canada).

The Agilent 1260 Infinity II System (Agilent, Waldbronn, Germany), equipped with an autosampler, column thermostat and diode-array detector (DAD), was used. The separation of nobiletin and tangeretin was performed on an Agilent Poroshell 120 SB-C18 column (4.6 × 150 mm, 4 μm) at 40 °C. The detection wavelengths were 280, 330 and 360 nm. The injected sample volume was 20 μL. The mobile phase was 2% formic acid (solvent A) and methanol (solvent B) at a flow rate of 0.8 mL/min. The solvent gradient in volume ratios was as follows: 0–10 min, 10–20% B; 10–20 min, 20–30% B; 20–30 min, 30–40% B; 30–35 min, 40% B; 35–42 min, 40–50% B; 42–52 min, 50–90% B; 52–53 min, 90–10% B; and 53–60 min, 10% B. Polymethoxyflavones were identified by matching the retention time of each chromatographic peak with external standards and the DAD spectrum. The quantification of individual PMF peaks was performed by the external standard method. Results are expressed as mg per g of dried mandarin peel. HPLC chromatograms are presented in Figure S1.

2.5. Characterization of Pectin

The physico-chemical characterization of pectin included the determination of yield, equivalent mass (EM), methoxyl content (MC), the degree of esterification (DE) and anhydrouronic acid content (AUA), as described in previous publications [40], along with Fourier transform infrared (FTIR) spectroscopy for functional group identification. All titrations were performed using standardized 0.01 M NaOH.

The pectin yield from both CSE and MAE was determined gravimetrically using Equation (2):

$$\text{Pectin yield}(\%) = \frac{\text{w(pectin)}}{\text{w(mandarin peel)}} \times 100 \quad (2)$$

where w is dry weight in grams.

For the determination of EM, the pectin sample (0.05 g) was moistened with 200 μL of 96% ethanol, dissolved in 10 mL of carbon dioxide-free water and left closed overnight in a magnetic stirrer to allow complete pectin dissolution. After the addition of 100 mg of NaCl and 1 drop of phenol red indicator, the mixture was titrated until the pink endpoint was reached. EM was calculated using Equation (3):

$$\text{EM}(\text{g/mol}) = \frac{\text{Weight of sample(g)} \times 1000}{\text{Volume of alkali(mL)} \times \text{Molarity of alkali}} \quad (3)$$

This neutralized solution was used for the determination of MC, by adding 2.5 mL of 0.25 M NaOH and leaving the mixture closed at room temperature. After 30 min, 2.5 mL 0.25 M HCl was added and titrated to the pink endpoint. MC was calculated from Equation (4):

$$\text{MC}(\%) = \frac{\text{Volume of alkali (mL)} \times \text{Molarity of alkali} \times 31}{\text{Weight of sample(g)} \times 1000} \times 100 \quad (4)$$

where 31 is the molecular weight of the methoxyl group.

For the determination of the DE, the pectin sample (0.05 g) was moistened with 500 μL of 96% ethanol, dissolved in 5 mL of distilled water and left closed overnight in a magnetic stirrer to allow complete pectin dissolution. After adding 1 drop of phenolphthalein, the solution was titrated until the pink endpoint was reached (initial titration volume). To neutralize polygalacturonic acid, 2.5 mL of 0.1 M NaOH was added, and the sample was vortexed for 30 s and left at room temperature for 2 h to allow pectin deesterification. Then,

2.5 mL of 0.1 M HCl was added along with 1 drop of phenolphthalein, and the mixture was titrated again until the pink endpoint was reached (final volume). The DE was calculated from Equation (5):

$$\mathrm{DE}(\%) = \frac{\text{Final titration volume (mL)}}{\text{Initial titration volume(mL)} + \text{Final titration volume(mL)}} \times 100 \quad (5)$$

AUA was calculated from the equation below using titration volumes obtained from the determination of EM and MC by Equation (6):

$$\mathrm{AUA}\ (\%) = \frac{176 \times 0.01z \times 100}{w \times 1000} + \frac{176 \times 0.01y \times 100}{w \times 1000} \quad (6)$$

where a molecular unit of AUA (1 unit) = 176 g, z = mL (titre) of standardized 0.01 M NaOH used in the determination of EM, y = mL (titre) of standardized 0.01 M NaOH used in the determination of MC and w = weight of the sample in grams.

The obtained pectin was analyzed using a FTIR spectrophotometer (Spectrum Two, Perkin Elmer, Waltham, MA, USA), over a spectral range of 500–4000 cm^{-1} with 16 scans and a spectral resolution of 4 cm^{-1}.

2.6. Energy Consumption

Total energy consumption for the optimized CSE and MAE protocols was calculated according to Equation (7):

$$\mathrm{E(kWh/kg)} = \frac{\mathrm{P(kW)} \times \mathrm{t(h)}}{\mathrm{K(kg)}} \quad (7)$$

where P is the power of the water bath/microwave extraction unit (kW); t is the time of heating/microwave radiation during extraction duration (h) and K is the capacity of the water bath/microwave extraction unit (kg), referring to the maximal mass of raw material that can be processed in one run due to the size/design of the water bath/microwave unit. The time of heating for CSE was the sum of the time needed for the water bath to heat to the targeted extraction temperature and the time the heater was working during the extraction process. In MAE, the instrument was at 100% power during the whole time of extraction. For CSE, the power of the water bath was 1.5 kW; K was 0.09 kg for pectin and 0.0018–0.0054 kg for antioxidants (depending on the conditions of the extraction procedure). For MAE, the power for pectin and antioxidants was 1.335 kW and 0.4 kW, respectively, while K was 0.0375 kg and 0.0008–0.0012 kg, respectively. Energy consumption for the CSE, calculated using Equation (7), was additionally corrected with the energy needed for the shaking of the water bath, approximated to 0.1 kW/h (data obtained from the producer).

2.7. Statistical Analysis

Design-expert 7.0.0 and Stat Ease 360 22.0.8 software were used for the RSM. GraphPad Prism 10.4.1 (GraphPad Software, San Diego, CA, USA) was used for conducting other statistical tests and for the graphical presentation of data. ANOVA and Student's *t*-test have been used for the calculation of significant differences between the obtained results. Analyses were conducted in 2–6 parallels (depending on the method) and obtained values were presented as means ± standard deviations.

3. Results

3.1. Optimization of Microwave-Assisted Extraction of Antioxidants

Response surface methodology was used to optimize the extraction parameters and obtain a model describing the yield of carotenoids, polyphenols, flavonoids and antioxidative activity (ABTS and DPPH) influenced by three independent variables. Single-factor and Box–Behnken designs were used for extraction optimization. Firstly, the effects of important aspects of the MAE process, like raw material, solvent ratio, power, time and temperature, on the yield of desired compounds were investigated in the single-factor experiment. Secondly, the Box–Behnken design was used to optimize the extraction process consisting of raw material (0.1–0.3%, *w*/*v*), ethanol/water solvent ratio (30–90%, *v*/*v*) and power (400–800 W). The experiment had 17 experimental runs, which were carried out in random order. Analysis of variance was used to assess the credibility of the model, and adequacy was assessed using the following criteria—*p*-value R2 (coefficient of determination), adjusted-R2, the coefficient of variation (CV), a lack of fit and adequate precision [41]—all of which are presented in Table S3. *p*-values were used to test the statistical significance of each term in the model. The five response variables presented in Table 3 are the means of the measurements (n = 5).

Table 3. Design of the experiment matrix for the microwave-assisted extraction of antioxidants and alongside responses.

	F1	F2	F3	R1	R2	R3	R4	R5
Run	**Power (W)**	**Solvent (%)**	**Raw Material (%)**	**TCC (μg Beta-Carotene/g)**	**TPC (mg GAE/g)**	**TFC (mg QE/g)**	**ABTS (mmol TE/g)**	**DPPH (mmol TE/g)**
1	600	60	0.2	71.98 ± 7.11	19.84 ± 0.89	74.06 ± 0.42	0.23 ± 0.02	0.03 ± 0.00
2	800	90	0.2	325.68 ± 4.79	12.31 ± 1.07	64.25 ± 1.58	0.31 ± 0.01	0.03 ± 0.00
3	600	60	0.2	75.94 ± 7.61	20.36 ± 1.60	73.46 ± 0.46	0.26 ± 0.02	0.03 ± 0.00
4	600	30	0.1	70.17 ± 7.07	21.10 ± 1.81	69.19 ± 2.45	0.27 ± 0.02	0.03 ± 0.00
5	800	30	0.2	48.68 ± 3.35	19.04 ± 0.43	70.59 ± 4.00	0.29 ± 0.02	0.03 ± 0.00
6	400	60	0.1	87.38 ± 2.99	21.83 ± 1.31	81.56 ± 3.33	0.37 ± 0.02	0.03 ± 0.00
7	600	30	0.3	45.57 ± 4.32	17.53 ± 0.87	62.61 ± 1.23	0.20 ± 0.01	0.02 ± 0.00
8	800	60	0.3	64.77 ± 2.48	20.00 ± 1.24	76.96 ± 3.38	0.29 ± 0.01	0.03 ± 0.00
9	600	60	0.2	60.47 ± 5.67	20.55 ± 1.10	79.62 ± 2.65	0.24 ± 0.02	0.03 ± 0.00
10	600	90	0.1	335.59 ± 10.79	19.29 ± 1.23	61.10 ± 0.81	0.25 ± 0.01	0.02 ± 0.00
11	800	60	0.1	84.14 ± 3.34	20.67 ± 0.74	71.95 ± 4.06	0.37 ± 0.02	0.03 ± 0.00
12	600	90	0.3	307.45 ± 14.17	15.94 ± 1.36	59.41 ± 0.98	0.19 ± 0.01	0.02 ± 0.00
13	400	90	0.2	352.39 ± 2.64	18.82 ± 0.98	73.83 ± 2.57	0.32 ± 0.01	0.02 ± 0.00
14	400	30	0.2	47.16 ± 2.50	19.13 ± 1.22	71.63 ± 1.70	0.31 ± 0.02	0.03 ± 0.00
15	400	60	0.3	70.04 ± 2.81	19.93 ± 1.17	82.94 ± 1.35	0.28 ± 0.01	0.02 ± 0.00
16	600	60	0.2	65.57 ± 2.99	20.94 ± 0.33	76.20 ± 0.17	0.25 ± 0.01	0.03 ± 0.00
17	600	60	0.2	77.73 ± 7.12	21.25 ± 1.43	77.77 ± 2.98	0.25 ± 0.02	0.03 ± 0.00

TCC—total carotenoid content; TPC—total phenolic content; TFC—total flavonoid content, ABTS—2,2-azino-bis (3-ethylbenzothiazoline-6-sulfonic acid) radical scavenging assay; DPPH—2,2-diphenyl-1-picrylhydrazyl radical scavenging assay; GAE—gallic acid equivalents; QE—quercetin equivalents; TE—Trolox equivalents.

$p < 0.0001$ implies the model for TCC is significant. Conversely, the lack of fit ($p = 0.1698$) was not significant. The signal-to-noise ratio is measured by "Adeq Precision", and a ratio greater than 4 is desirable [41]. The ratio of 40.87 indicates an adequate signal. A high value of R2 (0.9970) shows that the model successfully accounted for 99% of the variance of the observed dependent variable. The Adj R-Squared value (0.9931) indicates a high correlation between predicted and observed values, and the same indicates that the model can be applied to future data.

The second-order polynomial equation for TCC is presented in Table S2. It demonstrates that the yield of carotenoids is influenced by both first- and second-order terms. As shown, factors A (raw material) and C (power) have a negative impact on TCC, while factor B (solvent) has a positive one. A similar trend can be seen when analyzing the *p* values of the terms in the equation. Significant influence is assigned to factor A ($p = 0.0001$), B ($p < 0.0001$) and the quadratic term B2 ($p < 0.0001$). Interestingly, the quadratic nature of the solvent variable that follows a U-shaped curve means it reduces the TCC yield to a certain point when its influence is opposite and nonlinear, meaning that slight changes in the variable lead to a fast increase in TCC. This was expected, since ethanol is a less polar solvent compared to water and can be more effective for carotenoid extraction. Simply put, increasing the solvent ratio increases TCC, while an increase in power and raw material decreases TCC. This is visually represented by response surface plots (Figure 2). The highest yield was obtained with the highest ethanol ratio (90%). The interactions among independent variables were not shown to be significant; however, response surface plots do reveal some important trends. With the highest used ethanol ratio (90%) as a fixed parameter, increasing power up to 800 W resulted in a decrease in TCC, probably resulting in carotenoid degradation under strong microwave radiation [42]. When keeping the raw material fixed, it is obvious that the more ethanol, the more efficient the extraction, independent of the power used. As presented in Table 3 the obtained values of TCC ranged depending on the applied extraction conditions, from 45.57 to 352.39 μg β-carotene/g. Similar results were found in the research by Maslov Bandić et al., where TCC from mandarin peel ranged from 58.67 to 227.18 μg β-carotene/g [43]. Comparable yields were also obtained from citrus and orange peel by other authors [44,45].

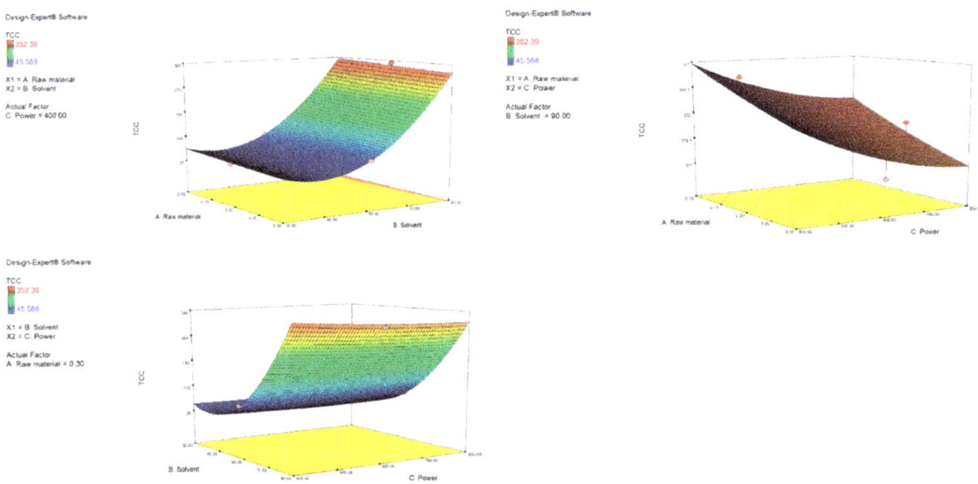

Figure 2. Response surface plots (3D) for TCC as a function of power, raw material and solvent.

For TPC extraction, a quadratic model was suggested (p = 0.0104). The lack of fit (p = 0.0304) was statistically significant; on the other hand, the residual plot was characterized by random scattering and constant variance (Figure S3B). A ratio of 11.064 indicates an adequate signal. The coefficient of variation (CV) is 5.86. In order to verify the model's repeatability, a CV of less than 10 is desirable, according to Beg et al. [46]. Almost 90% of the variation can be explained by the projected model proved by R2 0.8949. An Adj R-Squared value of 0.7599 indicates a good correlation between predicted and observed values. In the case of TFC, the suggested quadratic model is statistically significant (p = 0.0042). The lack of fit is not significant (p = 0.2790), and the signal is adequate, indicated by the ratio of 9.858. A CV of 4.14 is satisfactory. The model describes the relationship between the response and independent variables well, as can be seen from the high values of R2 (0.9207) and adj-R2 (0.8187) [47]. The final equation in terms of coded factors for TPC and TFC is presented in Table S2.

The model showed that all individual terms had a statistically significant negative effect: A—raw material (p = 0.0210), B—solvent (p = 0.0139) and C—microwave power (p = 0.0475). Furthermore, the BC interaction had a significant negative effect (p = 0.0252).

Term B2 also had a significant impact on the yield ($p = 0.0018$), where the term has a (-) sign, meaning it follows a reverse U-shaped curve. The increase in ethanol concentration leads to an increase in TPC up to a certain level, when that effect becomes reversed. The same was noticed in the case of TCC but in the opposite direction, which is logical when considering the different polarity of polyphenols and carotenoids [48].

Figure 3A visually describes the effects of independent variables and their interactions on TPC. With fixed raw material, an increase in ethanol ratio from 30 to 60% increased the TPC. Also, under fixed power, a lower raw material ratio (0.1%) resulted in a higher TPC (22.36 mg GAE/g d.w.), indicating that more solvent (compared to raw material) is needed to make the extraction of polyphenols efficient. As previously mentioned, it was visually confirmed that higher ethanol ratios significantly decrease the TPC yield (to 16.58 mg GAE/g). As seen in the third graph, with a fixed solvent, a decrease in power increases TPC. Shorter exposure intervals at low-to-moderate power may preserve or even increase TPC due to more suitable extraction conditions. On the other hand, longer exposure times at higher microwave power cause thermal degradation of phenolic compounds [49,50]. This model has shown that the highest yield of polyphenols can be obtained using 60% ethanol, with low power and a low amount of raw material. Similar findings were reported by García-Martín et al. [51], which determined the highest TPC with 50% ethanol.

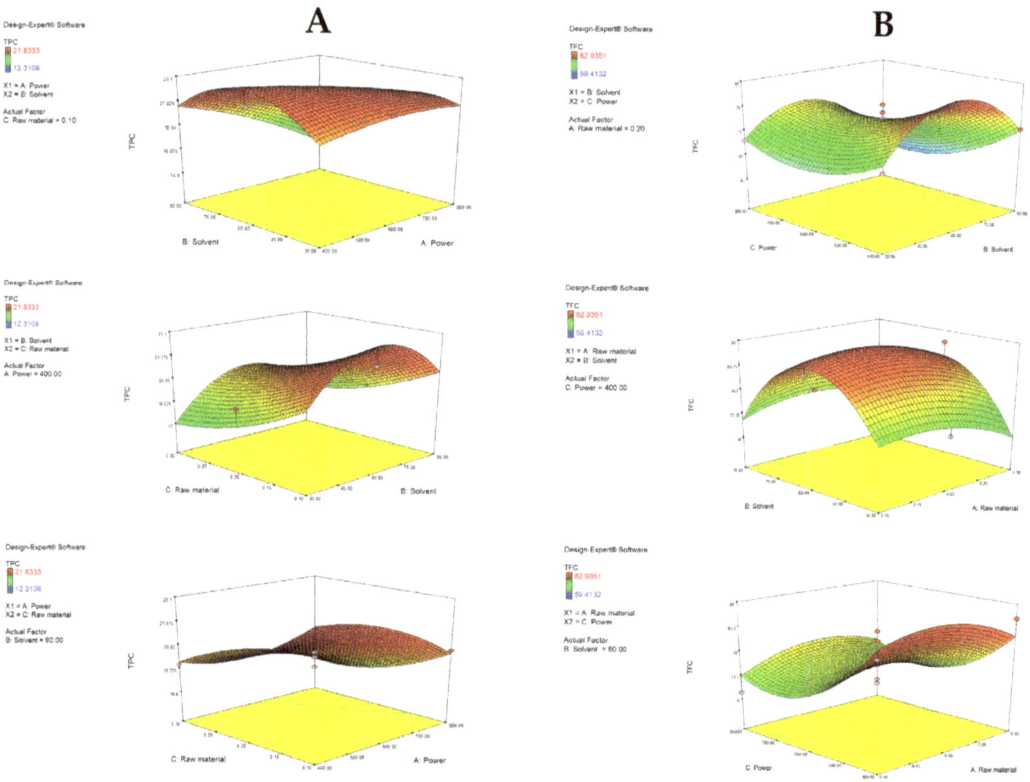

Figure 3. Response surface plots (3D) for TPC (**A**) and TFC (**B**) as a function of power, raw material and solvent.

When analyzing TFC, C (power) showed a statistically significant impact ($p = 0.0174$), specifically C2 ($p = 0.0166$), as well as solvent B2 (0.0003). The solvent showed a similar trend as described for TPC. Interestingly, the power had a more pronounced effect for TFC, where an increase from 600 to 800 W increased TFC slightly, while an increase in power from 400 to 600 W resulted in a decrease, clearly following the U-shaped curve of the quadratic term.

Figure 3B graphically demonstrates the effects of the tested variables on TFC. A rise in the yield of flavonoids was obtained with an increase in solvent up to 60%, while a further increase in the ethanol ratio resulted in a decrease in TFC. Additionally, more raw material, up to a central point (0.2%), resulted in a higher yield, while further addition of raw material resulted in a decrease. The highest TFC was determined with the lowest power (400 W), again emphasizing the sensitive chemical nature of flavonoids. With fixed power, raw material and solvent did not significantly influence TFC. Overall, TPC in the extracts ranged from 12.31 to 21.83 mg GAE/g, while TFC ranged from 59.41 to 82.94 mg QE/g, which is comparable to the results of other authors. Zhang et al. [23] determined TPC to be in the range from 22.80 to 32.76 mg GAE/g d.w., while Kumar et al. [52] quantified it at 22.88 to 43.61 mg GAE/g d.w. in Citrus reticulata peels. Furthermore, Maslov Bandić et al. [43] determined TPC in the range from 22.24 mg GAE/g to 28.77 mg GAE/g. On the other hand, the same authors obtained TFC in a range from 25.87 mg QE/g to 35.90 mg QE/g, depending on the mandarin variety. Similarly, Lee & Kim [53] found TFC in the range from 23.51 to 43.99 mg QE/g in mandarin peels of different maturation stages.

Furthermore, the impact of extraction conditions on ABTS antiradical activity was described using a quadratic model (p = 0.0001). The Lack of fit (p = 0.1576) was not significant, and the adequate precision was greater than 4 (16.953), which indicates an appropriate signal. R2 was 0.9671, with Adj R2 at 0.9249, confirming that the model successfully described the majority of variation in the dependent variable. The quadratic model for DPPH was significant (p = 0.0047), and the lack of fit (p = 0.0041) was statistically significant; however, the residual plot illustrates random scattering with no observable trends and constant variance (Figure S3D). A ratio of 10.457 indicates an adequate signal. Almost 92% of the variation could be explained by the projected model, according to the R2 value of 0.9181. An Adj R-Squared value of 0.8128 indicates a good correlation between predicted and observed values. The coefficients of variation (CVs) were satisfactory: 5.12 (ABTS) and 5.61 (DPPH). The final equations in terms of coded factors for antioxidative activity are shown in Table S2.

It can be observed that the increase in raw material significantly (p = 0.0001) decreases ABTS antiradical activity. Furthermore, the solvent follows a quadratic function (B), similar to the case of TFC. The term power also follows a quadratic function (C2). Figure 4A depicts response surface plots, and it can be seen that an increase in radical inhibition was achieved with an increase in ethanol from 30 to 60% (when the raw material is fixed), while a further increase resulted in the lowest antioxidant activity. This indicates that there is a central area that provides the most efficient extraction of antioxidants, probably due to the simultaneous extraction of both polar and less polar antioxidants [48]. The power increases to the middle point (600 W) resulted in a decrease in the antioxidative potential, while a further increase had a positive effect. With fixed power, a lower amount of raw material increases ABTS, and a higher ethanol ratio increases the antioxidative potential due to the greater capacity of the solvent to extract the antioxidants if it is present in a high ratio compared to the raw material. In that context, the highest ABTS values can be observed with the lowest power, the lowest raw material amount and 50% ethanol.

DPPH was significantly affected by the A—raw material (p = 0.0042), A2 (p = 0.0353), B—solvent (p = 0.0016) and C—power (p = 0.0480), along with the interaction of raw material and solvent (p = 0.0122) and raw material and power (p = 0.0248). Visualized in Figure 4B, the optimal raw material percentage for maximizing DPPH was 0.1%, and further increases had a negative impact on the yield. An increase in the ethanol ratio also decreased the DPPH antioxidative effect. Higher antioxidative activity was noted when power was increased, which is consistent with the results of Hayat et al. [14]. The interaction between raw material and solvent, as well as raw material and power, showed significant impact, meaning that if an increase in raw material occurs along with an increase in the ethanol ratio or power, a considerable amount of antioxidants can be extracted, which results in notable activity.

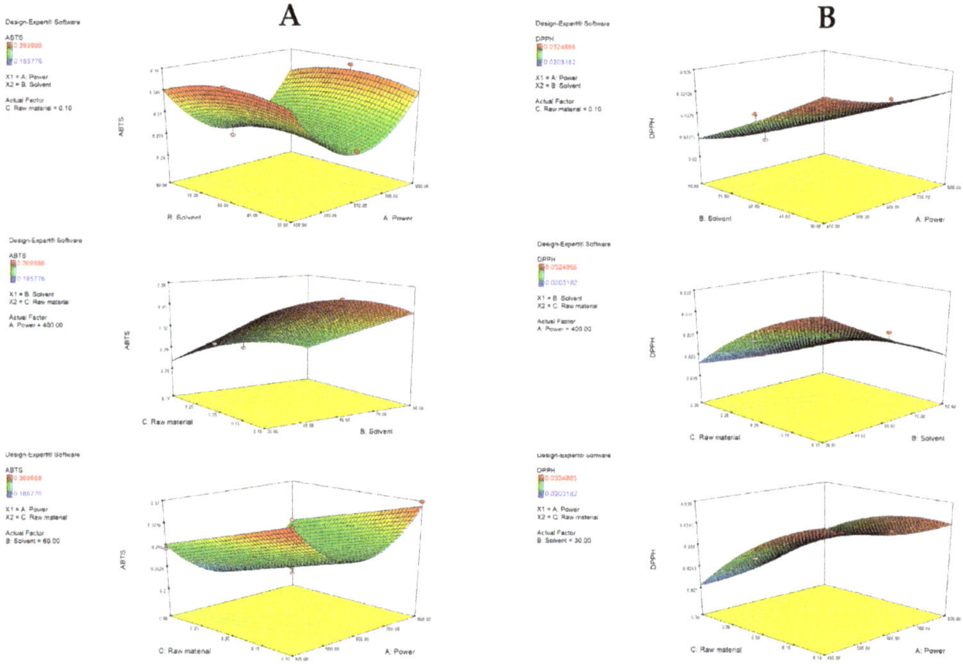

Figure 4. Response surface plots (3D) for ABTS (**A**) and DPPH (**B**) as a function of power, raw material and solvent.

Antioxidant activity ranged from 0.19 to 0.37 mmol TE/g and 0.02 to 0.03 mmol TE/g for ABTS and DPPH antiradical activity, respectively. The obtained results are comparable to the values obtained by other authors, although there is a high level of variation. This is probably due to variable extraction conditions and differences in mandarin genotypes, agroclimatic conditions and sample handling [23]. Despite the high variability, all available literature data show ABTS antioxidant activity to be significantly higher compared to DPPH, which is consistent with our results [21,54,55]. The abovementioned observations can be explained by the two radicals' different mechanisms of reaction [56,57]. DPPH radical reacts predominately with antioxidants with lipophilic characteristics (such as TCC), while ABTS reacts with both lipophilic and hydrophilic antioxidants (TPC, TFC and TCC) [23]. In the analyzed extracts, TCC was relatively low in relation to TPC and TFC, resulting in lower DPPH antiradical activity.

The optimal conditions obtained using these models were as follows: extract 1, in which TCC was maximized (raw material—0.11%, power—400 W, ethanol ratio—90%), extract 2, with the maximization of TPC and TFC (raw material—0.14%, power—400 W, ethanol ratio—54%), extract 3with maximized antioxidative activity (raw material—0.10%, power—400 W, ethanol ratio—41%), and extract 4, where all the responses were maximized (raw material—0.16%, power—400 W, ethanol ratio—77%). The temperature of extraction was always kept below 75 °C because flavonoids have been shown to be heat-sensitive [58]. Also, the oxidative degradation, free radical production and isomerization of carotenoids are influenced by extraction time and temperature [59].

Optimization and Validation of the Predicted Model

Experimental validation was performed to compare the predicted and experimentally obtained results. In that context, TCC values were in the range of 352.267 ± 17.402 µg β-carotene/g, which is comparable to the predicted ones (354.064 µg β-carotene/g) in optimal extract 1. In the case of TPC and TFC, the values were 21.764 ± 0.456 mg GAE/g and 83.128 ± 1.979 mg QE/g, compared to the predicted values according to the model (TFC—83.283 mg QE/g and TPC—21.878 mg GAE/g) for optimal extract 2. Values of ABTS and DPPH in optimal extract 3 were 0.366 ± 0.016 and 0.033 ± 0.001 mmol TE/g compared to the predicted values 0.367 and 0.032 mmol TE/g. For optimal extract 4, where all the input parameters were maximized, the experimentally obtained results were TCC—189.230 ± 16.498 µg β-carotene/g, TFC—77.050 ± 1.557 mg QE/g, TPC—21.230 ± 0.993 mg GAE/g, DPPH—0.026 ± 0.001 mmol TE/g and ABTS—0.244 ± 0.010 mmol TE/g, compared to the predicted ones of 201.245 µg β-carotene/g, 80.191 mg QE/g, 20.803 mg GAE/g, 0.025 mmol TE/g and 0.335 mmol TE/g, respectively. As shown, the adequacy of the model used was confirmed, with a good correlation between the predicted and experimentally obtained results.

The desirability function (DF), which provides a desirability grade, was used to assess an optimization technique based on the Harrington scale. The results in Table 4 indicate that the desirability in the case of optimal extract 1 and 2 was 1. The findings indicated that improvement beyond this point has no preference [60]. The quality evaluation of extract 3 is acceptable and excellent (0.991), and for extract 4, the desirability is 0.711, which is in the range of 0.80–0.63, evaluated as acceptable but good.

Table 4. Optimal yields of polyphenols, carotenoids and antioxidants depending on the target compound (extract 1–extract 4) and comparison of predicted and experimental data.

	TCC (µg β-Carotene/g d.w.)	TFC (mg QE/g d.w.)	TPC (mg GAE/g d.w.)	DPPH (mmol TE/g d.w.)	ABTS (mmol TE/g d.w.)	Desirability
Predicted TCC	354.064					1.000
Predicted TFC/TPC		83.283	21.878			1.000
Predicted DPPH/ABTS				0.032	0.367	0.991
Predicted TCC/TFC/TPC/DPPH/ABTS	201.245	80.191	20.803	0.025	0.335	0.711
Experimental TCC	352.267 ± 17.402					
Experimental FC/TPC		83.128 ± 1.979	21.764 ± 0.456			
Experimental DPPH/ABTS				0.033 ± 0.001	0.366 ± 0.016	
Experimental TCC/TFC/TPC/DPPH/ABTS	189.230 ± 16.498	77.050 ± 1.557	21.230 ± 0.993	0.026 ± 0.001	0.244 ± 0.010	
Predicted vs. experimental 1 (%)	0.508					
Predicted vs. experimental 2 (%)		0.186	0.521			
Predicted vs. experimental 3 (%)				−3.125	0.272	
Predicted vs. experimental 4 (%)	5.971	3.917	−2.053	−4.000	27.164	

TCC (raw material-0.11%/power-400 W/ethanol-90%); TFC/TPC (raw material-0.14%/power-400 W/ethanol-54%); DPPH/ABTS (raw material-0.10%/power-400 W/ethanol-41%); TCC/TFC/TPC/DPPH/ABTS (raw material-0.16%/power-400 W/ethanol 77%). Time of MAE in all optimal extracts-4 min.

To ensure that the results were reliable under optimal circumstances, validation tests were conducted. The model's consistency and dependability were demonstrated by the relative standard error (n = 5) between the experimental and projected values, which was less than 10% [61] and is presented in Table 4.

The chemical composition of extracts 1–4, obtained under optimized MAE conditions, is presented in Figure 5. The data show that the most observable effect of extraction variables is the effect of ethanol concentration on TCC yields. In extract 4, which maximized the yields of all antioxidants, the content of TCC was 1.8 times lower compared to the values obtained with extract 1 (189.2 µg β-carotene/g and 352.27 µg β-carotene/g, respectively). Furthermore, ABTS and DPPH values were the lowest in extract 1 compared to the other optimal extracts, which was related to the highest percentage of ethanol. The content of nobiletin and tangeretin in extracts 1–4 obtained under optimized MAE conditions is presented in Table 5—as mentioned previously, their concentration was determined as they are as the most abundant among citrus flavonoids and have proven health benefits.

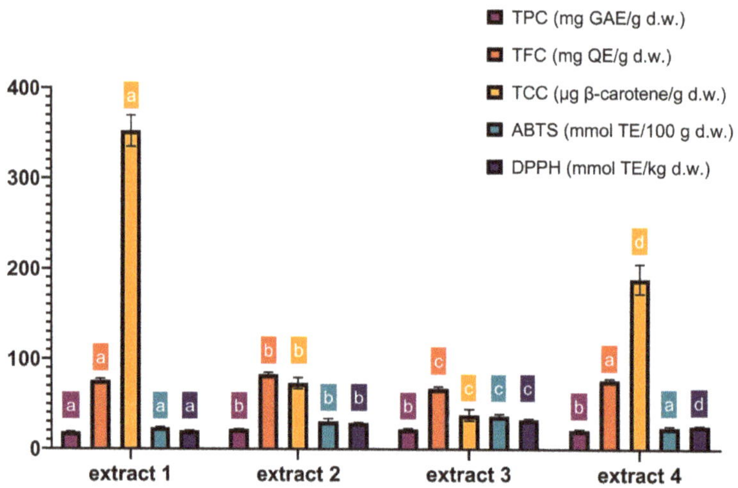

Figure 5. Characterization of TPC, TFC, TCC, ABTS and DPPH in four optimal extracts. TPC—total phenolic content; TFC—total flavonoid content; TCC—total carotenoid content; extract 1—maximized TCC (0.11% raw material/400 W power/90% ethanol); extract 2—maximized TPC and TFC (0.14% raw material/400 W power/54% ethanol); extract 3—maximized antioxidative activity (0.10% raw material/400 W power/41% ethanol); extract 4—maximized all responses (0.16% raw material/400 W power/77% ethanol). Time of MAE in all optimal extracts was 4 min. Columns marked with different letters belong to different statistical groups ($p < 0.05$). Columns and their corresponding statistical letters are colour-coded according to each antioxidant test.

Table 5. Content of nobiletin and tangeretin in optimal extracts.

Optimal Conditions	Nobiletin (µg/g d.w.)	Tangeretin (µg/g d.w.)
Extract 1	703.62 ± 51.72 [a]	134.22 ± 8.96 [a]
Extract 2	570.47 ± 25.00 [b]	138.24 ± 4.65 [a]
Extract 3	592.00 ± 4.86 [b]	139.7 ± 2.28 [a]
Extract 4	610.07 ± 2.06 [ab]	135.24 ± 0.51 [a]

Extract 1—maximized total carotenoid content(0.11% raw material/400 W power/90% ethanol); extract 2—maximized total phenolic and flavonoid content (0.14% raw material/400 W power/54% ethanol); extract 3—maximized antioxidative activity (0.14% raw material/400 W power/54% ethanol); extract 4—maximized all responses (0.16% raw material/400 W power/77% ethanol). Results in the same column marked with different letters belong to different statistical groups ($p < 0.001$).

Nobiletin was quantified in a range from 0.57 to 0.70 mg/g while the content of tangeretin was lower, ranging from 0.13 to 0.14 mg/g. The obtained results are similar to the results of Zhang et al. [62], who obtained 0.51–6.49 mg/g nobiletin and tangeretin in a range from 0.19 to 2.92 mg/g d.w. in different mandarin genotypes. Another study by Chen et al. [63] also showed similar results for nobiletin, at 0.39–7.79 mg/g, while tangeretin was determined in lower concentrations, at 0.15 to 3.37 mg/g. Table 5 shows that tangeretin yields were not significantly affected by different MAE conditions. On the other hand, nobiletin was significantly influenced by MAE conditions, and the highest yields were obtained in extracts 1 and 4 (and, as expected, not in extract 2, which contained the highest TFC). This shows that, due to variability in the chemical characteristics of flavonoids, maximizing total flavonoid content does not necessarily maximize the content of particular flavonoid compounds.

3.2. Microwave-Assisted Extraction of Pectin

Response surface methodology with Box–Behnken design was employed to optimize the MAE of pectin from mandarin peel. Independent variables were extraction time, microwave power and pH, while response variables pectin were yield, AUA and DE. The model that best fit the data for yield was higher-order quadratic ($p = 0.0167$, $R^2 = 0.8780$, adjusted $R^2 = 0.7211$). The model showed that reaction time was a key variable influencing pectin yield (A-time, $p = 0.0176$), but it also recognized the significance of the interaction between time and power (AB, $p = 0.0349$), indicating that reaction time and power modulate this influence and should be mutually considered when optimizing the yield of the extraction. Microwave irradiation within a limited timeframe can lead to increase in the yield; however, prolonged irradiation can lead to its deterioration. The statistical significance of the quadratic term (A^2, $p = 0.0039$) further shows that an increase in extraction time positively influences pectin yield to a specific point, after which that influence changes and starts to negatively impact yield.

AUA was described by a linear model ($p = 0.031$, $R^2 = 0.4828$, adjusted $R^2 = 0.3635$). pH ($p = 0.0081$) had a significant effect on the response variable. An acidic environment increases ester group hydrolysis, while keeping the AUA chains of the fibre stable, which may result in overall higher levels of AUA in pectin [64]. A similar phenomenon was observed for the DE (described by linear model ($p = 0.0414$, $R^2 = 0.4577$, adjusted $R^2 = 0.3326$), where pH also exhibited significant influence on the response variable. It is interesting to note that, although pH did not have a significant influence on yield in terms of statistical analysis of variance, it strongly affected the chemical characteristics of pectin. Model equations and additional statistical analyses can be found in the Supplementary Materials.

There were 17 runs in the optimization process (Table 6). The yield ranged from $4.19 \pm 0.17\%$ to $25.16 \pm 1.64\%$. It can be seen in Figure S2 that the conditions for the optimal yield are in the central part of the surface area. The plots also reveal additional interactions between the independent variables, which might remain unaccounted for if the focus is put solely on the model statistics. A lower pH can improve the yield if the extraction time is short (under constant optimal conditions of power). Under these conditions, the extraction time is not sufficient for the release of pectin molecules and additional acidification of the environment can compensate for that. The interaction between pH and power (under the optimal value for time) is shown in Figure S2.

An important variable in the extraction that was not included in the experimental design is the temperature (due to equipment shortages and the inability to precisely control both microwave power and temperature, as explained previously). It was monitored during extraction to evaluate its influence (alone and in interactions with other variables) on the pectin yield (Figure 6A). The relationship between the maximum achieved temperature, pH and yield is shown in Figure 6B.

Table 6. Design of the experiment matrix for the microwave-assisted extraction of pectin and alongside responses.

Run	F1	F2	F3	R1	R2	R3
	Time (min)	Power (W)	pH	Yield (%)	AUA (%)	DE (%)
1	3	1400	1.5	24.26 ± 3.46	59.74 ± 0.24	47.84 ± 0.62
2	3	1000	2	9.23 ± 0.54	55.70 ± 0.05	62.76 ± 1.25
3	5	1800	1.5	7.89 ± 1.04	60.52 ± 0.71	64.56 ± 0.41
4	5	1400	2	23.47 ± 0.94	59.39 ± 1.17	54.03 ± 0.75
5	3	1400	1.5	24.97 ± 1.33	63.11 ± 0.72	43.91 ± 0.75
6	3	1800	1	19.57 ± 1.19	78.84 ± 0.74	39.28 ± 0.35
7	3	1000	1	18.07 ± 1.09	61.25 ± 2.28	53.78 ± 1.78
8	1	1800	1.5	10.53 ± 0.18	60.97 ± 3.38	61.50 ± 1.92
9	3	1400	1.5	23.07 ± 2.27	66.83 ± 1.55	49.53 ± 1.19
10	1	1000	1.5	6.42 ± 0.02	64.88 ± 3.39	61.96 ± 1.14
11	3	1800	2	22.57 ± 2.43	63.86 ± 2.53	53.64 ± 2.46
12	1	1400	1	11.32 ± 0.86	64.25 ± 1.59	54.20 ± 0.86
13	3	1400	1.5	24.49 ± 3.85	68.96 ± 3.21	46.13 ± 3.30
14	3	1400	1.5	25.16 ± 1.64	65.76 ± 1.51	47.59 ± 0.93
15	5	1000	1.5	24.93 ± 0.67	65.99 ± 0.85	48.87 ± 0.45
16	1	1400	2	4.19 ± 0.17	60.15 ± 1.17	68.39 ± 2.45
17	5	1400	1	11.57 ± 1.23	78.69 ± 1.02	38.20 ± 0.38

AUA—anhydrouronic acid content; DE—degree of esterification.

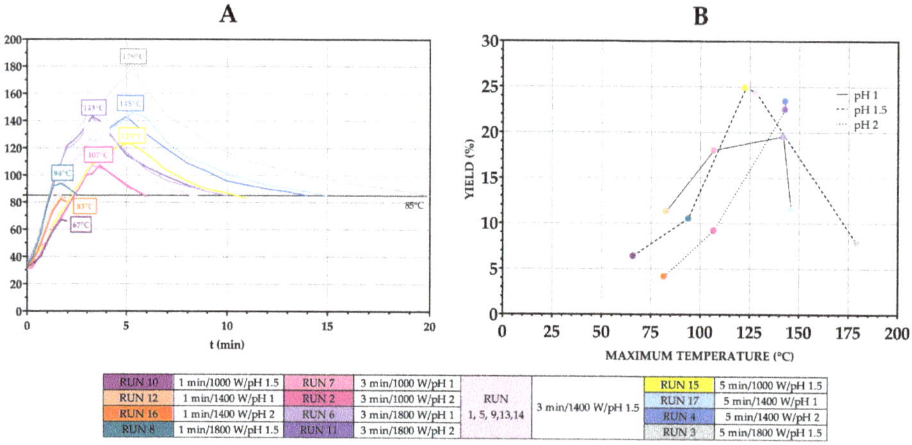

Figure 6. Impact of temperature on pectin yields. Temperature curves during microwave extractions (**A**) and yields achieved at maximum temperatures during runs (**B**).

Generally, at temperatures below 110 °C, the yield increased as the temperature increased. When comparing the yield from runs under identical power and time settings, it can be seen that acidic conditions may facilitate pectin extraction under mild thermal inputs: a higher yield was achieved with pH 1 compared to pH 2, at 11.32% vs. 4.19% (Runs 12 and 16) and 18.07% vs. 9.23% (Runs 7 and 2). This is in accordance with the interactions of pH and power/time as discussed previously (Figure S2). As temperature increased further, overall yield improved, reaching maximum values (above 20%) within an optimal temperature interval of 123–147 °C. In this range, the effect of pH reversed—a higher pH (pH 2) produced similar or better results compared to pH 1, 22.57% vs. 19.57% (Runs 11 and 6) and 23.47% vs. 11.57% (Runs 4 and 17), suggesting that a more acidic environment along with higher temperatures may accelerate degradation processes. Beyond this range, a further increase in temperature did not result in additional yield improvements, and there was noticeable decline in yield, likely due to thermal degradation. This was further supported by a visible colour change in pectin, obtained after Runs 3, 6 and 17, from light yellow-orange to darker orange/brown. Thus, while pH alone may not directly influence yield, its effect becomes pronounced in combination with heat, power and time, acting either as a facilitator of extraction or as a catalyst for degradation at elevated temperatures.

AUA was in the range of 55.7 ± 0.05 to 78.84 ± 0.74, as seen from Table 6, and DE from 38.20 ± 0.38 to 68.39 ± 2.45. Multiple-response optimization was performed on the following criteria: maximal yield (acceptable minimal value of 20% and maximal value of 30%), AUA in the range of 65–75% and a DE in the range of 42 to 62%. The optimal conditions for the extraction were 3.67 min, 1335 W and pH 1.49. The predicted and experimental results for the conformation run are represented in Table 7. It can be seen that the error in the prediction of AUA and yield was 10% or less, indicating satisfactory predictive potential of the model. The difference between the predicted and observed values was the highest for the DE, which is in accordance with the percentage of variability (R^2) that could be described by the model as stated above in the text. Additional statistical analysis can be found in Table S4.

Table 7. Predicted vs. experimental values of target parameters under optimal MAE conditions for pectin extraction.

	Yield (%)	AUA (%)	DE (%)
Predicted	25.072	65	51.089
Experimental	27.277	71.525	42.354
Predicted vs. experimental (%)	−8.794	−10.038	−20.623

AUA—anhydrouronic acid content; DE—degree of esterification.

Previous studies utilized surface response methodology to optimize the MAE orange peel-derived pectin. Prakash Maran et al. [47] applied the Box–Behnken design to model the influence of microwave power, time, pH and solid–liquid on pectin yield. They achieved a considerably lower yield compared to our results, with the optimal conditions (422 W, 169 s, pH 1.4, solid: liquid ratio = 1:69 g/mL) resulting in a 19.24% yield. The optimal microwave power was markedly lower compared to ours, which could be the reason for the reduction in the yield. Also, the protocol in their study included washing the pectin with ethanol to obtain a pure pectin fraction, which probably resulted in certain losses in the process. Hosseini et al. [65] utilized sour orange peel as a source of pectin and optimized MAE using the Box–Behnken design. They reported very high R^2 values (>0.9) for their models that explain the influence of time, power and pH on pectin yield and DE.

Similarly, Iñiguez-Moreno et al. [66] modelled the MAE of pectin using the central composite design. They tested the effects of time and temperature on extraction while keeping the microwave power at a constant value of 900 W. The optimal conditions were 4.9 min and 160.5 °C, resulting in 36.69% yield. These optimal conditions can be compared with those obtained in our study—the extraction time was higher compared to ours, due to the lower value of microwave power (900 W). The pectin obtained in their study had a DE above 50% in all tested conditions, while in our study, the DE ranged from a high- to lower-esterified form. Interestingly, they used a quadratic model to describe the influence of tested variables on the DE, while in our case, a linear model (pH having the main effect) was optimal to describe the behaviour of the mentioned variables. However, Iñiguez-Moreno et al. [66] did not include pH in their experimental design.

3.3. Comparison of MAE and CSE

3.3.1. Comparison of MAE and CSE for Antioxidant Extraction

As mentioned previously, MAE has generally been demonstrated to improve compound recovery in a shorter time with a lower volume of solvent and usually reduced extraction times. Table 8 compares the yields of target antioxidants in extract 4 obtained by optimized MAE (0.16% raw material, 77% ethanol and power of 400 W) and CSE (0.13% raw material, 80% ethanol and 50 °C).

Table 8. Comparison of CSE and MAE regarding the yields of antioxidants under the conditions optimized for extraction 4.

Extraction Method	Content of Observed Outputs (Extract 4)						
	TPC (mg GAE/g d.w.)	TFC (mg QE/g d.w.)	TCC (μg β-Carotene/g d.w.)	ABTS (μmol TE/g d.w.)	DPPH (μmol TE/g d.w.)	Nobiletin (μg/g d.w.)	Tangeretin (μg/g d.w.)
CSE	28.24 ± 1.16 [a]	82.91 ± 1.07 [a]	214.11 ± 15.49 [a]	189.61 ± 2.81 [a]	32.15 ± 1.15 [a]	881.28 ± 12.13 [a]	158.23 ± 2.30 [a]
MAE	21.23 ± 0.99 [b]	77.05 ± 1.56 [b]	189.21 ± 16.50 [a]	244.21 ± 9.69 [b]	26.07 ± 0.53 [b]	610.07 ± 2.06 [b]	135.24 ± 0.51 [b]

Extract 4—maximized all responses (0.16% raw material/400 W power/77% ethanol); TPC—total phenolic content; TFC—total flavonoid content; TCC—total carotenoid content; CSE—conventional solvent extraction; MAE—microwave-assisted extraction; ABTS—2,2-azino-bis (3-ethylbenzothiazoline-6-sulfonic acid) radical scavenging assay; DPPH—2,2-diphenyl-1-picrylhydrazyl radical scavenging assay; GAE—gallic acid equivalents; QE—quercetin equivalents; TE—Trolox equivalents. Results in the same column marked with different letters belong to different statistical groups ($p < 0.001$).

As shown, results obtained by both methods were comparable. Small, but statistically significant differences were obtained for polyphenolic compounds, while TCC was not influenced by extraction technique. Somewhat higher yields of TPP, TFC, DPPH, nobiletin and tangeretin were obtained by CSE while ABTS was significantly higher in MAE.

As can be observed from Table 9, the preparation of extracts using CSE requires from 5.0 to 16.8 times more energy when compared to the MAE (except in extract 3 where CSE is performed at room temperature). Furthermore, the CSE process was significantly longer.

Table 9. Comparison of the extraction times and energy consumption for the MAE and CSE preparation of extracts under optimized conditions.

	Energy Consumption (kWh/kg)		Time (min)	
	CSE	MAE	CSE	MAE
Extract 1	162	32.3	30	4
Extract 2	286	25.4	30	4
Extract 3	0.05	35.6	30	4
Extract 4	374	22.2	30	4
Pectin extract	29.6	2.2	120	3.7

CSE—conventional solvent extraction; MAE—microwave-assisted extraction; extract 1—raw material-0.11%/power-400 W/ethanol-90%; extract 2—raw material-0.14%/power-400 W/ethanol-54%; extract 3—raw material-0.10%/power-400 W/ethanol-41%; extract 4—raw material-0.16%/power-400 W/ethanol-77%.

3.3.2. Comparison of MAE and CSE for Pectin Extraction

Pectin obtained under optimal MAE conditions (3.67 min/1335 W/pH 1.49) was compared to pectin extracted by previously optimized CSE (120 min/85 °C/pH 1.49), as shown in Figure 7. Despite the significantly shorter extraction time, MAE achieved yields comparable to SLE (27.7 vs. 27.3%), highlighting its efficiency and potential as a rapid and effective alternative for pectin extraction. During MAE, the temperature peaked at 135 °C, in contrast to the constant 85 °C used in CSE. Higher microwave power and rapid heating contributed to efficient cell wall breakdown and high pectin yield achieved in a significantly shorter extraction time. This can be attributed to the mechanisms of microwave heating, which involve ionic conduction and dipole rotation. These processes rapidly generate heat within the solvent–sample matrix, promoting cell wall rupture and increasing the interaction between the solvent and plant material [67]. Previous studies have shown that microwave energy can cause the destruction of parenchymal cells, alter surface properties and inactivate enzymes that degrade pectin, all of which contribute to improved extraction efficiency [68].

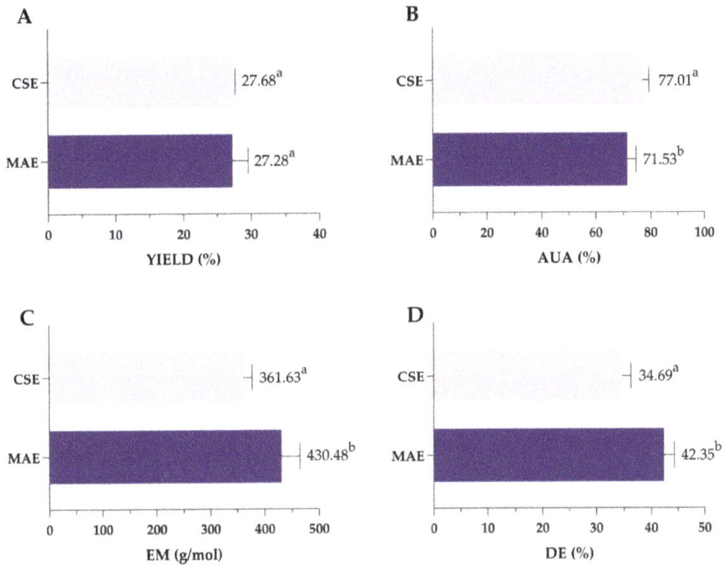

Figure 7. Comparison of yield (**A**), AUA (**B**), EM (**C**) and DE (**D**) of pectin obtained by optimized MAE and CSE. MAE—microwave-assisted extraction; CSE—conventional solvent extraction; AUA—anhydrouronic acid content; EM—equivalent mass; DE—degree of esterification. Columns marked with different letters belong to different statistical groups ($p < 0.05$).

Similar investigations that compared MAE and CSE for mandarin peel pectin extractions are scarce. The only available research on mandarin has been conducted by Kumar and co-workers [27] using the household microwave oven at 900 W (and not the closed-vessel system). In this work, both CSE and MAE resulted in significantly lower yields compared to our results, and MAE applied for 60 min showed yields comparable to CSE (18.58 vs. 14.85%). Investigations conducted on other types of citrus fruits are also partially in accordance with our results. Yeoh and co-workers [69] compared CSE (Soxhlet) and MAE for orange peel pectin extraction and obtained similar yields regardless of the applied extraction techniques. Rodsamran and Sothornvit [70] reported that MAE of lime peel at 700 W for 3 min, using citric acid and a 1:20 peel-to-extractant ratio, resulted in lower pectin yield compared to conventional heating. Unlike the mentioned studies, the present work used significantly higher microwave power (1335 W), which likely enhanced cell wall disruption and improved pectin release, resulting in fast and efficient extraction, which might explain observed differences. These findings suggest that microwave power plays a crucial role in optimizing extraction efficiency, which is in accordance with the results of our multiple-response optimization. However, higher pectin yields in this study might be due to the fact that we presented yields of raw pectin, which was not additionally purified after extraction (so that we could compare the impact of the extraction process on the purity of the obtained pectin). In previously mentioned research conducted by other authors, there are no specific data about conducting/omitting the purification step, so we cannot be sure if the yields reported refer to raw or purified pectin.

Pectin purity was also affected by the type of extraction—as shown in Figure 4B, both values of AUA exceeded the 65% threshold typically required for commercial-grade pectin, indicating high-quality extracts from both methods. However, AUA was significantly higher in pectin extracted by CSE (77.01%) compared to MAE (71.53%). Also, values of EM and the DE were significantly higher in pectin obtained by MAE; however, since all obtained values were lower than 50%, obtained pectin can be classified as low-methoxyl pectin regardless of the extraction type (Figure 7C,D).

The FTIR spectra of the Satsuma mandarin peel pectin extracted by CSE and MAE are shown in Figure 8. Both spectra showed comparable characteristic bands, indicating a similar structural composition. The broad band appearing between 3600 and 3000 cm^{-1} refers to the O-H stretching vibration due to the inter- and intramolecular hydrogen bonding of the galacturonic acid polymer. The band around 2950 cm^{-1} refers to the C-H stretching vibration, including CH, CH_2, and CH_3 groups [71]. The band observed in the areas of 1730 cm^{-1} corresponded to the C=O stretching vibration of esterified carboxyl groups, and the band at 1600–1630 cm^{-1} was related to the C=O stretching vibration of free carboxyl groups [69]. Both pectin samples had band values lower than 1741 cm^{-1}, which indicates that these pectin samples have low contents of hydrophobic groups [72]. The peaks at 1013 cm^{-1} and 1014 cm^{-1} refer to C–O, C–C and C–O–H stretching [73]. The area between 1200 cm^{-1} and 800 cm^{-1} is usually called the 'fingerprint' region, since the position and intensity of the individual band are unique for each polysaccharide and can be difficult to interpret [67]. Similar bands were observed in pectin extracted from Satsuma mandarin peel [25] and lime peel pectin [70].

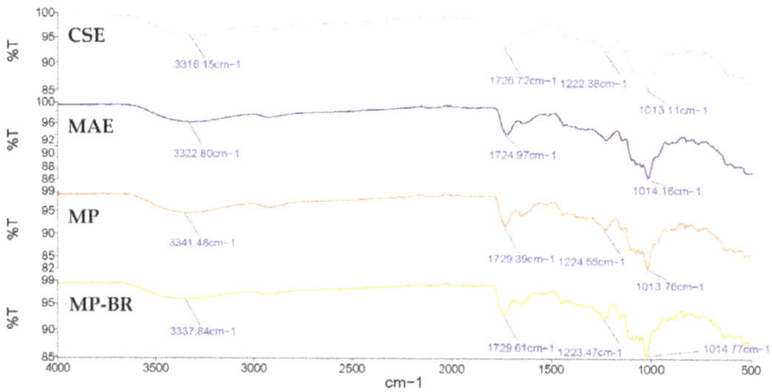

Figure 8. FTIR spectra of mandarin peel pectin extracted by different extraction methods. CSE—conventional solvent extraction; MAE—microwave-assisted extraction; MP—mandarin pectin obtained by optimized MAE from intact peel; MP-BR—mandarin pectin obtained using a biorefinery two-step process: optimized MAE of antioxidants from intact peel (extract 4, maximized all responses), followed by optimized MAE of pectin from the residue.

In addition to the possibility of higher yields, green extraction methods, such as MAE, are usually claimed to have a lower ecological footprint compared to CSE. Even though this aspect is often emphasized, when pointing out the advantages of green extraction techniques, the comparison of the actual ecological footprint (or one aspect of it) of the green extraction with the CSE is rarely addressed in the literature. Such data are lacking for citrus pectin but recently Golub and co-workers [74] utilized LCA for comparing CSE and MAE of pectin extracted from tomato pomace and showed that one conventional extraction treatment has higher environmental impacts compared to one microwave extraction treatment for all the analyzed indicators (climate change, freshwater eutrophication, human toxicity, ionizing radiation and ozone depletion), more than twice as much. Similarly, Joglekar and co-workers [75] conducted LCA to compare MAE and conventional pectin extraction form citrus waste and proved the significantly lower ecological footprint of MAE.

In this work, we compared the energy consumption per g of the raw material of the two processes (MAE and CSE), and the obtained results are presented in Table 9. The presented results clearly show the significant advantages of MAE, showing four times lower energy consumption compared to CSE.

3.4. Two-Step MAE of Antioxidants and Pectin—Development of Biorefinery Approach

As mentioned in the Section 1, an additional goal of this research was to investigate the possibility of a biorefinery approach that would integrate the antioxidant and pectin extractions from mandarin peel into a single two-step process where pectin is extracted from the residue remaining after the extraction of antioxidants. Despite the general advantages of this approach, to our knowledge, such investigations have not been carried out with mandarin peel, so the effects on the quality and yield of pectin are unknown. The obtained results comparing yields and characteristics of mandarin pectin obtained by optimized MAE from intact peel (MP) and mandarin pectin obtained using a biorefinery two-step process—comprising optimized MAE of antioxidants from intact peel (extract 4, maximized all responses) followed by optimized MAE of pectin from the residue (MP-BR)—are shown in Figure 9.

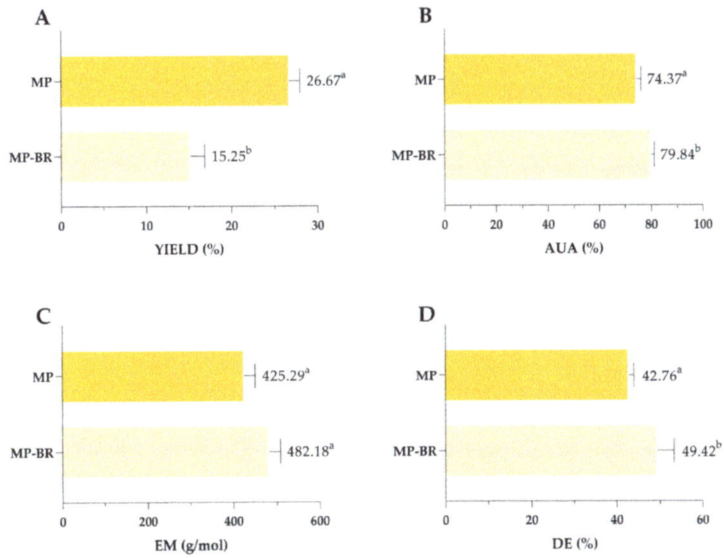

Figure 9. Comparison of yield (**A**), AUA (**B**), EM (**C**) and DE (**D**) of pectin obtained by MAE by integrated two-step procedure. MP—mandarin pectin obtained by optimized MAE from intact peel; MP-BR—mandarin pectin obtained using a biorefinery two-step process: optimized MAE of antioxidants from intact peel (extract 4, maximized all responses), followed by optimized MAE of pectin from the residue. Columns marked with different letters belong to different statistical groups ($p < 0.05$).

As shown in Figure 9, sequential extraction of polyphenols and pectin resulted in a 12% reduction in pectin yield compared to non-sequential extraction. However, this reduction was accompanied by improvements in pectin quality, including higher AUA, EM and DE values and a lighter colour (Figure 10).

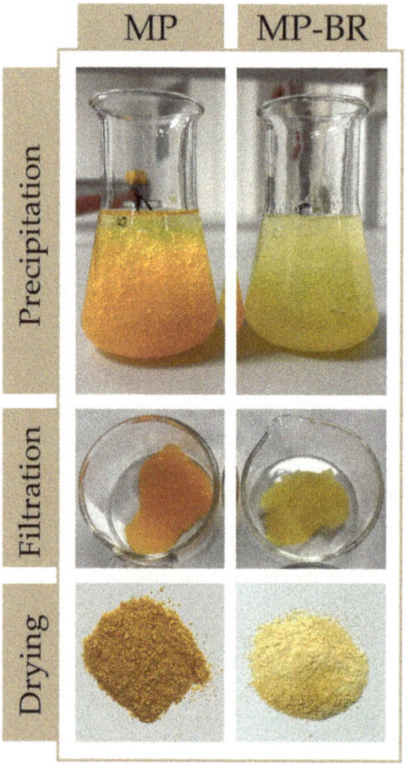

Figure 10. Comparison of the colour of mandarin peel pectin obtained by the single- or two-step extraction process. MP—mandarin pectin obtained by optimized MAE from intact peel; MP-BR—mandarin pectin obtained using a biorefinery two-step process: optimized MAE of antioxidants from intact peel (extract 4, maximized all responses), followed by optimized MAE of pectin from the residue.

The obtained results are in line with our expectations. Namely, for the extraction of antioxidants, 77% EtOH was used. Ethanol is usually used for the purification of raw pectin to achieve market-quality pectin (higher purity, lighter colour) as it removes remaining non-pectin polysaccharides and pigments from the protein fraction. In this two-step process, such purification of the raw material is conducted prior to pectin extraction, resulting in a lower yield but higher purity. This is obvious from the comparison of the organoleptic characteristics (colour) of MP and MP-BR presented in Figure 10—the ethanol pretreatment of mandarin peel caused the removal of pigments/coloured compounds (regarded as impurities in pectin extraction), which led to the colour change.

Even though the yield of MP-BR was lower compared to MP, the obtained values are still in accordance with the typical yields reported by other authors that used a purification step in pectin extraction. Duan and co-authors [25] extracted pectin from Satsuma mandarin peel by conventional extraction and high hydrostatic pressure, with a purification step involving washing the pectin with absolute ethanol and acetone three times, and achieved yields in the range of 15.34–18.99%, which is comparable to the yield of MP-BR.

Figure 8 also presents the FTIR spectra of MP and MP-BR, showing similar transmission patterns to the CSE and MAE pectin already discussed in Section 3.3.2. This confirms that pectin was successfully extracted from Satsuma mandarin peel using all applied methods.

Despite the mentioned advantages, such approaches are still rarely investigated and, to our knowledge, have only been applied to other citrus species, such as orange peel for the extraction of polyphenols, pectin and essential oils [76,77], while data on mandarin are still lacking.

As mentioned previously, investigations of the biorefinery approach for obtaining valuable products from secondary raw materials are scarce and are non-existent for mandarin peel. However, Guandalini and co-workers [78] also developed a two-step ultrasound-assisted extraction process for the sequential extraction of phenolics and pectin from mango peel. As in our work, they used the residue remaining after ethanolic extraction of polyphenols to extract pectin and obtained satisfactory yields (8.6%) of high-purity pectin. Other authors applied different sequences of extraction procedures but still managed to obtain a satisfactory yield and quality of targeted compounds. Figueira and co-workers [79] developed a two-step continuous process for the extraction of pectin and hesperidin from orange peel using CSE, with pectin yields varying from 17.23% to 20.61% and 1% of high-purity hesperidin (84%) in the subsequent extraction process. Similarly, Talekar and co-workers [80] applied a similar approach and optimized a low-temperature hydrothermal process that yielded high-methoxyl, food-quality pectin (18.8–20.9%) and high yields of punicalagin-rich phenolics (10.6–11.8%), while the solid residue was subsequently used for bio-ethanol production. The literature data are in consistent with our results justifying the validity of the biorefinery approach.

The existing literature shows that introducing a single two-step extraction process additionally offers significant economic and environmental advantages compared to using two separate extraction processes. It maximizes the valorization of agro-industrial waste by recovering high-value compounds in a single workflow, which reduces raw material losses and increases overall product yield while minimizing water use and shortening the time of extraction [81].

4. Conclusions

According to the obtained results, mandarin peel as an agro-industrial waste has great potential as a source of carotenoids, polyphenols, flavonoids and pectin. The obtained results show that the major advantage of MAE is a significantly shorter extraction time and lower energy consumption (except in the case of the extraction of antioxidants at room temperature) compared to CSE, while the yields of target compounds are, in most cases, comparable. The application of integrated polyphenols and pectin extraction resulted in slightly reduced pectin yields but significant improvements of pectin quality compared to non-sequential extraction. Future investigations should focus on exploring scale-up possibilities and more comprehensive assessments of the environmental and economic benefits of integrated extraction processes.

Supplementary Materials: The following supporting information can be downloaded at: https://www.mdpi.com/article/10.3390/antiox14060722/s1, Figure S1: HPLC chromatograms at 280 nm and 330 nm.; Figure S2: Response surface plots (3D) for pectin as a function of power, time and pH; Figure S3. Normal plots of residuals for A (TCC), B (TPC), C (TFC), D (ABTS) and E (DPPH); Table S1: The model equations for the CSE of antioxidants; Table S2: The model equations for the MAE of antioxidants and pectin; Table S3. ANOVA for response surface quadratic model for antioxidants; Table S4. ANOVA for response surface quadratic model for pectin.

Author Contributions: Conceptualization, D.V.Č.; methodology, E.G. and K.R.; formal analysis, M.J., N.G. and E.G.; investigation, M.J., N.G., E.G. and L.M.B.; resources, L.M.B.; data curation, E.G., K.R.; writing—original draft preparation, M.J., N.G. and D.V.Č.; writing—review and editing, D.V.Č.; visualization, N.G.; supervision, D.V.Č. project administration, L.M.B.; funding acquisition, L.M.B. All authors have read and agreed to the published version of the manuscript.

Funding: This research was funded by Croatian Science Foundation through the project "Mandarins from Neretva Valley—Chemical Characterization and Innovative Postharvest Treatments" (HRZZ-UIP-2020-02-7496) and by the project FarmInova (KK.01.1.1.02.0021) funded by the European Regional Development Fund. The work of doctoral students Marina Jurić and Nikolina Golub was supported through "Young Researchers' Career Development Project—Training New Doctoral Students" (HRZZ-DOK-09-2018; HRZZ-DOK-2021-02-6801).

Institutional Review Board Statement: Not applicable.

Informed Consent Statement: Not applicable.

Data Availability Statement: The original contributions presented in this study are included in the article/Supplementary Materials. Further inquiries can be directed to the corresponding author.

Conflicts of Interest: The authors declare no conflicts of interest.

Abbreviations

The following abbreviations are used in this manuscript:

AUA	Anhydrouronic acid content
ABTS	2,2-azino-bis (3-ethylbenzothiazoline-6-sulfonic acid) radical scavenging assay
CSE	Conventional solvent extraction
DAD	Diode-array detector
DE	Degree of esterification
DPPH	2,2-diphenyl-1-picrylhydrazyl radical scavenging assay
EM	Equivalent mass
FTIR	Fourier transform infrared spectroscopy
GAE	Gallic acid equivalents
HPLC	High-performance liquid chromatography
MAE	Microwave-assisted extraction
MC	Methoxyl content
MP	Mandarin pectin obtained by optimized MAE from intact peel
MP-BR	Mandarin pectin obtained using a biorefinery two-step process: optimized MAE of antioxidants from intact peel (extract 4, maximized all responses), followed by optimized MAE of pectin from the residue
PMFs	Polymethoxyflavones
QE	Quercetin equivalents
RSM	Response surface methodology
TCC	Total carotenoid content
TE	Trolox equivalents
TFC	Total flavonoid content
TPC	Total phenolic content
UAE	Ultrasound-assisted extraction

References

1. Mahato, N.; Sharma, K.; Sinha, M.; Baral, E.R.; Koteswararao, R.; Dhyani, A.; Hwan Cho, M.; Cho, S. Bio-Sorbents, Industrially Important Chemicals and Novel Materials from Citrus Processing Waste as a Sustainable and Renewable Bioresource: A Review. *J. Adv. Res.* **2020**, *23*, 61–82. [CrossRef] [PubMed]
2. Državni Zavod Za Statistiku. Available online: https://podaci.dzs.hr/hr/search?q=proizvodnja%20vo%C4%87a (accessed on 9 May 2025).
3. Medved, I.; Gaurina-Medimurec, N.; Mavar, K.N.; Mijić, P. Waste Mandarin Peel as an Eco-Friendly Water-Based Drilling Fluid Additive. *Energies* **2022**, *15*, 2591. [CrossRef]
4. Anticona, M.; Blesa, J.; Frigola, A.; Esteve, M.J. High Biological Value Compounds Extraction from Citruswaste with Non-Conventional Methods. *Foods* **2020**, *9*, 811. [CrossRef]
5. Polyphenols Market Size, Share, Growth & Trends Report, 2030. Available online: https://www.grandviewresearch.com/industry-analysis/polyphenols-market-analysis (accessed on 9 May 2025).

6. Polyphenols Market Size, Share, Growth Forecast | 2030. Available online: https://www.vynzresearch.com/food-beverages/polyphenols-market (accessed on 9 May 2025).
7. Radić, K.; Galić, E.; Vinković, T.; Golub, N.; Vitali Čepo, D. Tomato Waste as a Sustainable Source of Antioxidants and Pectins: Processing, Pretreatment and Extraction Challenges. *Sustainability* **2024**, *16*, 9158. [CrossRef]
8. Pectin Market Size, Share & Trends | Industry Growth Forecast, 2025. Available online: https://www.grandviewresearch.com/industry-analysis/pectin-market (accessed on 9 May 2025).
9. Carotenoids Market Size, Share, Analysis & Forecast 2031. Available online: https://www.transparencymarketresearch.com/carotenoids-market.html (accessed on 9 May 2025).
10. Teigiserova, D.A.; Hamelin, L.; Thomsen, M. Review of High-Value Food Waste and Food Residues Biorefineries with Focus on Unavoidable Wastes from Processing. *Resour. Conserv. Recycl.* **2019**, *149*, 413–426. [CrossRef]
11. Kaur, S.; Singh, V.; Chopra, H.K.; Panesar, P.S. Extraction and Characterization of Phenolic Compounds from Mandarin Peels Using Conventional and Green Techniques: A Comparative Study. *Discov. Food* **2024**, *4*, 60. [CrossRef]
12. Inoue, T.; Tsubaki, S.; Ogawa, K.; Onishi, K.; Azuma, J.-i. Isolation of Hesperidin from Peels of Thinned Citrus Unshiu Fruits by Microwave-Assisted Extraction. *Food Chem.* **2010**, *123*, 542–547. [CrossRef]
13. Nishad, J.; Saha, S.; Dubey, A.K.; Varghese, E.; Kaur, C. Optimization and Comparison of Non-Conventional Extraction Technologies for *Citrus paradisi* L. Peels: A Valorization Approach. *J. Food Sci. Technol.* **2019**, *56*, 1221–1233. [CrossRef]
14. Hayat, K.; Zhang, X.; Chen, H.; Xia, S.; Jia, C.; Zhong, F. Liberation and Separation of Phenolic Compounds from Citrus Mandarin Peels by Microwave Heating and Its Effect on Antioxidant Activity. *Sep. Purif. Technol.* **2010**, *73*, 371–376. [CrossRef]
15. Ethos X Microwave Extraction System—ATS Scientific. Available online: https://ats-scientific.com/products/ethos-ex-microwave-extraction (accessed on 9 May 2025).
16. Liu, L.; Xu, X.; Cheng, D.; Yao, X.; Pan, S. Structure-Activity Relationship of Citrus Polymethoxylated Flavones and Their Inhibitory Effects on Aspergillus Niger. *J. Agric. Food Chem.* **2012**, *60*, 4336–4341. [CrossRef]
17. Stuetz, W.; Prapamontol, T.; Hongsibsong, S.; Biesalski, H.K. Polymethoxylated Flavones, Flavanone Glycosides, Carotenoids, and Antioxidants in Different Cultivation Types of Tangerines (*Citrus reticulata* Blanco Cv. Sainampueng) from Northern Thailand. *J. Agric. Food Chem.* **2010**, *58*, 6069–6074. [CrossRef] [PubMed]
18. Mitani, R.; Tashiro, H.; Arita, E.; Ono, K.; Haraguchi, M.; Tokunaga, S.; Sharmin, T.; Aida, T.M.; Mishima, K. Extraction of Nobiletin and Tangeretin with Antioxidant Activity from Peels of *Citrus poonensis* Using Liquid Carbon Dioxide and Ethanol Entrainer. *Sep. Sci. Technol.* **2021**, *56*, 290–300. [CrossRef]
19. Rey, F.; Zacarías, L.; Rodrigo, M.J. Carotenoids, Vitamin C, and Antioxidant Capacity in the Peel of Mandarin Fruit in Relation to the Susceptibility to Chilling Injury during Postharvest Cold Storage. *Antioxidants* **2020**, *9*, 1296. [CrossRef] [PubMed]
20. Kadi, A.; Boudries, H.; Bachir-Bey, M.; Teffane, M.; Taibi, A.; Arroul, Y.; Boulekbache-Makhlouf, L. Optimisation of Ultrasound-Assisted Extraction of Carotenoids and Antioxidant Activity from *Citrus reticulata* Blanco Peels (Wilking Mandarin). *Acta Aliment.* **2023**, *52*, 378–389. [CrossRef]
21. Anticona, M.; Blesa, J.; Lopez-Malo, D.; Frigola, A.; Esteve, M.J. Effects of Ultrasound-Assisted Extraction on Physicochemical Properties, Bioactive Compounds, and Antioxidant Capacity for the Valorization of Hybrid Mandarin Peels. *Food Biosci.* **2021**, *42*, 101185. [CrossRef]
22. Maslov Bandić, L.; Vlahoviček Kahlina, K.; Jurić, S. Optimization of Solid–Liquid Extraction Technique for Carotenoids from Mandarin Peels Using Green Solvents. *J. Anal. Chem.* **2023**, *78*, 1480–1486. [CrossRef]
23. Zhang, H.; Yang, Y.-F.; Zhou, Z.Q. Phenolic and Flavonoid Contents of Mandarin (*Citrus reticulata* Blanco) Fruit Tissues and Their Antioxidant Capacity as Evaluated by DPPH and ABTS Methods. *J. Integr. Agric.* **2018**, *17*, 256–263. [CrossRef]
24. Suri, S.; Singh, A.; Nema, P.K. Current Applications of Citrus Fruit Processing Waste: A Scientific Outlook. *Appl. Food Res.* **2022**, *2*, 100050. [CrossRef]
25. Duan, X.; Zhu, Y.; Shu, C.; Gao, J.; Liu, F.; Pan, S. Extraction of Pectin from Satsuma Mandarin Peel: A Comparison of High Hydrostatic Pressure and Conventional Extractions in Different Acids. *Molecules* **2022**, *27*, 3747. [CrossRef]
26. Karbuz, P.; Tugrul, N. Microwave and Ultrasound Assisted Extraction of Pectin from Various Fruits Peel. *J. Food Sci. Technol.* **2021**, *58*, 641–650. [CrossRef]
27. Kumar, S.; Kumar, R.; Sharma, P.C.; Nambi, V.E. Aqueous and Microwave Assisted Extraction of Pectin from Grapefruit and Nagpur Mandarin. *Int. J. Curr. Microbiol. Appl. Sci.* **2020**, *9*, 1938–1949. [CrossRef]
28. Herrero, M.; Ibañez, E. Green Extraction Processes, Biorefineries and Sustainability: Recovery of High Added-Value Products from Natural Sources. *J. Supercrit. Fluids* **2018**, *134*, 252–259. [CrossRef]
29. Chen, X.; Ding, J.; Ji, D.; He, S.; Ma, H. Optimization of Ultrasonic-Assisted Extraction Conditions for Bioactive Components from Coffee Leaves Using the Taguchi Design and Response Surface Methodology. *J. Food Sci.* **2020**, *85*, 1742–1751. [CrossRef] [PubMed]

30. Zhou, G.; Ma, J.; Tang, Y.; Wang, X.; Zhang, J.; Yao, X.; Jiang, W.; Duan, J.A. Optimization of Ultrasound-Assisted Extraction Followed by Macroporous Resin Purification for Maximal Recovery of Functional Components and Removal of Toxic Components from Ginkgo Biloba Leaves. *Biomed Res. Int.* **2018**, *2018*, 4598067. [CrossRef]
31. Fakayode, O.A.; Aboagarib, E.A.A.; Yan, D.; Li, M.; Wahia, H.; Mustapha, A.T.; Zhou, C.; Ma, H. Novel Two-Pot Approach Ultrasonication and Deep Eutectic Solvent Pretreatments for Watermelon Rind Delignification: Parametric Screening and Optimization via Response Surface Methodology. *Energy* **2020**, *203*, 117872. [CrossRef]
32. Salazar Ripoll, C.S.; Hincapié-Llanos, G.A. Evaluation of Sources and Methods of Pectin Extraction from Fruit and Vegetable Wastes: A Systematic Literature Review (SLR). *Food Biosci.* **2023**, *51*, 102278. [CrossRef]
33. Patil, B.; Patel, D.; Patil, J.; Nibe, R.L. Extraction of Pectin from Citrus Peels—A Review. *Int. J. Adv. Res. Sci. Commun. Technol.* **2022**, *2*, 631–637. [CrossRef]
34. Casas-Orozco, D.; Villa, A.L.; Bustamante, F.; González, L.M. Process Development and Simulation of Pectin Extraction from Orange Peels. *Food Bioprod. Process.* **2015**, *96*, 86–98. [CrossRef]
35. Barros, L.; Cruz, T.; Baptista, P.; Estevinho, L.M.; Ferreira, I.C.F.R. Wild and Commercial Mushrooms as Source of Nutrients and Nutraceuticals. *Food Chem. Toxicol.* **2008**, *46*, 2742–2747. [CrossRef]
36. Ainsworth, E.A.; Gillespie, K.M. Estimation of Total Phenolic Content and Other Oxidation Substrates in Plant Tissues Using Folin-Ciocalteu Reagent. *Nat. Protoc.* **2007**, *2*, 875–877. [CrossRef]
37. Ivanova, V.; Stefova, M.; Chinnici, F. Determination of the Polyphenol Contents in Macedonian Grapes and Wines by Standardized Spectrophotometric Methods. *J. Serb. Chem. Soc* **2010**, *75*, 45–59. [CrossRef]
38. Re, R.; Pellegrini, N.; Proteggente, A.; Pannala, A.; Yang, M.; Rice-Evans, C. Antioxidant Activity Applying an Improved ABTS Radical Cation Decolorization Assay. *Free Radic. Biol. Med.* **1999**, *26*, 1231–1237. [CrossRef] [PubMed]
39. Brand-Williams, W.; Cuvelier, M.E.; Berset, C. Use of a Free Radical Method to Evaluate Antioxidant Activity. *LWT—Food Sci. Technol.* **1995**, *28*, 25–30. [CrossRef]
40. Khamsucharit, P.; Laohaphatanalert, K.; Gavinlertvatana, P.; Sriroth, K.; Sangseethong, K. Characterization of Pectin Extracted from Banana Peels of Different Varieties. *Food Sci. Biotechnol.* **2018**, *27*, 623–629. [CrossRef]
41. Boateng, I.D.; Kumar, R.; Daubert, C.R.; Flint-Garcia, S.; Mustapha, A.; Kuehnel, L.; Agliata, J.; Li, Q.; Wan, C.; Somavat, P. Sonoprocessing Improves Phenolics Profile, Antioxidant Capacity, Structure, and Product Qualities of Purple Corn Pericarp Extract. *Ultrason. Sonochem.* **2023**, *95*, 106418. [CrossRef]
42. Nonglait, D.L.; Gokhale, J.S. Review Insights on the Demand for Natural Pigments and Their Recovery by Emerging Microwave-Assisted Extraction (MAE). *Food Bioprocess Technol.* **2024**, *17*, 1681–1705. [CrossRef]
43. Maslov Bandić, L.; Vlahoviček-Kahlina, K.; Sigurnjak Bureš, M.; Sopko Stracenski, K.; Jalšenjak, N.; Fruk, G.; Antolković, A.M.; Jurić, S. Fruit Quality of Satsuma Mandarins from Neretva Valley and Their Flavonoid and Carotenoid Content. *Horticulturae* **2023**, *9*, 383. [CrossRef]
44. Wang, Y.C.; Chuang, Y.C.; Hsu, H.W. The Flavonoid, Carotenoid and Pectin Content in Peels of Citrus Cultivated in Taiwan. *Food Chem.* **2008**, *106*, 277–284. [CrossRef]
45. Murador, D.C.; Salafia, F.; Zoccali, M.; Martins, P.L.G.; Ferreira, A.G.; Dugo, P.; Mondello, L.; de Rosso, V.V.; Giuffrida, D. Green Extraction Approaches for Carotenoids and Esters: Characterization of Native Composition from Orange Peel. *Antioxidants* **2019**, *8*, 613. [CrossRef]
46. Beg, Q.K.; Sahai, V.; Gupta, R. Statistical media optimization and alkaline protease production from Bacillus mojavensis in a bioreactor. *Process Biochem* **2003**, *39*, 203–209. [CrossRef]
47. Prakash Maran, J.; Sivakumar, V.; Thirugnanasambandham, K.; Sridhar, R. Optimization of Microwave Assisted Extraction of Pectin from Orange Peel. *Carbohydr. Polym.* **2013**, *97*, 703–709. [CrossRef] [PubMed]
48. Lovrić, V.; Putnik, P.; Bursać Kovačević, D.; Jukić, M.; Dragović-Uzelac, V. The Effect of Microwave-Assisted Extraction on the Phenolic Compounds and Antioxidant Capacity of Blackthorn Flowers. *Food Technol. Biotechnol.* **2017**, *55*, 243–250. [CrossRef] [PubMed]
49. Almaiman, S.A.; Albadr, N.A.; Alsulaim, S.; Alhuthayli, H.F.; Osman, M.A.; Hassan, A.B. Effects of Microwave Heat Treatment on Fungal Growth, Functional Properties, Total Phenolic Content, and Antioxidant Activity of Sorghum (*Sorghum bicolor* L.) Grain. *Food Chem.* **2021**, *348*, 128979. [CrossRef] [PubMed]
50. Chowdhury, A.; Kumar, A.Y.N.; Kumar, R.; Maurya, V.K.; Mahesh, M.S.; Singh, A.K.; Yadav, P.K.; Ghosh, M. Optimization of Microwave Parameters to Enhance Phytochemicals, Antioxidants and Metabolite Profile of de-Oiled Rice Bran. *Sci. Rep.* **2024**, *14*, 23959. [CrossRef]
51. García-Martín, J.F.; Feng, C.H.; Domínguez-Fernández, N.M.; Álvarez-Mateos, P. Microwave-Assisted Extraction of Polyphenols from Bitter Orange Industrial Waste and Identification of the Main Compounds. *Life* **2023**, *13*, 1864. [CrossRef]
52. Kumar, A.; Rout, R.K.; Rao, P.S. Effect of Drying Methods on Physico-Chemical and Bioactive Compounds of Mandarin (*Citrus reticulata*) Peel. *Int. J. Food Eng.* **2022**, *18*, 689–700. [CrossRef]

53. Lee, S.; Kim, H.J. Antioxidant Activities of Premature and Mature Mandarin (*Citrus unshiu*) Peel and Juice Extracts. *Food Sci. Biotechnol.* **2022**, *31*, 627–633. [CrossRef]
54. Chen, Q.; Wang, D.; Tan, C.; Hu, Y.; Sundararajan, B.; Zhou, Z. Profiling of Flavonoid and Antioxidant Activity of Fruit Tissues from 27 Chinese Local Citrus Cultivars. *Plants* **2020**, *9*, 196. [CrossRef]
55. Marey, S.; Shoughy, M. Effect of Temperature on the Drying Behavior and Quality of Citrus Peels. *Int. J. Food Eng.* **2016**, *12*, 661–671. [CrossRef]
56. Liyana-Pathirana, C.M.; Shahidi, F.; Alasalvar, C. Antioxidant Activity of Cherry Laurel Fruit (*Laurocerasus* Officinalis Roem.) and Its Concentrated Juice. *Food Chem.* **2006**, *99*, 121–128. [CrossRef]
57. Zhang, H.; Xi, W.; Yang, Y.; Zhou, X.; Liu, X.; Yin, S.; Zhang, J.; Zhou, Z. An On-Line HPLC-FRSD System for Rapid Evaluation of the Total Antioxidant Capacity of Citrus Fruits. *Food Chem.* **2015**, *172*, 622–629. [CrossRef] [PubMed]
58. Chaaban, H.; Ioannou, I.; Chebil, L.; Slimane, M.; Gérardin, C.; Paris, C.; Charbonnel, C.; Chekir, L.; Ghoul, M. Effect of Heat Processing on Thermal Stability and Antioxidant Activity of Six Flavonoids. *J. Food Process. Preserv.* **2017**, *41*, e13203. [CrossRef]
59. Ricarte, G.N.; Coelho, M.A.Z.; Marrucho, I.M.; Ribeiro, B.D. Enzyme-Assisted Extraction of Carotenoids and Phenolic Compounds from Sunflower Wastes Using Green Solvents. *3 Biotech* **2020**, *10*, 405. [CrossRef]
60. Bezerra, M.A.; Ferreira, S.L.C.; Novaes, C.G.; dos Santos, A.M.P.; Valasques, G.S.; da Mata Cerqueira, U.M.F.; dos Santos Alves, J.P. Simultaneous Optimization of Multiple Responses and Its Application in Analytical Chemistry—A Review. *Talanta* **2019**, *194*, 941–959. [CrossRef]
61. Akpabli-Tsigbe, N.D.K.; Ma, Y.; Ekumah, J.N.; Osabutey, J.; Hu, J.; Xu, M.; Johnson, N.A.N. Novel Solid-State Fermentation Extraction of 5-O-Caffeoylquinic Acid from Heilong48 Soybean Using *Lactobacillus helviticus*: Parametric Screening and Optimization. *LWT* **2021**, *149*, 111809. [CrossRef]
62. Zhang, Y.; Sun, Y.; Xi, W.; Shen, Y.; Qiao, L.; Zhong, L.; Ye, X.; Zhou, Z. Phenolic Compositions and Antioxidant Capacities of Chinese Wild Mandarin (*Citrus reticulata* Blanco) Fruits. *Food Chem.* **2014**, *145*, 674–680. [CrossRef]
63. Chen, X.M.; Tait, A.R.; Kitts, D.D. Flavonoid Composition of Orange Peel and Its Association with Antioxidant and Anti-Inflammatory Activities. *Food Chem.* **2017**, *218*, 15–21. [CrossRef]
64. Pérez, J.; Gómez, K.; Vega, L. Optimization and Preliminary Physicochemical Characterization of Pectin Extraction from Watermelon Rind (*Citrullus lanatus*) with Citric Acid. *Int. J. Food Sci.* **2022**, *2022*, 3068829. [CrossRef] [PubMed]
65. Hosseini, S.S.; Khodaiyan, F.; Yarmand, M.S. Optimization of Microwave Assisted Extraction of Pectin from Sour Orange Peel and Its Physicochemical Properties. *Carbohydr. Polym.* **2016**, *140*, 59–65. [CrossRef]
66. Iñiguez-Moreno, M.; Pizaña-Aranda, J.J.P.; Ramírez-Gamboa, D.; Ramírez-Herrera, C.A.; Araújo, R.G.; Parra-Saldívar, R.; Melchor-Martínez, E.M. Multitarget Optimization of Citrus Pectin Extraction Using Microwave-Assisted Technique and Citric Acid. *Biomass Convers. Biorefinery* **2025**, 1–15. [CrossRef]
67. Mahmud, M.M.; Belal, M.; Ahmed, S.; Hoque, M.M.; Zzaman, W. Microwave-Assisted Extraction and Characterization of Pectin from Citrus Fruit Wastes for Commercial Application. *Food Res.* **2021**, *5*, 80–88. [CrossRef]
68. Putnik, P.; Bursać Kovačević, D.; Režek Jambrak, A.; Barba, F.J.; Cravotto, G.; Binello, A.; Lorenzo, J.M.; Shpigelman, A. Innovative "Green" and Novel Strategies for the Extraction of Bioactive Added Value Compounds from Citruswastes—A Review. *Molecules* **2017**, *22*, 680. [CrossRef]
69. Yeoh, S.; Shi, J.; Langrish, T.A.G. Comparisons between Different Techniques for Water-Based Extraction of Pectin from Orange Peels. *Desalination* **2008**, *218*, 229–237. [CrossRef]
70. Rodsamran, P.; Sothornvit, R. Microwave Heating Extraction of Pectin from Lime Peel: Characterization and Properties Compared with the Conventional Heating Method. *Food Chem.* **2019**, *278*, 364–372. [CrossRef]
71. Gnanasambandam, R.; Proctor, A. Determination of Pectin Degree of Esterification by Diffuse Reflectance Fourier Transform Infrared Spectroscopy. *Food Chem.* **2000**, *68*, 327–332. [CrossRef]
72. Baraiya, K.; Yadav, V.K.; Choudhary, N.; Ali, D.; Raiyani, D.; Chowdhary, V.A.; Alooparampil, S.; Pandya, R.V.; Sahoo, D.K.; Patel, A.; et al. A Comparative Analysis of the Physico-Chemical Properties of Pectin Isolated from the Peels of Seven Different Citrus Fruits. *Gels* **2023**, *9*, 908. [CrossRef] [PubMed]
73. Spinei, M.; Oroian, M. Microwave-Assisted Extraction of Pectin from Grape Pomace. *Sci. Rep.* **2022**, *12*, 12722. [CrossRef]
74. Golub, N.; Galić, E.; Radić, K.; Smigic, N.; Djekic, I.; Pedisic, S.; Vitali Čepo, D. Microwave-Assisted Valorization of Tomato Pomace for Pectin Recovery: Improving Yields and Environmental Footprint. *Foods* **2025**, *14*, 1516. [CrossRef]
75. Joglekar, S.N.; Pathak, P.D.; Mandavgane, S.A.; Kulkarni, B.D. Process of Fruit Peel Waste Biorefinery: A Case Study of Citrus Waste Biorefinery, Its Environmental Impacts and Recommendations. *Environ. Sci. Pollut. Res.* **2019**, *26*, 34713–34722. [CrossRef]
76. Boukroufa, M.; Boutekedjiret, C.; Petigny, L.; Rakotomanomana, N.; Chemat, F. Bio-Refinery of Orange Peels Waste: A New Concept Based on Integrated Green and Solvent Free Extraction Processes Using Ultrasound and Microwave Techniques to Obtain Essential Oil, Polyphenols and Pectin. *Ultrason. Sonochem.* **2015**, *24*, 72–79. [CrossRef]
77. Ángel Siles López, J.; Li, Q.; Thompson, I.P. Biorefinery of Waste Orange Peel. *Crit. Rev. Biotechnol.* **2010**, *30*, 63–69. [CrossRef] [PubMed]

78. Guandalini, B.B.V.; Rodrigues, N.P.; Marczak, L.D.F. Sequential Extraction of Phenolics and Pectin from Mango Peel Assisted by Ultrasound. *Food Res. Int.* **2019**, *119*, 455–461. [CrossRef] [PubMed]
79. Figueira, O.; Pereira, V.; Castilho, P.C. A Two-Step Approach to Orange Peel Waste Valorization: Consecutive Extraction of Pectin and Hesperidin. *Foods* **2023**, *12*, 3834. [CrossRef] [PubMed]
80. Talekar, S.; Patti, A.F.; Vijayraghavan, R.; Arora, A. An Integrated Green Biorefinery Approach towards Simultaneous Recovery of Pectin and Polyphenols Coupled with Bioethanol Production from Waste Pomegranate Peels. *Bioresour. Technol.* **2018**, *266*, 322–334. [CrossRef]
81. Podetti, C.; Riveros-Gomez, M.; Román, M.C.; Zalazar-García, D.; Fabani, M.P.; Mazza, G.; Rodríguez, R. Polyphenol-Enriched Pectin from Pomegranate Peel: Multi-Objective Optimization of the Eco-Friendly Extraction Process. *Molecules* **2023**, *28*, 7656. [CrossRef]

antioxidants

MDPI

Article

Supercritical Fluid Extraction of Bioactive Components from Apple Peels and Their Modulation of Complex I Activity in Isolated Mitochondria

Antonella Aresta [1,*], Nicoletta De Vietro [1], Pietro Cotugno [2], Ciro Leonardo Pierri [3], Lucia Trisolini [1] and Carlo Zambonin [1]

1 Department of Biosciences, Biotechnology and Environment, University of Bari "Aldo Moro", Via Orabona 4, 70125 Bari, Italy; nicoletta.devietro@uniba.it (N.D.V.); l.trisolini@ibiom.cnr.it (L.T.); carlo.zambonin@uniba.it (C.Z.)

2 Department of Chemistry, University of Bari "Aldo Moro", Via Orabona 4, 70125 Bari, Italy; pietro.cotugno@uniba.it

3 Department of Pharmacy, Pharmaceutical Sciences, University of Bari "Aldo Moro", Via Orabona 4, 70125 Bari, Italy; ciro.pierri@uniba.it

* Correspondence: antonellamaria.aresta@uniba.it

Abstract: Supercritical fluid extraction (SFE) was used to extract bioactive compounds from apple (*Malus domestica*) peel waste from three different Italian cultivars. The bioactive fractions were extracted applying a temperature of 60 °C and a pressure of 250 bar for 15 min with 20% ethanol as co-solvent, at a flow rate of 2 mL/min. The total polyphenol (TP), anthocyanin (TA), ascorbic acid (AA), and antioxidant activity contents (TACs) were measured, while chromatographic analyses were performed to highlight the differences between the extracts. The Stark cultivar had the highest levels of polyphenols, anthocyanins, and ascorbic acid, while the Royal Gala cultivar showed the highest total antioxidant activity. SFE extracts were then tested for their effect on the mitochondrial NADH–ubiquinone oxidoreductase (Complex I) activity on mitochondria isolated from human embryonic kidney cells (HEK239). The Stark extract showed the most positive response in terms of NADH oxidation. The results obtained in this work highlight the potential of apple peel waste as a source of functional phytocompounds and suggest that Stark cultivar extracts may be exploited for pharmacological applications. This study supports the circular bioeconomy by promoting the use of waste products as a valuable resource.

Keywords: SFE; HPLC; apple peels; bioactive compounds; in vitro activity

1. Introduction

Bioactive compounds are present in small amounts in foods and other natural matrices [1] and provide an extra-nutritional contribution to diet due to their beneficial effects on health. Scientific research has recently been focused on the development of new and more advantageous methods for their extraction from food waste [2–10], a potential source of useful molecules, in the attempt to provide the food industry with an efficient, cheap, and environmentally friendly solution for waste disposal.

Apple (*Malus domestica* (Suckow) Borkh) is a type of fruit available all year round and is widespread throughout the world for economic and cultural reasons [11–13]. According to a "Food and Agriculture Organization" report, the 2020 world apple production was estimated at ~86 million tons. Approximately 18% of global production was used to produce transformed foods, generating large amounts of by-products whose disposal represents an environmental problem and which add additional costs to food producers [13,14]. However, due to the high content of compounds useful for human health, apple waste constitutes a potential resource [14–21]. For instance, apple peel [21,22] contains fibers [19,21], minerals [18], flavonoids [16,19], phenolic acids [16,19], and vitamins, such as C, B1, B2, B3, and A [23,24], possessing great potential in functional food development and exerting a positive influence on the prevention of various diseases. The distribution of bioactive compounds varies between the peel, pulp, and seed [2,16,25], even if the peel is characterized by higher concentrations, and notable differences can also be observed in fruits of the same cultivar.

Polyphenols, likely the most important bioactive compounds in apple peels, are naturally present as acetyl-, malonyl-, and β-glucosides, conjugated precursor forms characterized by greater hydrophilicity and lower biological activity compared to the molecules that represent their core. The free polyphenolic forms therefore represent their least abundant hydrophobic active fraction [26].

Traditionally, extractions on apple peel were based on conventional techniques, which were neither applicable to large-scale samples nor environmentally friendly, as they used large amounts of organic solvents on fresh or dried peels [20], and nowadays green extraction technologies are preferred to process apple peel into products of added value [2,3,14]. Among them, supercritical fluid extraction (SFE) constitutes a simple, cost-effective, eco-friendly approach, which can even be applied to systems on different scales. In fact, it can be used in laboratories on small amounts of samples for analytical or preparative purposes, or to treat quantities of raw material in the order of kilograms (pilot systems) up to tons (industrial sector) [3,20]. The use of small amounts of organic solvent, such as methanol or ethanol, with supercritical CO_2 was successfully used for the extraction of polar compounds, such as polyphenols and water-soluble vitamins, allowing the simultaneous recovery of compounds of different polarities [27].

In this study, CO_2 was used as a supercritical fluid with ethanol as a modifier to extract bioactive compounds from apple peel. The waste apple peels were obtained from three of the most widespread cultivars in Italy, two from organic farming (Royal Gala and Stark) and one from non-organic farming (Gala). Each SC-CO_2 extract was characterized in terms of total phenolic content, flavonoid, anthocyanin, vitamin C, and antioxidant activity, while chromatographic analyses were also performed to highlight the differences between the extracts.

Since several mitochondrial diseases and mitochondrial dysfunction associated with ageing and some cancers [28] may depend on NADH–ubiquinone oxidoreductase (Complex I) impairment [29,30], it is crucial to find small molecules that are able to stimulate Complex I activity and/or mitochondrial function. Thus, each extract was subjected for the first time to in vitro tests on mitochondria from human embryonic kidney cell lines (HEK293) [31] to evaluate their abilities in stimulating the oxidation of NADH and mitochondrial function for possible future pharmacological applications.

2. Materials and Methods

2.1. Apple Collection and Apple Peel Preparation

Apples from Stark, Gala, and Royal Gala cultivars were obtained from apple orchards in Italy and acquired by local suppliers in the period August–September 2021. Royal Gala and Stark cultivars were both from Italian organic farms and purchased from local suppliers in the same period.

The fruits were washed with tap water, thin peels were obtained from each cultivar and cut into small pieces, put on Petri plates, weighed, and immediately covered with paper to avoid light exposure. Samples were frozen at −20 °C for 24 h and finally freeze-dried for 48 h in a ScanVac cool safe lyophilizer supplied by Chemie (BA, Italy), operating at a temperature of −50 °C and a pressure of 0.5 torr. Freeze-dried peel samples were stored in a dryer at room temperature in the dark until use.

2.2. Supercritical Fluid Extraction

SC-CO_2 extraction was carried out according to Aresta et al. [5], with modifications. The SC-CO_2 system was a Spe-ed SFE from Applied Separations (Allentown, PA, USA) connected in-line with a 40P pump from Knauer Wissenschaftliche Geräte GmbH (Berlin, Germany) capable of introducing the modifier into the SC-CO_2 line via a pressurization branch and a T-valve. One gram of each freeze-dried peel sample was mixed with a small quantity of a dispersing material, Ottawa sand (O_2Si, 50–70 mesh particle size, Applaied Separation), to facilitate the contact between the supercritical fluid and the sample particles. The mixture was placed into a 10 mL extraction cell, which was sealed under pressure before being introduced into the oven at 60 °C.

Carbon dioxide (supercritical fluid grade, SCF) from Rivoira (Milan, Italy) was used as extraction solvent with 20% ethanol (liquid chromatographic grade, LC; Sigma-Aldrich, Milan, Italy) as co-solvent. Before each extraction, manual purging of the co-solvent pump was necessary to ensure the correct flow at the same stage and to prevent the pump from undergoing a pressure stroke during extraction. Then, a static period of 3 min was applied before starting the extraction by activating the co-solvent pump. Subsequently, the dynamic extraction process was carried out at 60 °C and 250 bar for 15 min, with carbon monoxide and ethanol (0.4 mL/min) at a total flow rate of 2 mL/min. The extracts were collected in amber vials using the heated micrometric valve, set at 70 °C. At the end of each extraction cycle, an ethanol cleaning cycle was carried out using a stainless-steel by-pass instead of the jar, for 3 min, to remove all residues.

The extracts were then filtered through a syringe filter device with a 25 mm diameter and 0.45 μm PTFE (polytetrafluoroethylene) membrane (Sigma-Aldrich) before analysis.

2.3. *Total Antioxidant Capacity (TAC) Assay*

The assay was performed according to slightly modified previous literature protocols [32]. An aliquot (10 μL) of SC-CO_2 extract (S) was transferred into a test tube containing 0.99 mL of 0.1 mM 2,2-diphenyl-1-picrylhydrazyl (DPPH; Sigma Aldrich) or ethanol (EtOH). The solutions were kept in the dark for 1 h at room temperature. The absorbances were read at 517 nm against EtOH using a UV–Visible spectrophotometer (UV-1650 PC; Shimadzu, Kyoto, Japan). The radical scavenging activity (*RSA*) was expressed as the percentage of the DPPH consumed, which was calculated using the following formula:

$$\%RSA = 100 - [(AS - AEtOH) \div ADPPH] \times 100$$

where *AS* is the absorbance of the extract with DPPH, *AEtOH* is the absorbance of the extract without DPPH, and *ADPPH* is the absorbance of the DPPH solution. The calibration curve was prepared with standard solutions of (±)-6-Hydroxy-2,5,7,8-tetramethylchromane-2-carboxylic acid (Trolox; Sigma Aldrich) in the range 1–100 mM. The TAC was expressed as the Trolox equivalent antioxidant capacity (TEAC) (mmole of Trolox/100 g of freeze-dried material, f.d.m.) [33].

2.4. *Quantification of Antioxidant Compounds*

2.4.1. Total Phenol (TP) Determination

The TP content was evaluated by using 4-benzoylamino-2,5-dimethoxybenzenediazonium chloride hemi [zinc chloride] salt, namely Fast Blue BB diazonium salt (FB BB D; Sigma Aldrich), according to Medina et al.'s protocol [33]. Briefly, 0.1 mL of 0.1% (*w*/*v*) FB BB D reagent in 0.1% ethanol was added at 1 mL of SC-CO_2 extract previously diluted 1:10 in water. Samples were accurately mixed and 0.1 mL of 20% (*w*/*v*) Na_2CO_3 in 1 M NaOH was added to each test tube. The absorbances of samples were measured at 420 nm at 0 and 30 min and the difference between two measurements was used for the estimation. Gallic acid (GA; Sigma Aldrich) was used as the standard compound (calibration curve in the range 0.02–20 μg/mL) for the quantification of TPs, expressed as mg of GA/100 g of f.d.m. Each measurement was performed in triplicate.

2.4.2. Total Flavonoid (TF) Determination

The content of TFs was carried out following the method proposed by Zhishen et al. [34], with a few modifications. Briefly, 50 μL of SC-CO_2 extract was dried in a test tube and 0.5 mL of distilled water (suitable for HPLC; Sigma-Aldrich) was added to the residue. After accurate mixing, 37.5 mL of 5% (*w*/*v*) $NaNO_2$ (Sigma-Aldrich) was added to each test tube, which was then kept for 5 min at room temperature. Subsequently, 37.5 mL of 10% (*w*/*v*) $AlCl_3$ (Sigma-Aldrich) was added. After 6 min, 250 mL of 1 M NaOH was added, mixed, and then each tube received another 300 mL of distilled water. The absorbance at 510 nm of the mixture was finally measured against a blank sample obtained in the same mode. GA was used as the standard compound for the quantification of TFs, expressed as mg of GA/100 g of f.d.m. Each measurement was performed in triplicate.

2.4.3. Total Anthocyanin (TA) Determination

The monomeric anthocyanin content of the SC-CO_2 extract from apple peel was measured using a spectrophotometric pH differential protocol [35]. An aliquot (0.1 mL) of apple peel extract was mixed thoroughly with 0.9 mL of 0.025 M KCl pH 1 buffer. The absorbance of the mixture was measured at 515 and 700 nm against a distilled water blank. Another aliquot was combined similarly with 25 mM sodium acetate buffer pH 4.5, and the absorbance of the solution was measured at the same wavelengths. Finally, the differences between ($A_{515nm} - A_{700nm}$) pH 1 and ($A_{515nm} - A_{700nm}$) pH 4.5 were used for the determination of total anthocyanins. Cyanidin-3-glucoside chloride (CG, Reference Substance; Sigma-Aldrich) was used as the standard compound for the quantification of anthocyanin content in each apple peel extract. Total anthocyanins were expressed as mg of CG/100 g of f.d.m. Each measurement was performed in triplicate.

2.4.4. Ascorbic Acid (AA) Determination

The quantification of AA was performed according to Kschonsek et al. [22]. Briefly, an aliquot (0.2 mL) of SC-CO_2 extracts, previously diluted 1:10 with ultra-pure water, was mixed with 0.3 mL of trichloroacetic acid (0.31 M; Sigma Aldrich) and centrifuged (5 min, 17,000× *g*). Then, 0.3 mL of supernatant was mixed with 0.1 mL of DNP reagent [one volume of thiourea solution (0.83 M in distilled water), one volume of copper sulfate solution (24 mM in distilled water), and 20 volumes of 2,4-dinitrophenylhydrazine solution (0.11 M in 4.5 M sulfuric acid). All reagents were provided by Sigma Aldrich]. The mixture was heated in a thermomixer for 1 h at 60 °C. The samples were cooled in an ice bath for 5 min. Then, 0.4 mL of sulfuric acid (9 M; Sigma Aldrich) was added and mixed. The samples were kept in the dark for 20 min. Finally, each sample was transferred into a semi-micro cuvette and measured at 520 nm. Each measurement was performed in triplicate. In the same way, a calibration line was obtained with six standard solutions of AA (Reference Standard; Sigma Aldrich) covering the concentration range of 0.06 to 6 mg/mL.

2.5. HPLC/DAD Analysis

Chromatographic analyses were performed using an HPLC system (LC20ADXR; Shimadzu, Milan, Italy) equipped with a binary pump (LC20ADXR; Shimadzu), an auto sampler (SIL20ACXR; Shimadzu), and a UV-diode array detector (PDA-1; Shimadzu) with a flow cell (10 mm, 1/1600, steel, 2.4 mL, LWL). The chromatographic column was an Accucore XLC18 (150 × 4.6 mm, 4 μm; Thermo Scientific, Milan, Italy) equipped with an Accucore XLC18 precolumn (10 × 4 mm, 4 μm; Thermo Scientific).

The mobile phase used was (A) 0.1% formic acid in water, (B) acetonitrile (Sigma Aldrich) with a flow rate of 1.2 mL/min. The gradient elution program was as follows: B (8%) (2 min), 8% B to 15% B (3 min), 15% B to 25% B (5 min), 25% B to 35% (5 min), 35% B to 50% B (5 min), B (50%) (15 min), and re-equilibration of the column (5 min). The total chromatographic run time was 45 min. Injection volume was 20 μL.

Spectra were acquired in the range of 220–500 nm, while meticulous composite chromatograms were obtained using the Max Plot software 5.17 of the PDA-1 detector, which automatically selects and stores the maximum absorbances for each peak, thus providing the maximum signal for all compounds detected. The phenolic compounds were identified by comparing their retention times and UV–visible spectrum with those obtained from standard compounds (10 mg/mL; all Sigma-Aldrich), when available. Otherwise, compounds were tentatively identified by comparing the obtained information with the available data reported in the literature.

An enzymatic deconjugation was also performed as follows: 0.1 mL of enzymatic solution for glycoside hydrolysis [obtained by dissolving 10 mg of β-Glucuronidase from bovine liver (type B-1, ≥1,000,000 units/g solid; Sigma Aldrich) in 13 mL of 0.1 M acetate buffer, pH 5.0] was added to 0.05 mL of SC-CO_2 extract and the resulting mixture was immediately incubated overnight (i.e., approximately 17 h) at 37 °C. Before being subjected to chromatographic analysis, the mixture was filtered through a syringe filter device with a 13 mm diameter (0.45 µm PTFE; Sigma-Aldrich). The experiments were performed in triplicate.

2.6. *Evaluating Biological Activity*

2.6.1. Cell Cultures

HEK293 cells were obtained from the American Type Culture Collection (https://www.atcc.org/products/crl-1573) accessed on 12 September 2022. For the proposed analyses, HEK293 cells were maintained in Dulbecco's Modified Eagle's Medium (DMEM), which has high glucose with sodium pyruvate and stable glutamine (Euroclone, Pero (MI), Italy), and supplemented with 10% (*v*/*v*) fetal bovine serum (FBS; Euroclone ECS0180L, Pero, Milan, Italy) and 1% (*v*/*v*) penicillin-streptomycin (Euroclone, *ECM0010*, Pero, Milan, Italy). The cells were cultured in a humidified atmosphere with 5% CO_2 and 37 °C.

2.6.2. Mitochondrial Isolation

Cells were grown in T75 flasks. At confluence, cells were detached by trypsin and centrifuged at 125× *g* for 5 min, the supernatant was discarded, and the pelleted cells were resuspended in Ringer NaCl buffer (135 mM NaCl, 20 mM HEPES, 0.8 mM $MgSO_4$, 3 mM KCl, 1.8 mM CaCl2, 11 mM D-glucose, pH = 7.5) according to Palacino et al. [36]. Afterwards, cells were centrifuged at 125× *g* for 5 min and the obtained pellet was suspended in 2 mL of A buffer (sucrose 320 mM, Tris-HCl 5 mM, EGTA 2 mM, pH = 7.4) and homogenized with a glass–Teflon grinder kept in ice. Thus, the homogenate underwent a centrifugation step at 4 °C for 6 min at 2000× *g* to remove nuclei and tissue particles, while the supernatant was collected for further centrifugation at 4 °C for 15 min at 12,000× *g* to pellet mitochondria. The entire isolation procedure of subcellular fractions was carried out according to Palacino et al. [36]. The mitochondria amount was determined according to Bradford methods [37].

2.6.3. Complex I Activity Measurements

Rotenone-sensitive NADH (β-Nicotinamide adenine dinucleotide) ubiquinone oxidoreductase (Complex I) activity was measured spectrophotometrically following the decrease in NADH absorbance at 340 nm as described by Spinazzi et al. [38], with some modifications. We used a reaction mix containing a 25 µg sample of mitochondria, TNS buffer 3% (*w*/*v*), 50 mM potassium phosphate buffer pH 7.5, 600 mM KCN (Sigma Aldrich), and 90 mM NADH (≥97% pure, grade HPLC; Sigma Aldrich). The mitochondria were incubated for 2 min with apple peel extracts diluted 1:100, 1:1000, or 1:10,000 in H_2O or with only ethanol used as a control (at the same dilutions in water) before starting the reaction. The reaction was started by adding 30 mM Decilubiquinone (≥97% pure, grade HPLC; Sigma Aldrich). NADH (β-Nicotinamide adenine dinucleotide) ubiquinone oxidoreductase (Complex I)-specific activity was checked by adding an excess of Rotenone 100 µM. In parallel, as a further control test, we prepared a cuvette containing the same quantity of extract (ethanol) dilutions and the mitochondrial sample in the presence of 100 µM Rotenone (≥95% pure; Sigma Aldrich), which is a Complex I selective inhibitor.

2.6.4. Statistical Analysis

All analyses related to the quantification of antioxidant compounds were performed in triplicate and the results expressed as mean values ± standard deviation. MedCalc statistical software ver 22.021 for Windows was used to calculate the difference between the averages observed in two independent samples. A significance value (p value) < 0.05 was used to assess the difference. For NADH–ubiquinone oxidoreductase activity in HEK cell mitochondria, a nonparametric Wilcoxon test was used to calculate the difference ($p < 0.05$) between mitochondria incubated with diluted SC-CO_2 extract diluted from Stark, Gala, and Royal Gala wastes and nontreated mitochondria in the corresponding ethanol obtained from at least four independent experiments.

3. Results and Discussion

3.1. Supercritical Fluid Extraction

The parameters applied during supercritical fluid extraction (SFE) were found in the literature [1–4,36]. Ethanol with a percentage of 20% was selected as the extraction co-solvent to help CO_2, which has a low polarity, to favor the extraction of compounds with different polarities from apple peel [5,27].

Additionally, a mild temperature (60 °C) was selected to avoid thermal degradation of the compounds and preserve the antioxidant properties of the extracts [4,36]. Given these observations, the samples were prepared according to the protocol optimized by Aresta et al. for the determination of polyphenols and vitamins in winemaking by-products by extraction with SC-CO_2 [5].

3.2. Quantification of Antioxidant Compounds

The specific spectrophotometric assays for the determination of the total antioxidant capacity and the quantification of the antioxidant compounds present in the extracts of Stark, Gala, and Royal Gala apple peels obtained by SFE (Section 2.2) were selected from the literature [33] considering specific features, such as sensitivity, specificity, and ease of execution. TPs were detected using the FB BB D reagent, which, unlike the more common Folin–Ciocalteu reagent, is not sensitive to reducing sugars which can be naturally present in extracts and determine overestimates with Folin–Ciocalteu [33].

Table 1 shows the average values of the complete set of determinations (TAC, TPs, TFs, TAs, and AA) performed on each apple peel SC-CO_2 extract. The data obtained were in good agreement with the existing literature for all the analytes except for ascorbic acid, which was found in all extracts at concentration levels lower than expected, since Kschonsek et al. [22] reported that peel levels for TPs and AA range from 99.6 ± 5.4 to 495.3 ± 44.0 mg/100 g and 99.2 ± 10.0 to 300.9 ± 10.8 mg/100 g, respectively.

Table 1. TAC, TPs, TFs, TAs, and AA apple peel SC-CO_2 extract contents. For every cultivar, three replicates were performed (n = 3).

Cultivar	TAC mmole Trolox/100 g (n = 3)	TPs mg GA/100 g (n = 3)	TFs mg GA/100 g (n = 3)	TAs mg CG/100 g (n = 3)	AA mg/100 g (n = 3)
Stark	5.74 ± 0.07	379 ± 68	120 ± 2	7.0 ± 0.3	43.75 ± 6.05
Gala	2.20 ± 0.04	152 ± 25	90 ± 1	5.0 ± 0.3	9.02 ± 1.65
Royal Gala	5.95 ± 0.89	136 ± 14	115 ± 2	4.8 ± 0.1	25.59 ± 1.96

T-tests showed some statistically significant differences between the extracts of the three cultivars in the five assays ($p < 0.05$). Stark extracts were higher in TPs, TAs, and AA than the other two. Instead, they showed no significant differences in comparison with Royal Gala for TAC. Gala and Royal Gala were similar in TP and TA. On the other hand, vitamin C contents were very different between the three extracts. In particular, the Gala apples were characterized by lower levels and lower antioxidant activity. Then, phytochemicals can contribute in different ways to the antioxidant activity of the extracts and the poor correlation between the estimated amounts of the analytes and the antioxidant power of the samples.

3.3. HPLC/DAD Analysis

Chromatographic analyses confirmed the existence of differences between samples deriving from apple waste of different origins. Figure 1 shows chromatograms relevant to the three SC-CO_2 extracts (Stark, Gala, and Royal Gala). The chromatograms appear rather poor, although apple peel is a rich source of polyphenols.

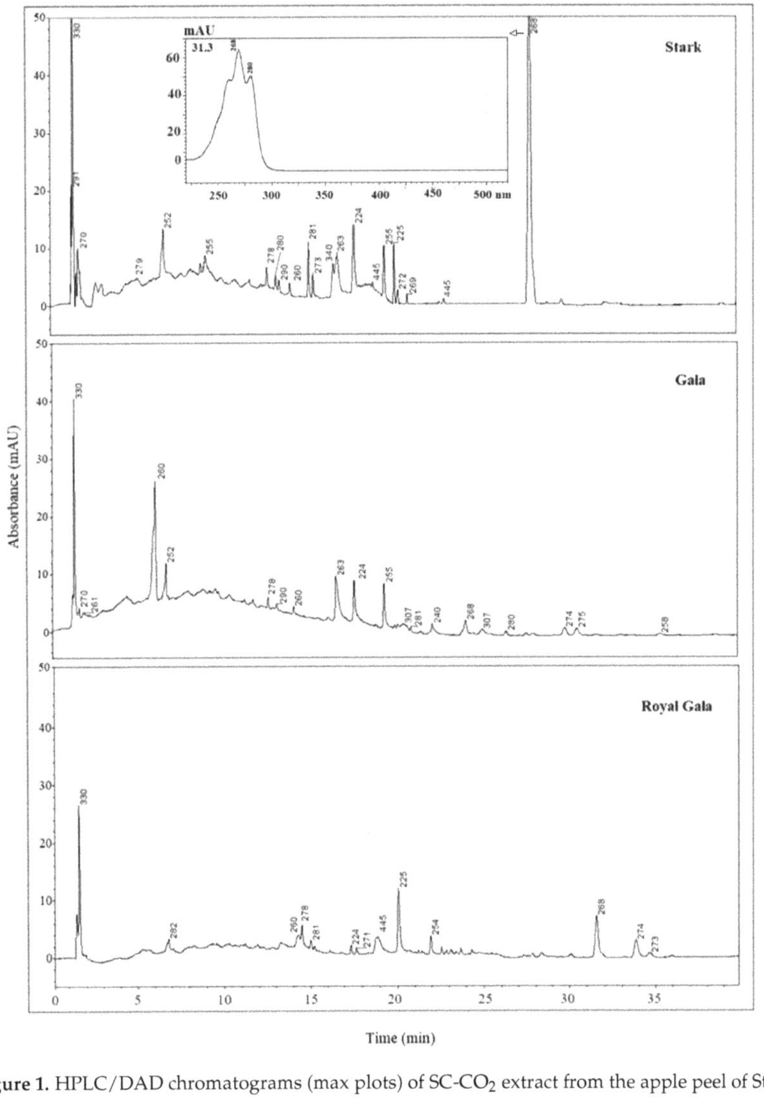

Figure 1. HPLC/DAD chromatograms (max plots) of SC-CO_2 extract from the apple peel of Stark, Gala, and Royal Gala cultivars. The numbers refer to the λ_{max} detected for each peak. Chromatographic and acquisition conditions are described in Section 2.5.

However, some polyphenols were identified by comparing both the chromatographic retention times and the UV–Visible spectra taken at the apex of each peak with those obtained from standard compounds analyzed under the same conditions.

Table 2 lists the standards that were subjected to chromatographic analysis, their retention times (RT, min), the λ_{max} recorded by the detector, and the presence or absence in the considered cultivar.

Table 2. Retention times of standard compounds, λ_{max} detected, and presence in SC-CO_2 extract.

RT (min)	Compound	λ_{max} (nm)	Presence in SC-CO_2 Extract
2.0 ± 0.1	Gallic acid	270	Stark and Gala
5.0 ± 0.1	(+)-Catechin	279	Stark
5.6 ± 0.1	Vanillic acid	260	Gala
9.1 ± 0.1	Rutin	255	Stark
12.4 ± 0.1	trans-Resveratrol	307	
13.8 ± 0.1	Quercetin	370	
14.3 ± 0.2	Cinnamic acid	278	Royal Gala

For analyte recognition, the purity of each peak was determined. The spectra acquired at the apex and in the ascending and descending tracts of each peak during elution were superimposed with the spectrum of the standard acquired in the same peak, always obtaining results better than 99%.

Rutin is a glycoside of the flavonol quercetin, in which the aglycone is bound to the disaccharide α-L-rhamnopyranosyl-(1→6)-β-D-glucopyranose. It is found in a wide variety of plants and apple peels and is believed to be a rich source of flavonoids [8]. However, it was unexpectedly detected only in Stark extracts.

Then, all the SC-CO_2 extracts were subjected to enzymatic hydrolysis to obtain the respective aglycones. The glycosylated deconjugates were then subjected to LC analysis in order to check their presence. Figure 2 shows, for instance, an LC chromatogram of a deconjugate Stark sample. Both the retention time and the UV–Visible spectrum of the peak eluting at 13.9 min were found to be clearly comparable to those of the standard of quercetin analyzed using the same chromatographic conditions. On the contrary, analysis of the deconjugates related to the other two cultivars confirmed the absence of the flavonol.

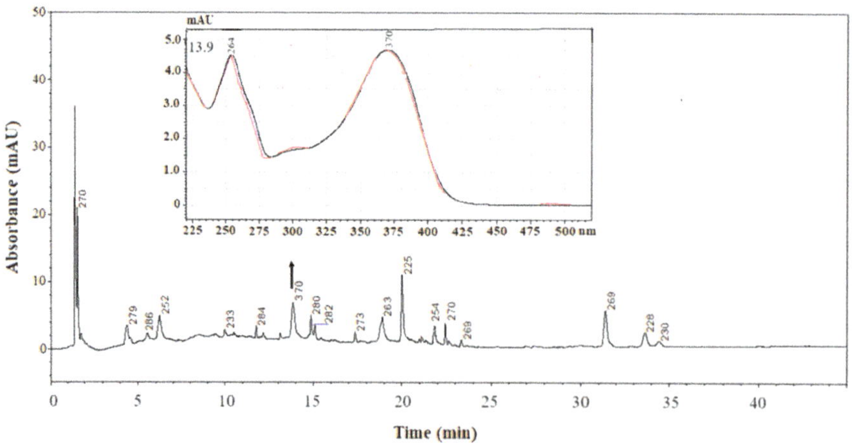

Figure 2. LC-UV-DAD chromatograms (max plots) of enzymatically hydrolyzed SC-CO_2 extract from the apple peel of the Stark cultivar. The numbers refer to the λ_{max} detected for each peak. The figure shows the spectrum of the compound at 13.9 min, coincident with quercetin standard (red line). Chromatographic and acquisition conditions are described in Section 2.5.

To evaluate the quercetin levels in the sample, a calibration curve was generated with five standard solutions that was linear in the range 0.06–20 µg/mL, with a determination coefficient (R^2) of 0.9998. The detection and quantification limits obtained by interpolation of the calibration curve were 0.02 and 0.06 µg/mL, respectively, according to European Commission recommendations [39].

The method had good repeatability, with RSD values of 5.9 and 9.7% for within days (n = 3) and between days (n = 15), respectively. In relation to the concentration of quercetin in deconjugated samples, it was undetectable at 50 µg/mL.

The careful inspection of retention times and spectra and the provisional identification, also compared with the obtained information from the literature data, showed the probable presence of catechins (λ_{max} 280 nm), caffeic acid (238 nm), cyanidins (278 nm), chlorogenic acid (324 nm), isoflavones (260 nm), retinoid (340 nm), and carotenoids (445 nm) [40,41].

In the chromatograms relative to the SC-CO_2 extracts of Stark samples, the presence of a very abundant peak is evident at the retention time of 31.3 min, whose UV–Visible spectrum is reported in Figure 1. Interestingly, this spectrum is shared with other peaks of the same chromatogram, namely the one with RTs of 18.9, 22.5, and 23.4 min. Comparing the chromatographic data relevant to this extract with those of the other cultivar analyzed, only one peak in the chromatogram relevant to the Royal Gala extract showed a peak eluting at 18.9 min, also characterized by the same UV–Visible spectrum. It is worth noting that the Royal Gala and Stark cultivars were both from organic farms.

3.4. *Evaluating Biological Activity*

To examine the effect of each apple peel extract on mitochondria, the NADH oxidoreductase activity was measured on mitochondria isolated from HEK293 cells in the presence of different dilutions of the investigated extracts.

Firstly, it was noticed that the Complex I activity measured from mitochondria extracted from the cultured selected cells after the addition of the three apple peel extracts at 1:100 dilution was unchanged with respect to the ethanol control. Instead, we observed an increase in Complex I activity in the presence of the Stark apple peel extract at 1:1000 and above all at 1:10,000 dilution, with respect to the ethanol control at the same dilution, whereas the Complex I activity in the presence of Gala and Royal Gala apple peel extracts was unchanged (Figure 3).

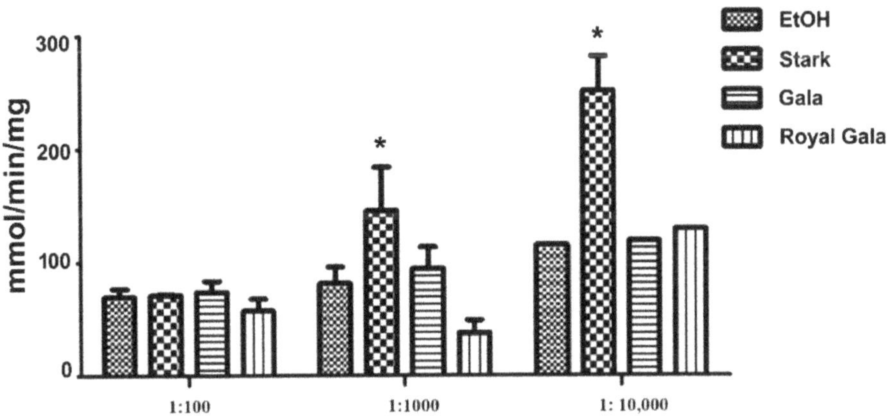

Figure 3. NADH–ubiquinone oxidoreductase activity in HEK cell mitochondria incubated with SC-CO_2 extract diluted from Stark, Gala, and Royal Gala waste. Values represent mean rates (nmol/min/mg) ± SEM obtained from at least four independent experiments. * $p < 0.05$, nonparametric Wilcoxon test between mitochondria administered with 1:100, or 1:1000, or 1:10,000 and nontreated mitochondria in the corresponding ethanol (EtOH). Dilution in water (1:100, 1:1000, or 1:10,000).

As is evident, ethanol does not affect mitochondrial function, as observed by Tempio et al. [42], while only SC-CO_2 Stark extracts were able to induce a significant stimulation of Complex I activity at higher dilutions, probably due to their higher concentration of bioactive molecules (almost double the concentration of AA, TP, and TA) compared to the other cultivars studied. Furthermore, the increased Complex I activity in the presence of diluted Stark extracts could be ascribed either to the minimum concentration of bioactive molecules able to produce a positive effect without causing any toxicity, or to a combination of AA, TPs, and TAs able to exert a protective effect on mitochondria at specific concentration levels.

Moreover, Stark extracts were well tolerated by mitochondria, as well as comparable to the other investigated extracts, even if an excess of antioxidant molecules, which may counteract ROS formation into mitochondria, can alter the endogenous ROS signaling between the cytosol and mitochondria, and can even result in toxicity [43,44]. Indeed, apple peels are rich in vitamins (i.e., vitamin E and vitamin K [45,46]) that can be structurally related to ubiquinone and can target either mitochondrial proteins of the inner membrane or other FAD/NADH/ubiquinone-dependent dehydrogenases widely expressed in other cell compartments [43].

More generally, the hypothesis of a protective role of the tested extracts on mitochondrial function is consistent with Carrasco-Pozo [47], who proposed a protective role of dietary polyphenols on mitochondria. It was also shown that quercetin, resveratrol, and rutin protected Caco-2 cells against indomethacin-induced mitochondrial dysfunction due to the ability of the molecules to enter cells and accumulate in mitochondria. In addition, a structural similarity between quercetin and ubiquinone has been proposed by some authors as a possible explanation for the protective effect [45]. Furthermore, Skemiene et al. [48] proposed that anthocyanins can behave as electron acceptors in Complex I, resulting in increased ATP production in pathological conditions, such as after ischemia.

Based on the experimental results obtained, which are coherent with analogous findings described in the literature, Stark apple peel extracts appear to be a potentially advantageous dietary supplement for human health. Thus, they will be the subject of further studies aimed at determining the individual polyphenol concentrations. The role of each compound in terms of antioxidant capacity and in terms of protective activity on mitochondria in the presence of pro-apoptotic molecules will be explored by performing mitochondrial respiration assays on mitochondria extracted from different cell lines.

4. Conclusions

In this work, it has been shown that bioactive molecules can be extracted simultaneously from apple peels by means of SFE. In particular, the waste apple peels obtained from an Italian cultivar from an organic farm (Stark) seem the most promising both for the higher content of total polyphenols, anthocyanins, and vitamin C, but also for the greater presence of lipophilic substances, the nature of which is being investigated. The ratio between the constituents, however, is the most balanced among the three investigated to preserve or stimulate mitochondrial function without inducing any toxicity.

Author Contributions: Conceptualization, A.A. and C.Z.; Methodology, A.A., P.C. and C.L.P.; Validation, A.A., P.C. and C.L.P.; Investigation, A.A., N.D.V., P.C. and L.T.; Resources, A.A.; Data Curation, A.A.; Writing—Original Draft Preparation, A.A., N.D.V. and C.L.P.; Writing—Review and Editing, A.A.; Supervision, C.Z.; Funding Acquisition, A.A. and C.Z. All authors have read and agreed to the published version of the manuscript.

Funding: This work was carried out within the framework of the research activities envisaged by the Project funded under the National Recovery and Resilience Plan (NRRP), Mission 4 Component 2 Investment 1.3—Call for tender No. 341 of 15 March 2022 of the Italian Ministry of University and Research funded by the European Union—NextGenerationEU; Project code PE00000003, Concession Decree No. 1550 of 11 October 2022 adopted by the Italian Ministry of University and Research, CUP D93C22000890001, Project title "ON Foods—Research and innovation network on food and nutrition Sustainability, Safety and Security—Working ON Foods".

Institutional Review Board Statement: Not applicable.

Informed Consent Statement: Not applicable.

Data Availability Statement: The data presented in this study are available on request from the corresponding author.

Conflicts of Interest: The authors declare no conflicts of interest.

References

1. Carpena, M.; da Pereira, R.; Garcia-Perez, P.; Otero, P.; Soria-Lopez, A.; Chamorro, F.; Alcaide-Sancho, J.; Fraga-Corral, M.; Prieto, M.A.; Simal-Gandara, J. An Overview of Food Bioactive Compounds and Their Properties. In *Membrane Separation of Food Bioactive Ingredients. Food Bioactive Ingredients*; Jafari, S.M., Castro-Muñoz, R., Eds.; Springer: Cham, Switzerland, 2021.
2. Cai, H.L.; You, S.Y.; Xu, Z.Y.; Li, Z.M.; Guo, J.J.; Ren, Z.Y.; Fu, C.L. Novel extraction methods and potential applications of polyphenols in fruit waste: A review. *J. Food Meas. Charact.* **2021**, *15*, 3250–3261. [CrossRef]
3. Putra, N.R.; Rizkiyah, D.N.; Abdul Aziz, A.H.; Che Yunus, M.A.; Veza, I.; Harny, I.; Tirta, A. Waste to Wealth of Apple Pomace Valorization by Past and Current Extraction Processes: A Review. *Sustainability* **2023**, *15*, 830. [CrossRef]
4. Vetralla, M.; Ferrentino, G.; Zambon, A.; Spilimbergo, S. A Study about the Effects of Supercritical Carbon Dioxide Drying on Apple Pieces. *Int. J. Food Eng.* **2018**, *4*, 186–190. [CrossRef]
5. Aresta, A.; Cotugno, P.; De Vietro, N.; Massari, F.; Zambonin, C. Determination of Polyphenols and Vitamins in Wine-Making by-Products by Supercritical Fluid Extraction (SFE). *Anal. Lett.* **2020**, *53*, 2585–2595. [CrossRef]
6. Garofulic, I.E.; Zoric, Z.; Pedisic, S.; Brncic, M.; Dragovic-Uzelac, V. UPLC-MS_2 profiling of blackthorn flower polyphenols Isolated by ultrasound-assisted extraction. *J. Food Sci.* **2018**, *83*, 2782–2789. [CrossRef] [PubMed]
7. Ma, G.L.; Chen, Y.T. Polyphenol supplementation benefits human health via gut microbiota: A systematic review via meta-analysis. *J. Fuoncional. Food* **2020**, *66*, 103829. [CrossRef]
8. Fernandes, P.A.R.; Wessel, D.F.; Coimbra, M.A.; Cardoso, S.M. Apple (*Malus domestica*) By-products: Chemistry, Functionality and Industrial Applications. In *Mediterranean Fruits Bio-Wastes*; Ramadan, M.F., Farag, M.A., Eds.; Springer: Cham, Switzerland, 2022.
9. De la Peña-Armada, R.; Mateos-Aparicio, I. Sustainable Approaches Using Green Technologies for Apple By-Product Valorisation as A New Perspective into the History of the Apple. *Molecules* **2022**, *27*, 6937. [CrossRef] [PubMed]
10. Martău, G.A.; Teleky, B.-E.; Ranga, F.; Pop, I.D.; Vodnar, D.C. Apple Pomace as a Sustainable Substrate in Sourdough Fermentation. *Front. Microbiol.* **2021**, *12*, 742020. [CrossRef]
11. Chen, Z.; Yu, L.; Liu, W.; Zhang, J.; Wang, N.; Chen, X. Research progress of fruit color development in apple (*Malus domestica* Borkh.). *Plant Physiol. Biochem.* **2021**, *162*, 267–279. [CrossRef] [PubMed]
12. Vasylieva, N.; James, H. Production and trade patterns in the world apple market. *Innov. Mark.* **2021**, *17*, 16–25. [CrossRef]
13. Fotirić Akšić, M.; Dabić Zagorac, D.; Gašić, U.; Tosti, T.; Natić, M.; Meland, M. Analysis of apple fruit (*Malus* × *domestica* Borkh.) quality attributes obtained from organic and integrated production systems. *Sustainability* **2022**, *14*, 5300. [CrossRef]
14. Rabetafika, H.N.; Bchir, B.; Blecker, C.; Richel, A. Fractionation of apple by-products as source of new ingredients: Current situation and perspectives. *Trends Food Sci. Technol.* **2014**, *40*, 99–114. [CrossRef]
15. Rupasinghe, V.H.P.; Wang, L.; Huber, M.G.; Pitts, L.N. Effect of baking on dietary fibre and phenolics of muffins incorporated with apple skin powder. *Food Chem.* **2008**, *107*, 1217–1437. [CrossRef]
16. Shehzadi, K.; Rubab, Q.; Asad, L.; Ishfaq, M.; Shafique, B.; Nawaz Ranjha, M.M.A.; Mahmood, S.; Mueen-Ud-Din, G.; Javaid, T.; Sabtain, B.; et al. Critical Review on Presence of Polyphenols in Commercial Varieties of Apple Peel, their Extraction and Health Benefits. *J. Bio. Sci. Res.* **2020**, *6*, 1–8.
17. Hidalgo, A.; Brandolini, A.; Čanadanovic-Brunet, J.; Ćetkovic, G.; Tumbas-Šaponjac, V. Microencapsulates and extracts from red beetroot pomace modify antioxidant capacity, heat damage and colour of pseudocereals-enriched einkorn water biscuits. *Food Chem.* **2018**, *268*, 40–48. [CrossRef] [PubMed]
18. Mendoza-Wilson, A.M.; Castro-Arredondo, I.S.; Espinosa-Plascencia, A.; Robles-Burgueño, M.R.; Balandrán-Quintana, R.R.; Bermúdez-Almada, M.C. Chemical composition and antioxidant-prooxidant potential of a polyphenolic extract and a proanthocyanidin-rich fraction of apple skin. *Heliyon* **2016**, *2*, e00073. [CrossRef] [PubMed]
19. Henríquez, C.; Speisky, H.; Chiffelle, I.; Valenzuela, T.; Araya, M.; Simpson, R.; Almonacid, S. Development of an ingredient containing apple peel, as a source of polyphenols and dietary fiber. *J. Food Sci.* **2010**, *75*, 172–181. [CrossRef] [PubMed]
20. Massini, L.; Rico, D.; Martin-Diana, A.B.; Barry-Ryan, C. Valorisation of apple peels. *Eur. J. Food Res. Rev.* **2013**, *3*, 1–15.
21. Kaur, M.; Kaur, M.; Kaur, H. Apple peel as a source of dietary fiber and antioxidants: Effect on batter rheology and nutritional composition, textural and sensory quality attributes of muffins. *J. Food Meas. Charact.* **2022**, *16*, 2411–2421. [CrossRef]
22. Kschonsek, J.; Wolfram, T.; Stöckl, A.; Böhm, V. Polyphenolic compounds analysis of old and new apple cultivars and contribution of polyphenolic profile to the in vitro antioxidant capacity. *Antioxidants* **2018**, *7*, 20. [CrossRef]
23. Vicki Brower, V. An Apple a Day May Be Safer Than Vitamins. *J. Natl. Cancer Inst.* **2008**, *100*, 770–772. [CrossRef]
24. Lemmens, E.; Alos, E.; Rymenants, M.; De Storme, N.; Keulemans, W. Dynamics of ascorbic acid content in apple (*Malus* × *domestica*) during fruit development and storage. *Plant Physiol. Biochem.* **2020**, *151*, 47–51. [CrossRef]

25. Awad, M.A.; De Jager, A.; Van Westing, L.M. Flavonoid and chlorogenic acid levels in apple fruit: Characterisation of variation. *Sci. Hortic.* **2000**, *83*, 249–263. [CrossRef]
26. Wiczkowski, W.; Piskuła, M.K. Food flavonoids. *Pol. J. Food Nutr. Sci.* **2004**, *13*, 101–114.
27. Aizpurua-Olaizola, O.; Ormazabal, M.; Vallejo, A.; Olivares, M.; Navarro, P.; Etxebarria, N.; Usobiaga, A. Optimization of supercritical fluid consecutive extractions of fatty acids and polyphenols from Vitis vinifera grape wastes. *J. Food Sci.* **2015**, *80*, E101–E107. [CrossRef] [PubMed]
28. Punzi, G.; Porcelli, V.; Ruggiu, M.; Hossain, M.F.; Menga, A.; Scarcia, P.; Castegna, A.; Gorgoglione, R.; Pierri, C.L.; Laera, L.; et al. SLC25A10 biallelic mutations in intractable epileptic encephalopathy with complex I deficiency. *Hum. Mol. Genet.* **2018**, *27*, 499–504. [CrossRef] [PubMed]
29. Wallace, D.C. Mitochondrial DNA in aging and disease. *Sci. Am.* **1997**, *277*, 40–47. [CrossRef] [PubMed]
30. Di Mauro, S.; Schon, E.A. Mitochondrial DNA mutations in human disease. *Am. J. Med. Genet.* **2001**, *106*, 18–26. [CrossRef] [PubMed]
31. Hu, J.W.; Han, J.Z.; Li, H.R.; Zhang, X.; Liu, L.L.; Chen, F.; Zeng, B. Human Embryonic Kidney Cells: A Vehicle for Biopharmaceutical Manufacturing, Structural Biology, and Electrophysiology. *Cell Tissues Organs* **2018**, *205*, 1–8. [CrossRef] [PubMed]
32. Al-Duais, M.; Müller, L.; Böhm, V.; Jetschke, G. Antioxidant capacity and total phenolics of cyphostemma digitatum before and after processing: Use of different assays. *Eur. Food. Res. Technol.* **2009**, *228*, 813–821. [CrossRef]
33. Medina, B. Simple and rapid method for the analysis of phenolic compounds in beverages and grains. *J. Agric. Food Chem.* **2011**, *59*, 1565–1571. [CrossRef] [PubMed]
34. Zhishen, J.; Mengcheng, T.; Jianming, W. The determination of flavonoid contents in mulberry and their scavenging effects on superoxide radicals. *Food Chem.* **1999**, *64*, 555–559. [CrossRef]
35. Lee, J.; Durst, R.W.; Wrolstad, R.E. Determination of total monomeric anthocyanin pigment content of fruit juices, beverages, natural colorants, and wines by the pH differential method: Collaborative study. *J AOAC Int.* **2005**, *88*, 1269–1278. [CrossRef] [PubMed]
36. Palacino, J.J.; Sagi, D.; Goldberg, M.S.; Krauss, S.; Motz, C.; Wacker, M.; Klose, J.; Shen, J. Mitochondrial Dysfunction and Oxidative Damage in parkin-deficient Mice. *J. Biol. Chem.* **2004**, *279*, 18614–18622. [CrossRef] [PubMed]
37. Bradford, M.M. A rapid and sensitive method for the quantitation of microgram quantities of protein utilizing the principle of protein-dye binding. *Anal. Biochem.* **1976**, *72*, 248–254. [CrossRef] [PubMed]
38. Spinazzi, M.; Casarin, A.; Pertegato, V.; Salviati, L.; Angelini, C. Assessment of mitochondrial respiratory chain enzymatic activities on tissues and cultured cells. *Nat. Protoc.* **2012**, *31*, 1235–1246. [CrossRef]
39. Gegenschatz, S.A.; Chiappini, F.A.; Teglia, C.M.; Munoz de la Pena, A.; Goicoechea, H.C. Binding the gap between experiments, statistics, and method comparison: A tutorial for computing limits of detection and quantification in univariate calibration for complex samples. *Anal. Chim. Acta* **2021**, *1209*, 339342. [CrossRef]
40. Da Porto, C.; Natolino, A. Supercritical fluid extraction of polyphenols from grape seed (*Vitis vinifera*): Study on process variables and kinetics. *J. Supercrit. Fluids* **2017**, *130*, 239–245. [CrossRef]
41. Pandey, J.; Bastola, T.; Tripathi, J.; Tripathi, M.; Kumar, R.; Rokaya, R.K.; Dhakal Bhawana, R.; Ravin, D.C.; Bhandari, R.; Poudel, A. Estimation of Total Quercetin and Rutin Content in *Malus domestica* of Nepalese Origin by HPLC Method and Determination of Their Antioxidative Activity. *J. Food Qual.* **2020**, *2020*, 8853426. [CrossRef]
42. Tempio, A.; Niso, M.; Laera, L.; Trisolini, L.; Favia, M.; Ciranna, L.; Marzulli, D.; Petrosillo, G.; Pierri, C.L.; Lacivita, E.; et al. Mitochondrial Membranes of Human SH-SY5Y Neuroblastoma Cells Express Serotonin 5-HT7 Receptor. *Int. J. Mol. Sci.* **2020**, *21*, 9629. [CrossRef]
43. Tragni, V.; Primiano, G.; Tummolo, A.; Cafferati Beltrame, L.; La Piana, G.; Sgobba, M.N.; Cavalluzzi, M.M.; Paterno, G.; Gorgoglione, R.; Volpicella, M.; et al. Personalized Medicine in Mitochondrial Health and Disease: Molecular Basis of Therapeutic Approaches Based on Nutritional Supplements and Their Analogs. *Molecules* **2022**, *27*, 3494. [CrossRef] [PubMed]
44. Gęgotek, A.; Skrzydlewska, E. Antioxidative and Anti-Inflammatory Activity of Ascorbic Acid. *Antioxidants* **2022**, *11*, 1993. [CrossRef] [PubMed]
45. Chun, J.; Lee, J.; Ye, L.; Exler, J.; Eitenmiller, R.R. Tocopherol and tocotrienol contents of raw and processed fruits and vegetables in the United States diet. *J. Food Compos. Anal.* **2006**, *19*, 196–204. [CrossRef]
46. Dismore, M.L.; Haytowitz, D.B.; Gebhardt, S.E.; Peterson, J.W.; Booth, S.L. Vitamin K content of nuts and fruits in the US diet. *Res. Prof. Brief* **2003**, *103*, 1650–1652. [CrossRef]
47. Carrasco-Pozo, C.; Mizgier, M.L.; Speisky, H.; Gotteland, M. Differential protective effects of quercetin, resveratrol, rutin and epigallocatechin gallate against mitochondrial dysfunction induced by indomethacin in Caco-2 cells. *Chem.-Biol. Interact.* **2012**, *195*, 199–205. [CrossRef]
48. Skemiene, K.; Liobikas, J.; Borutaite, V. Anthocyanins as substrates for mitochondrial complex I—Protective effect against heart ischemic injury. *FEBS J.* **2015**, *282*, 963–971. [CrossRef]

antioxidants

MDPI

Article

Advanced Solubilization of Brazilian Cerrado Byproduct Extracts Using Green Nanostructured Lipid Carriers and NaDESs for Enhanced Antioxidant Potentials

Victor Carlos Mello [1,2,*], Giovanna Oliveira de Brito [3], Marina Arantes Radicchi [1,2], Isadora Florêncio [1,2], Tathyana Benetis Piau [4], Eduardo Antonio Ferreira [5], Leonardo Fróes de Azevedo Chang [1,2], Ariane Pandolfo Silveira [1,2], Marina Mesquita Simões [1,2], Karen Letycia Rodrigues de Paiva [1,2], Mac-Kedson Medeiros Salviano Santos [6], Nicole Santana Alves [1,2], Cesar Koppe Grisolia [4], Sônia Nair Báo [2] and Eliana Fortes Gris [3,*]

[1] Cooil Cosmetics, Brasília 72622-401, Brazil; maradicchi.bep@gmail.com (M.A.R.); isadoraflorenciofs@gmail.com (I.F.); nicolesalves18@gmail.com (N.S.A.); leonardochang93@gmail.com (L.F.d.A.C.); pandolfo.ariane@gmail.com (A.P.S.); marinamesquita3007@gmail.com (M.M.S.); karendepaiva@gmail.com (K.L.R.d.P.)
[2] Laboratory of Microscopy and Microanalysis, Department of Cell Biology, Institute of Biological Sciences, University of Brasília, Brasília 70910-900, Brazil; snbao@unb.br
[3] Graduate Program in Health Sciences and Technologies, Faculty of Health Sciences and Technologies, University of Brasilia, Centro Metropolitano, Conjunto A, Lote 01, Brasilia 72220-275, Brazil; giovanna.odebrito@gmail.com
[4] Laboratory of Genetic Toxicology, Department of Genetics and Morphology, Institute of Biological Sciences, University of Brasília, Brasília 70910-900, Brazil; tathyanabenetis@gmail.com (T.B.P.); grisolia@unb.br (C.K.G.)
[5] Faculty of Health Sciences and Technologies, University of Brasilia, Centro Metropolitano, Conjunto A, Lote 01, Brasilia 72220-275, Brazil; eduardoferreira@unb.br
[6] Green Nanotechnology Group, University of Brasilia, Brasília 70910-900, Brazil; mackedson@hotmail.com
* Correspondence: victor.silva@unb.br (V.C.M.); elianagris@unb.br (E.F.G.)

Abstract: This study explores the development and characterization of lipid nanostructures (NLCs) containing natural deep eutectic solvents (NaDESs) derived from taperebá peel extract (*Spondias mombin*), a by-product rich in bioactive phenolic compounds, including ellagic acid and quercetin. The taperebá extract exhibited a high polyphenol content (2623 mg GAE/L) and notable antioxidant activity, as demonstrated by DPPH (258 mM TEAC/100 mL) and ABTS (495 mM TEAC/100 mL) assays. NLCs were developed using NaDESs to enhance the stability and bioavailability of the antioxidant compounds. Physicochemical characterization confirmed the formation of stable, nanometric, and monodispersed formulations with efficient encapsulation. Biological evaluation of the NLC-TAP-NaDES formulation demonstrated its remarkable capacity to mitigate oxidative stress in cells subjected to H_2O_2-induced ROS generation. Fluorescence imaging revealed a significant reduction in intracellular ROS levels in treated cells compared to untreated controls, confirming the antioxidant efficacy of the formulation. This outcome underscores the synergy between NaDESs and NLC systems in protecting and delivering phenolic compounds. This study highlights the potential of utilizing underexplored by-products, such as taperebá peels, to develop sustainable and effective antioxidant delivery systems. The NLC-TAP-NaDES platform combines nanotechnology with green chemistry principles, presenting significant implications for the treatment of oxidative stress-related conditions and broader applications in pharmaceutical and nutraceutical sciences. These findings contribute to advancing sustainable innovations in antioxidant therapies, leveraging the dual benefits of bioeconomy and high-performance nanomaterials.

Keywords: nanostructured lipid carriers; natural deep eutectic solvents; *Spondias mombin*; phenolic compounds; bioactive encapsulation; sustainability; green nanotechnology; circular economy; agricultural byproducts

1. Introduction

The Brazilian Cerrado, a vast and ecologically rich tropical savanna, is globally recognized as one of the most significant biodiversity hotspots [1]. This biome harbors an extraordinary variety of plant species, many of which are rich in bioactive compounds, particularly phenolic compounds with remarkable therapeutic potential. Phenolic compounds belong to a diverse group of chemical structures characterized by an aromatic ring attached to a hydroxyl group. These compounds are well documented for their potent antioxidant and anti-inflammatory activities, which have been extensively studied due to their significant therapeutic potential. They are widely distributed in the Kingdom Plantae, occurring in a variety of species found in both leaves and fruits, where they play critical roles in defense mechanisms against oxidative stress, pathogens, and environmental stressors [2,3].

Among the numerous endemic fruits of the Cerrado, *Spondias mombin* L., commonly known as taperebá, cajá, or cajá-mirim, stands out for its promising biological activities, including gastroprotective effects demonstrated in animal models [4,5] and cytotoxic effects on ovarian cancer cell lines [6].

While the pulp of *S. mombin* is widely utilized in the food industry, the peel is often discarded as waste despite its high concentration of bioactive phenolic compounds, which are well known for their antioxidant properties and potential health benefits [7,8]. Previous research conducted by this group chemically characterized the phenolic compounds found in the peels of *S. mombin* using UPLC-MS/MS. The results demonstrated a significant content of polyphenolic compounds in the peels, emphasizing the high content of ellagic acid and quercetin, alongside considerable antioxidant potential. Moreover, this study successfully identified and quantified certain compounds in the *Spondias* genus for the first time [7]. These secondary metabolites play essential ecological roles in plants, such as by protecting them against pathogens, mitigating UV radiation damage, and reducing oxidative stress [9,10]. However, the clinical application of phenolic compounds is often limited due to their poor stability in gastric environments, low intestinal absorption, and susceptibility to degradation during storage [11,12].

To address these challenges, advanced delivery systems such as nanoencapsulation have garnered increasing attention. Nanostructured lipid carriers (NLCs) are lipid-based nanoparticles composed of a mixture of solid and liquid lipids at room temperature, such as oils and butters. Their structure, characterized by a solid matrix interspersed with more fluid regions, enhances overall structural flexibility and provides a versatile platform for the controlled release of bioactive compounds, with particles typically smaller than 100 nm, offering protection against environmental factors such as light and temperature [13–15]. Moreover, the surface properties of NLCs can be precisely tailored to support diverse therapeutic applications, ensuring stability and biocompatibility [16].

Simultaneously, the demand for sustainable and biocompatible encapsulation systems has driven the exploration of Natural Deep Eutectic Solvents (NaDESs). NaDESs represent a class of green solvents resulting from the combination of natural organic compounds, such as acids, sugars, amino acids, and choline derivatives. When mixed in specific proportions, these compounds interact through hydrogen bonding, forming a eutectic mixture with a melting point lower than that of the individual components. Due to this characteristic, NaDESs exhibit unique solubilization properties, enabling the dissolution of a wide range of bioactive molecules [17–19]. These solvents are not only non-toxic but also possess cryoprotective capabilities, stabilizing sensitive compounds during processes such as lyophilization, thereby enhancing their stability and storage potential [18,19]. Recent studies have highlighted the synergistic effects of integrating NaDESs with NLC formulations, resulting in improved stability and industrial scalability of nanoparticle systems [20,21].

Despite the rich antioxidant profile of *Spondias mombin* peel, its poor water solubility poses a significant challenge for formulation and bioavailability. In this context, its encapsulation within an NLC system using NaDESs as a solubilization medium for phenolic compounds extracted from *S. mombin* peel represents an innovative strategy to valorize this often-overlooked byproduct. NaDESs not only enhance the dissolution and stabilization of phenolic compounds but also contribute to the development of a more sustainable and biocompatible encapsulation system. This work sets a precedent for the development of scalable and environmentally friendly nanoformulations with potential applications in treating oxidative stress-related diseases, such as certain cancers, thereby expanding the therapeutic use of bioactives from Brazilian flora in global health applications [20].

The developed NLC-NaDES platform offers a versatile solution with potential applications in the pharmaceutical, nutraceutical, and cosmetic industries, driven by its capacity to stabilize and enhance the bioavailability of bioactive compounds. The synergy between nanostructured lipid carriers and NaDESs ensures efficient encapsulation and controlled release of phenolic compounds, making it particularly valuable for the treatment of oxidative stress-related pathologies, including neurodegenerative diseases, cancer, and chronic inflammatory disorders. The potent antioxidant properties demonstrated by the NLC-TAP-NaDES formulation underscore its suitability for therapeutic interventions aimed at mitigating oxidative cellular damage.

Furthermore, the system's biocompatibility and cryoprotective capabilities expand its potential for cosmetic applications, such as anti-aging products and skin protectants, where oxidative stress plays a central role in cellular aging. In the nutraceutical field, this platform offers a promising vehicle for the delivery of natural antioxidants, thereby enhancing the functional value of dietary supplements. Additionally, the use of agricultural byproducts, such as *S. mombin* peels, aligns with the principles of a circular economy, promoting sustainability and resource efficiency. This green nanotechnology, therefore, bridges scientific innovation with environmental responsibility, opening new avenues for the valorization of underutilized natural resources while contributing to bioeconomy development.

2. Materials and Methods

2.1. Materials, Reagents and Samples

Analytical standard anhydrous sodium carbonate ($\geq$99% purity) was obtained from Dinâmica Química Contemporânea Ltda., Indaiatuba, São Paulo, Brazil. Murumuru butter (*Astrocaryum murumuru*) and buriti oil (*Mauritia flexuosa*) were provided by Amazon Oil, Ananindeua, Pará, Brazil. Folin–Ciocalteu reagent, ethanol ($\geq$99.5% purity), dimethyl sulfoxide (DMSO, $\geq$99.9% purity), Roswell Park Memorial Institute medium (RPMI-1640), Dulbecco's Modified Eagle Medium (DMEM), 2,2-diphenyl-1-picrylhydrazyl (DPPH), 2,2′-Azino-bis(3-ethylbenzothiazoline-6-sulfonic acid) diammonium salt (ABTS), glycerol analytical standard, and Brij® O10 were purchased from Sigma-Aldrich, St. Louis, MO, USA. Analytical standard choline chloride ($\geq$98% purity) and anhydrous citric acid ($\geq$99.5% purity) were obtained from Êxodo Científica, Sumaré, São Paulo, Brazil. Fetal bovine serum (FBS), penicillin-streptomycin solution (100 U/mL penicillin and 100 µg/mL streptomycin), and trypsin-EDTA (0.25%) were purchased from Gibco (Thermo Fisher Scientific), Waltham, MA, USA. The MTT reagent [3-(4,5-dimethylthiazol-2-yl)-2,5-diphenyl tetrazolium bromide] was obtained from Invitrogen (Thermo Fisher Scientific), Waltham, MA, USA. Phosphate-buffered saline (PBS, pH 7.4) was supplied by LaborClin, Pinhais, Paraná, Brazil.

2.2. Obtaining the Taperabá Fruits and Extract

The fruits of taperebá (*Spondias mombin* L.) were collected when they were ripe by the Brazilian Agricultural Research Corporation (Embrapa Cerrados (CPAC), located in Planaltina, Federal District—DF (15°54′16.50″ South and 47°22′37.49″ (West, at 855 m altitude). The characteristics of the area fall within the Cerrado biome. This project is registered in the National Genetic Heritage and Associated Traditional Knowledge Management System (SisGen) under numbers A002D4B and A235193. The fruits were peeled in a manual process, and the peels dried naturally at room temperature, protected from light, for 24 h. The extract was prepared according to Brito et al. (2022) [7].

2.3. Quantification of Phenolic Compounds and the In Vitro Antioxidant Activity of the Extract

The quantification of phenolic compounds in the extract was carried out through spectrophotometric analysis, being evaluated using the Folin–Ciocalteau method [22]. Calculations were made according to the gallic acid standard curve ($y = 0.0012x + 0.0273$, $R^2 = 0.9979$) and the results were expressed as gallic acid equivalent (GAE) per L of taperebá peel extract.

Previous studies by this group have analyzed the phenolic compounds profile in these peels of *S. mombin* using ultra-performance liquid chromatography coupled with tandem mass spectrometry (UPLC-MS/MS), data previously described by De Brito et al. [7]. Chromatographic separation was carried out on a Waters Acquity UPLC system (Milford, MA, USA), and mass spectrometry detection was performed using a Waters Xevo TQMS instrument (Milford, MA, USA) equipped with an electrospray ionization (ESI) source using the method previously described by Vrhovsek et al. (2012) [22]. Multiple reaction monitoring (MRM) conditions were optimized using flow injections of individual metabolites; for most compounds, the Waters Intellistart software (version 4.1) performed automatic optimization, while for certain analytes, optimal cone voltages and collision energies were determined manually through collision-induced dissociation (CID) experiments

The in vitro antioxidant activity of the extract was evaluated through DPPH [23] and ABTS [24] free radical capture analysis. The results were expressed as Trolox equivalents (mM TEAC/100 mL extract of taperebá peel) and calculated from a standard curve.

2.4. Preparation of NaDESs

The natural analogs of deep eutectic solvents (NaDESs) were made with choline chloride, glycerol and citric acid (1:4:1), with 25% water. The mixture was heated to 80 °C until the reagents were completely dissolved [25]. After concentrating the ethanolic extract in a rotary evaporator, the concentrated extract was dissolved using the prepared NaDESs.

2.5. Development and Optimization of Formulations

To develop a formulation capable of nanoencapsulating the phenolic compounds extracted from taperebá peel, different proportions of surfactants and lipids were tested, following the methodology described by Silva [26], with specific adaptations for this study. Both systems with and without NaDESs were evaluated for their colloidal properties, thermal stability, and encapsulation efficiency.

2.6. Preparation of Lipidic and Aqueous Phases

Initially, formulations were prepared to standardize the individual components. For the lipidic phase, murumuru butter was used as the solid lipid, while buriti oil was included as the liquid lipid to enhance nanoparticle fluidity and stability. For the aqueous phase, the surfactant Brij® O10 (Sigma-Aldrich, St. Louis, MI, USA) was dissolved in distilled water, with its concentration varied to minimize toxicity while optimizing colloidal stability.

2.7. Extract Solubilization

For non-NaDES formulations, the concentrated taperebá peel extract, obtained via rotary evaporation, was directly incorporated into the lipidic phase due to its poor water solubility. In contrast, for NaDES-based formulations, the extract was pre-diluted in a NaDES solution at a ratio of 1:6 (*w*/*v*), composed of choline chloride, citric acid, and glycerol. The resulting mixture was added to the lipidic phase after melting the murumuru butter, ensuring enhanced solubility and uniform dispersion.

2.8. Nanoformulation Production

The nanostructured lipid carriers (NLCs) were produced using a hot emulsification method. The lipidic and aqueous phases were heated separately to specific temperatures (70, 75, and 80 °C) to ensure homogeneity. After heating, the phases were combined and subjected to high-shear stirring to form an emulsion. Finally, the emulsion was rapidly cooled in an ice bath to solidify the lipid matrix and stabilize the nanoparticles.

2.9. Formulation Optimization

The formulations were evaluated based on their polydispersity index (PDI), measured by dynamic light scattering (Zetasizer, Malvern Panalytical), with acceptable values set at <0.25. Particle size was also measured to ensure dimensions below 200 nm, and macroscopic stability was assessed visually to check for phase separation or emulsion instability. Different proportions of the concentrated extract were tested to determine the optimal amount to incorporate, both in its pure form and when diluted in NaDESs. Additionally, the impact of varying NaDES volumes on the colloidal characteristics of the formulations was analyzed.

2.10. Assessment of Colloidal Properties

The Dynamic Light Scattering (DLS) technique was used to determine the mean particle hydrodynamic diameters and dispersion of the chosen NLCs formulations, using a ratio of 1:10 (*v*/*v*) in distilled water, and results expressed as an average of triplicates using the ZetaSizer (Nano ZS®, Malvern Instruments, Malvern, UK) at 25 °C.

The Zeta potential (mV) values of the selected NLCs were determined using the ZetaSizer equipment (Nano ZS®, Malvern Instruments, Malvern, UK) at 25 °C. The formulations were added to distilled water in a ratio of 1:10 (*v*/*v*).

2.11. Study of the Colloidal Stability of Formulations

The formulations described in Figure 1 were subjected to a colloidal stability study, evaluating hydrogen-ion potential (pH) at 25 °C (pHmeter DM-22, Digimed, Sao Paulo, Brazil), as well as particle diameter, polydispersity, and zeta potential at 25 °C (Nano ZS®, Malvern Instruments, Malvern, UK), over time. These parameters were assessed on the day of formulation, after 24 h, and subsequently after 7, 15, and 30 days under different temperature conditions: room temperature (25 °C), high temperature (37 °C), refrigerated (−4 °C), and frozen (−20 °C).

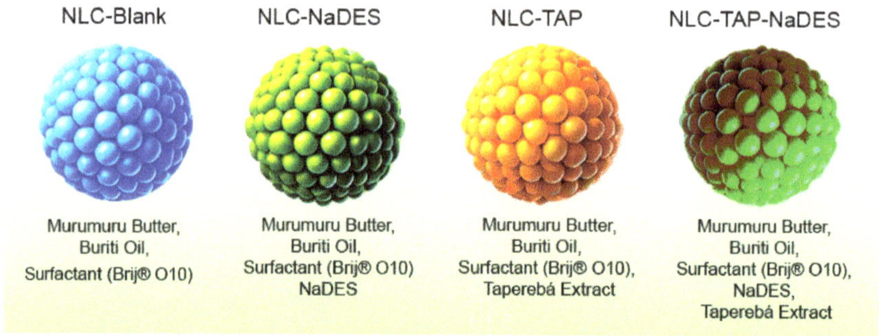

Figure 1. Composition of nanostructured lipid carrier (NLC) formulations. The table details the specific combinations of components used in each formulation, including murumuru butter (solid lipid), buriti oil (liquid lipid), surfactant Brij® O10, natural deep eutectic solvents (NaDESs), and taperebá extract. Each formulation was designed to assess the individual and combined effects of these components on the physicochemical properties, stability, and bioactivity of the NLCs.

2.12. Morphology of Nanoparticles (NPs)

The morphology of NLCs was evaluated by transmission electron microscopy (TEM) using the Transmission Electron Microscope JEM 1011 (JEOL, Tokyo, Japan), which was operated with an acceleration voltage of 80 kV. Suspensions were diluted 1:10 (*v:v*) with Milli-Q® water and deposited directly onto carbon-coated grids used for observing the samples using an osmium tetroxide contrast. The microscope was operated in bright field mode with magnification above 10,000 times [27].

2.13. Assessment of Physicochemical Properties and Thermodynamic Stability of NLCs

The evaluation of physicochemical properties and thermodynamic stability of NCLs was carried out using thermogravimetric analysis (TGA). The NLCs that presented the most appropriate PDI and size results were analyzed. The contribution of NaDESs was also evaluated in NaDES samples without extract, and NLCs with murumuru butter, surfactants, and buriti oil (NLC-NaDES). In addition to NLC with extract dissolved in NaDES (NLC-TAP-NaDES) and NLC with extract without NaDESs (NLC-TAP), the pure lyophilized extract was also analyzed. The measurements were conducted using a differential thermal analysis (DTG-60, Shimadzu, Kyoto, Japan). A heating rate of 10 °C/min was used, with a temperature range of 30–600 °C, under a nitrogen atmosphere with flow rate of 50 mL/min. The samples were previously lyophilized (L101 Liotop Lyophilizer, LABIOM São Carlos, Brazil) and analyzed in a platinum pan as a reference, using approximately 10 mg of material.

2.14. Study of the Stability of Total Polyphenols Contained in NLCs

The NLC formulations were subjected to study of the concentration stability of total polyphenols using spectrophotometric analysis, being evaluated using the Folin–Ciocalteau method [22,28] with adaptations. The nanostructures were subjected to agitation for 24 h in a 1% acetic acid solution, and then used for the Folin–Ciocalteau reaction. Before being evaluated in a spectrophotometer (U-3900H, Hitachi) at 750 nm, the reaction was centrifuged at 3500 rpm for 10 min.

The stability of the phenolic compounds was carried out on the day of formulation (day 0), and subsequently after 7, 15 and 30 days (days 7, 15 and 30). The samples were stored at different storage temperatures: ambient (25 °C), high (37 °C), refrigerated (−4 °C) and frozen (−20 °C).

2.15. Encapsulation Efficiency of Nanoparticles (NPs)

After standardization, the NLCs were subjected to phenolic quantification. The effectiveness of the process was calculated as a percentage [28], according to Equation (1):

$$EE\% = \frac{\text{Qobtained}}{\text{Qtheoretical}} \times 100 \quad (1)$$

EE% is the encapsulation efficiency of phenolic compounds in the nanoparticle, Qobtained is the amount of total polyphenols present after nanoencapsulation and Qtheoretical is the amount of total polyphenols that was added.

2.16. Fourier Transform Infrared Spectroscopy (FT-IR)

FT-IR spectra were acquired using a Vertex 70 spectrometer (Bruker Corporation, Billerica, MA, USA) in attenuated total reflectance (ATR) mode, with samples in liquid state. For analysis, 2 µL of each sample (without dilution) were deposited in a diamond crystal and the spectra were obtained in the region between 4.000 and 500 cm^{-1}, with a resolution of 4 cm^{-1} and 64 scans, in absorbance mode. Data were acquired with OPUS 7.2 software (Bruker Corporation, Ettlingen, Germany) and processed with Origin Pro 2015 software (OriginLab Corporation, Northampton, MA, USA).

2.17. Cell Maintenance

Fibroblasts (L929) were obtained from *Banco de Células do Rio de Janeiro* (BCRJ) and were cultured in RPMI medium, supplemented with 10% (v/v) fetal bovine serum (FBS) and 1% (v/v) antibiotic solution. The cells were maintained in an incubator under a humidified atmosphere with 5% CO_2 at 37 °C throughout the entire experiment, ensuring stable culture conditions from cell seeding to the final analysis. Regular monitoring was performed to maintain cell viability and consistency during the experimental procedures.

2.18. Cultivation System and Obtaining of Zebrafish Embryos

The *Danio rerio* embryos utilized in the embryotoxicity test were supplied by the Zebrafish facility (Techniplast, Italy) of the Laboratory of Toxicologic Genetic of University of Brasília. The adults of zebrafish are maintained in an automated recirculating water system, stocked with filtered water by activated coal. The physical and chemical characteristics of the water are maintained in: pH 7.2–7.6; hardness 6.70 dH; temperature of 26 ± 1 °C; conductivity of 728 µS. The facility room disposes of a photoperiod of 12:12 h light/dark. The fishes are fed two to three times a day with commercial feed (SERAVipan©; Tetramin©) and live feed (nauplii de *Artemia salina*). The zebrafish embryotoxicity test does not require an animal ethic approval, because the embryogenesis up to 96 h is considered similar as an in vitro test, since the sensory system is not completely formed.

2.19. Viability of Fibroblasts (L929)

The 3-(4,5-dimethylthiazol-2-yl)-2,5-diphenyltetrazolium bromide (MTT) [29] assay was performed to analyze cell viability. The concentrations used were: 0.002 mg/mL; 0.008 mg/mL; 0.040 mg/mL; 0.200 mg/mL; 1.000 mg/mL; 5.002 mg/mL; and 25.008 mg/mL (mg NLC/mL).

Cell lines were plated in 96-well plates and treated for 24 h. In all groups, after the time points, the treatment was withdrawn and 150 µL of the MTT solution (0.5 mg/mL in culture medium) was added and incubated for 4 h at 37 °C. After incubation, this solution was removed and 200 µL of DMSO was added to dissolve the formazan crystals. The absorbance was measured at 540 nm using a microplate reader (SpectraMax®, Molecular Devices, San Jose, CA, USA) operated with the SoftMax Pro program (version 7.1, Molecular Devices).

2.20. Toxicity Test with Zebrafish Embryos (FET)

The embryo bioassays were based on the OECD protocol n. 236 [30] for toxicity assessment: Fish Embryo Toxicity—FET test. After collecting the embryos from the pawn breeding system, they were washed and immediately distributed into microplates with "test solutions" to ensure the beginning of exposure in the early stages. Exposure was carried out in 96-well microplates with 200 µL of each concentration. The tested concentrations were: 0 (control); 0.59 µg/mL; 1.18 µg/mL; 2.35 µg/mL; 4.70 µg/mL; 9.41 µg/mL; 18.81 µg/mL; and 37.63 µg/mL. The exposures were conducted in a climatic chamber with conditions identical to the culture room. The test solutions were prepared using zebrafish culture water (physical and chemical characteristics previously described). All bioassays were performed in triplicate with a total of 60 organisms per concentration and for 96 h.

2.21. Reactive Oxygen Species (ROS) Production Assay

L929 cells (1×10^3 cells per well), both control and treated for 4 h with 10 µM of NLC-TAP-NaDES, were exposed to H_2O_2 to induce oxidative stress. After the treatments, the cells were gently washed with PBS (1×) and fixed with 3.5% formaldehyde for 15 min at room temperature. Subsequently, the cells were stained with 500 nM DAPI for nuclear labeling and with 5 µM CellROX® Green Reagent (ThermoFisher®, Waltham, MA, USA) to detect intracellular reactive oxygen species (ROS).

Confocal images were captured using a Leica CS SP5 microscope, employing different z-stacks to acquire three-dimensional images of the cells. Wide-field images were obtained to analyze nuclear localization and the fluorescence of the CellROX® Green Reagent (ThermoFisher®, Waltham, MA, USA) across the cell population. Quantitative analysis was performed on the fluorescence intensity of CellROX® Green Reagent to evaluate whether NLC-TAP-NaDES treatment would reduce ROS production compared to control cells.

2.22. Statistical Analysis

Quantification of total phenolic, antioxidant activity and encapsulation efficiency of taperebá pell extract were calculated from a standard curve and the results were expressed as a mean of triplicates and standard deviation. ANOVA, Correlation Analysis and Tukey HSD Test were performed in the STATISTICA 10.0 program with a significance level of 5% ($p < 0.05$).

Therefore, the results of the FET were statistically analyzed using Sigma Plot 14.0. For normally distributed datasets, two-way ANOVA was used to detect intergroup differences. In cases of non-normal distributions, the Kolmogorov–Smirnov test for normality and Levene's test for variance homogeneity were applied, followed by the Kruskal–Wallis test. Significant differences between tested concentrations and controls were determined using Dunnett's or Dunn's test for parametric or non-parametric data, respectively ($p < 0.05$).

The results of the formulation and stability of NLCs were expressed as a mean of triplicates and standard deviation. The MTT assay was performed in quadruplicate and in three independent experiments. The results obtained were analyzed using the Graphpad Prism 5.0 program and subjected to specific tests with statistical confidence of 95%. The Two Way Anova test was used.

3. Results and Discussion

3.1. Synthesis and Characterization

3.1.1. Characterization of the Taperebá Pell Extract

Our work determined that the ethanolic extract of taperebá peels exhibits a remarkable total polyphenol content, corresponding to 2623 mg of gallic acid equivalents (EAG) per liter of fresh peel extract, which was subsequently utilized in the development of lipid nanostructures. The antioxidant capacity of this extract was rigorously evaluated using both DPPH and ABTS assays, yielding values of 258 mM TEAC and 495 mM TEAC per 100 mL of peel extract, respectively.

Complementary to these findings, previous investigations by our group employed UPLC-MS/MS to chemically characterize and quantify a diverse array of phenolic compounds in the peels of *Spondias mombin*. This comprehensive profiling revealed a substantial polyphenolic content, notably high in ellagic acid and quercetin, and marked the first successful identification and quantification of certain compounds within the *Spondias* genus [7]. In detail, the UPLC-MS/MS analysis enabled the quantification of several classes of phenolic compounds, including flavonols, phenylpropanoids, benzoic acid derivatives, coumarins, stilbenes, dihydrochalcones, flavones, and flavanones (Table 1).

Table 1. Quantification of metabolites from taperebá peel (μg/g) by UPLC-MS/MS Table adapted from De Brito et al. [7].

Category	Compound	Concentration (μg/g)
Benzoic acid derivatives	2,5-Dihydroxybenzoic acid	0.102 ± 0.090
Benzoic acid derivatives	Cinnamic acid	1.254 ± 0.040
Benzoic acid derivatives	Ellagic acid	79.080 ± 3.272
Benzoic acid derivatives	Gallic acid	21.994 ± 0.361
Benzoic acid derivatives	Methyl anthranilate	0.003 ± 0.002
Benzoic acid derivatives	Methyl gallate	0.031 ± 0.010
Benzoic acid derivatives	Syringaldehyde	0.136 ± 0.053
Benzoic acid derivatives	Vanillic acid	0.006 ± 0.003
Benzoic acid derivatives	Vanillin	0.869 ± 0.080
Coumarins	Daphnetin	0.377 ± 0.121
Coumarins	Esculin	4.016 ± 0.371
Coumarins	Fraxin	0.088 ± 0.030
Coumarins	Scopoletin	0.382 ± 0.161
Phenylpropanoids	Caffeic acid	0.239 ± 0.031
Phenylpropanoids	Chlorogenic acid	10.236 ± 0.211
Phenylpropanoids	Cryptochlorogenic acid	0.141 ± 0.012
Phenylpropanoids	Ferulic acid	0.163 ± 0.025
Phenylpropanoids	Neochlorogenic acid	0.129 ± 0.011
Phenylpropanoids	p-Coumaric acid	1.868 ± 0.211
Phenylpropanoids	Sinapyl alcohol	1.142 ± 0.042
Phenylpropanoids	trans-Coutaric acid	0.036 ± 0.031
Stilbenes	cis-Piceid	21.106 ± 1.330
Stilbenes	trans-Piceid	3.577 ± 0.181
Stilbenes	trans-Resveratrol	0.650 ± 0.022
Dihydrochalcones	Phloretin	0.017 ± 0.004
Dihydrochalcones	Phloridzin	0.215 ± 0.041
Dihydrochalcones	Trilobatin	0.051 ± 0.011
Flavones	Apigenin	0.035 ± 0.011
Flavones	Hesperidin	0.129 ± 0.071
Flavones	Luteolin	0.214 ± 0.011
Flavones	Luteolin-7-O-Glucoside	1.185 ± 0.081
Flavones	Sinensetin	1.453 ± 0.031
Flavanones	Naringenin	1.037 ± 0.061
Flavonols	Isorhamnetin	0.769 ± 0.051
Flavonols	Isorhamnetin-3-O-glucoside	1.788 ± 0.081
Flavonols	Kaempferol	0.374 ± 0.061
Flavonols	Kaempferol-3-O-glucoside	2.997 ± 0.091
Flavonols	Kaempferol-3-O-rutinoside	0.089 ± 0.011
Flavonols	Myricetin	8.137 ± 0.141
Flavonols	Quercetin	66.402 ± 1.131
Flavonols	Quercetin-3-Glc-Ara	0.065 ± 0.021
Flavonols	Quercetin-3-O-glucuronide	0.078 ± 0.021
Flavonols	Quercetin-3-O-rhamnoside	0.305 ± 0.041
Flavonols	Rhamnetin	0.150 ± 0.071
Flavonols	Rutin	1.326 ± 0.081
Flavonols	Syringetin	1.811 ± 0.051
Flavonols	Syringetin-3-O-glucoside	0.023 ± 0.011
Hydroquinone derivative	Arbutin	1.279 ± 0.071

Within the flavonol category, 14 distinct compounds were quantified, with quercetin being the most abundant, followed by myricetin and kaempferol-3-glucoside; noteworthy levels of syringetin and isorhamnetin-3-glucoside were also observed. The phenylpropanoid group was represented by cinnamic acid and its derivatives—encompassing various hydroxycinnamic acids and sinapyl alcohol—with chlorogenic acid present in the highest concentration, followed by p-coumaric and cinnamic acids. Among the benzoic acid derivatives, ellagic acid predominated over gallic acid in the taperebá peel extract. Additionally, the coumarin esculin was prominently detected, while among the stilbenes, cis-piceid was quantified at notably high levels, accompanied by significant amounts of trans-piceid and trans-resveratrol. The flavone fraction was characterized by the predominance of sinensetin and luteolin-7-O-glucoside, and the analysis further identified glycosylated hydroquinone (arbutin) [7].

In the quantitative analysis presented in Table 1, the phenolic composition of the extract reveals a pronounced heterogeneity across several compound classes. Among the benzoic acid derivatives, ellagic acid exhibits an exceptionally high concentration, followed by gallic acid and cinnamic acid, underscoring their potential pivotal role in mediating the extract's antioxidant properties. Within the coumarin group, esculin is notably predominant. The phenylpropanoid fraction is characterized by a high level of chlorogenic acid, with p-coumaric acid and sinapyl alcohol further enhancing the spectrum of bioactive compounds. Notably, the stilbene category is distinguished by a substantial amount of cis-piceid, which contrasts with the lower concentrations of trans-piceid and trans-resveratrol, potentially indicating isomer-specific functional differences. The flavonoid spectrum is further diversified, with flavones like sinensetin and luteolin-7-O-glucoside and the flavanone naringenin playing notable roles. The flavonol group is particularly prominent, with quercetin and myricetin dominating the profile, complemented by significant levels of kaempferol-3-O-glucoside and isorhamnetin-3-O-glucoside, while additional compounds such as rutin and syringetin further contribute to the complexity. Moreover, the detection of arbutin as a hydroquinone derivative introduces an additional bioactive moiety to the extract. Collectively, these data illustrate a rich and diverse phenolic profile that is likely to underpin the extract's multifaceted biological activities, thereby supporting its potential application in advanced therapeutic and cosmetic formulations [7].

This integrated characterization not only underscores the rich and diverse polyphenolic profile of taperebá peels but also highlights the extract's potent antioxidant capacity and its potential applicability in the design of bioactive nanostructured lipid systems. Such findings pave the way for further exploration into the utilization of natural phenolic compounds in advanced material and pharmaceutical applications [7].

3.1.2. Design of NLC's

Prior to the formulation of NLCs, the extract was concentrated using a rotary evaporator to reduce its volume and increase the concentration of bioactive compounds, thereby facilitating its subsequent incorporation into the nanoparticles. After concentration, the extract exhibited physical characteristics that made direct dissolution in water or conventional solvents challenging. To address this limitation, the concentrated extract was diluted in a pre-heated NaDES solvent, enabling more efficient incorporation into the lipid phase. As reported in the literature, NaDESs are known for their ability to solubilize phenolic compounds from natural extracts [20].

The NLC formulations were comprehensively evaluated using macroscopic analysis and detailed colloidal characterization, focusing on the influence of key variables such as lipid composition, surfactant concentration, extract content, and the incorporation of NaDESs containing the extract (Figure 2). Colloidal properties analyzed included the polydispersity index (PDI) and particle size, measured as the hydrodynamic diameter (HD). The PDI, ranging from 0 to 1, serves as an indicator of the uniformity in nanoparticle size distribution, with values closer to 0 signifying a more homogeneous system [31]. Particle size was precisely determined in nanometers (nm) using hydrodynamic measurements, providing a reliable metric for assessing the stability and scalability of the formulations.

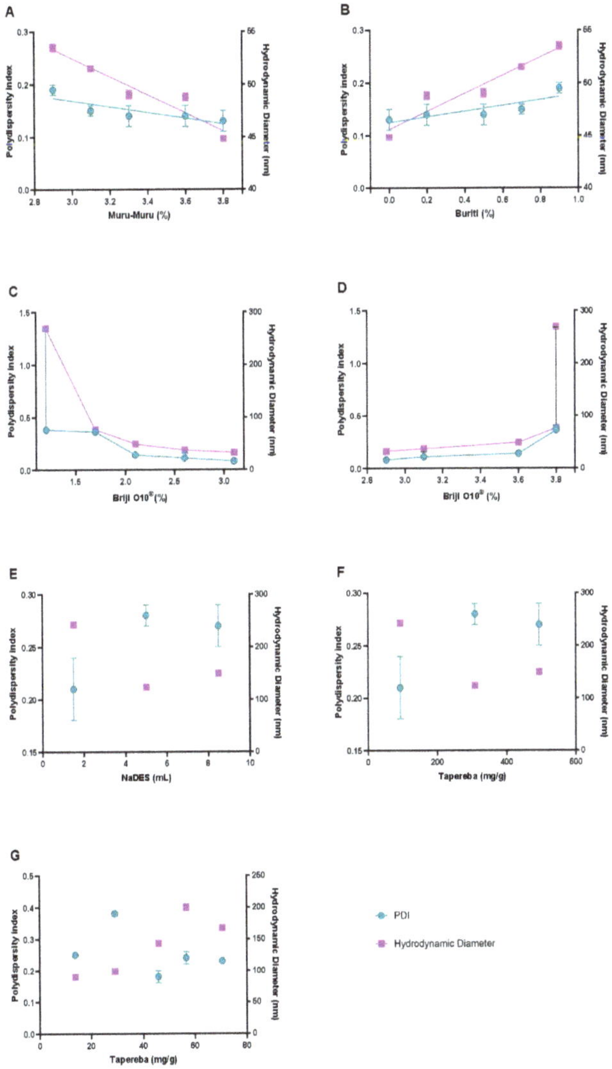

Figure 2. Influence of formulation parameters on the colloidal properties of nanostructured lipid carriers (NLCs). The graphs illustrate the effect of key variables, including murumuru butter percentage (**A**), buriti oil percentage (**B**), surfactant (Brij® O10) concentration in different ranges (**C**,**D**), NaDES volume (**E**), and *Spondias mombin* extract concentration in NaDESs (**F**,**G**) on the polydispersity index (PDI) and hydrodynamic diameter (HD).

Nanostructured lipid carriers (NLCs) represent the second generation of lipid nanoparticles and are systems for encapsulating drugs and active compounds, with a core structure formed by the combination of solid and liquid lipids at room temperature, stabilized by a surfactant layer. This characteristic provides the NLCs with greater fluidity in the lipid matrix, resulting in enhanced solubilization and stabilization of active compounds, as well as enabling their controlled release [32].

In this context, the formulation process for NLCs involves a careful selection of solid and liquid lipids to ensure the creation of small-sized, homogeneous particles. In this context, murumuru butter was selected as the solid lipid due to its high thermal stability and capacity to form crystalline lipid matrices, which are crucial for maintaining the structural integrity of the nanoparticles during storage and application [33,34].

The inclusion of buriti oil as the liquid lipid serves to enhance fluidity and improve the stability of the nanoparticles. Buriti oil is rich in monounsaturated fatty acids and antioxidants, such as tocopherols, which contribute to its stability and nutritional value [35,36]. The optimal ratio of murumuru butter to buriti oil is determined through systematic experiments that assess various parameters, including the polydispersity index (PDI), hydrodynamic diameter, and visual stability of the emulsions. Studies have shown that combinations with lower proportions of buriti oil and higher amounts of murumuru butter yield smaller and more stable particles, as indicated by PDI values remaining below 0.25, which is a benchmark for good emulsion stability.

The stability of emulsions is significantly influenced by the viscosity associated with the concentration of the dispersed phase, where higher viscosity can lead to improved stability [37]. Furthermore, the fatty acid profile of buriti oil, which includes a high content of oleic acid, contributes to its effectiveness in stabilizing emulsions and enhancing the overall performance of the NLCs [38,39]. The presence of antioxidants in buriti oil not only aids in the stability of the nanoparticles but also provides additional health benefits, making it a suitable candidate for various applications, including drug delivery systems [40]. These findings from systematic experiments underscore the importance of lipid selection and formulation parameters in achieving desirable characteristics in NLCs.

The integration of surfactants, such as Brij® O10 (Sigma-Aldrich, St. Louis, MI, USA), was also critical for stabilizing the NLCs. This nonionic surfactant was selected for its compatibility with biological systems and low toxicity, essential features for health applications. Surfactant concentrations were adjusted to minimize toxicity without compromising colloidal stability. Analysis of the results revealed that lower surfactant levels increased particle size and PDI, indicating greater heterogeneity, whereas intermediate concentrations produced more uniform and stable particles.

A major innovation of this study was the incorporation of natural deep eutectic solvents (NaDESs) into the formulation of nanostructured lipid carriers (NLCs). Composed of glycerol, choline chloride, and citric acid, NaDESs were employed as a sustainable and biocompatible alternative to traditional solvents [41,42]. Beyond enhancing the solubility of phenolic compounds extracted from *Spondias mombin* peel, NaDESs contributed significantly to nanoparticle stabilization. This dual role was evidenced through improved colloidal stability and validated by infrared spectroscopy (FTIR), highlighting robust molecular interactions and protective effects that will be further detailed in subsequent sections [43,44].

Another pivotal aspect of the NLC development was the production method, which utilized hot emulsification followed by rapid cooling. This approach ensured the solidification of the lipid matrix, leading to the formation of nanoparticles with homogeneous sizes while effectively encapsulating phenolic compounds in a protective environment [45]. Key variables in the process, including extract concentration and NaDES percentage, significantly influenced the final properties of the NLCs [46]. Results demonstrated that higher emulsification temperatures (~80 °C) enhanced dispersion and reduced particle size in certain formulations. However, lower temperatures (~70 °C) were more appropriate for formulations containing NaDESs, accommodating the thermal sensitivity of these solvents and ensuring optimal nanoparticle stability [47,48].

The physicochemical characterization of the NLCs was another strength of the study. Zeta potential analyses demonstrated that the particles exhibited negative surface charges, promoting greater colloidal stability through electrostatic repulsion. Below, in Table 2, are the parameters of the final formulation with and without NaDESs (NLC-TAP-NaDES), which were defined as the main formulations used in this study. These data provide a comprehensive overview of the physicochemical and structural characteristics that underpin the functional properties of each formulation, enabling detailed comparisons and highlighting the effects of NaDESs' presence on the systems analyzed.

Table 2. Physicochemical properties of nanostructured lipid carrier (NLC) formulations, including polydispersity index (PDI), hydrodynamic diameter (HD), zeta potential (ZP), total phenolic content (TP), and encapsulation efficiency (EE%).

Formulation	PDI	HD (nm)	ZP (mV)	TP (mg GAE/mL NLC)	EE%
NLC-Blank	0.14 ± 0.02	46.71 ± 0.20	-19.39 ± 0.76	-	-
NLC-NaDES	0.26 ± 0.02	196.73 ± 2.37	-2.83 ± 0.27	-	-
NLC-TAP	0.23 ± 0.01	199.13 ± 0.91	-4.31 ± 0.16	27.05 ± 0.97	83.95
NLC-TAP-NaDES	0.21 ± 0.03	159.00 ± 0.66	-2.35 ± 0.35	20.64 ± 0.58	85.81

3.1.3. Nanoparticles (NPs) Morphology

The microscopic images in Figure 3 illustrate the morphology of NLCs without NaDESs (Figure 3A) and with NaDESs (Figure 3B). Both formulations exhibit a spherical shape, but Figure 3A displays a more organized structure, while Figure 3B reveals a diffuse morphology, likely influenced by NaDESs. This suggests that NaDESs interfere with the formation of lipid crystals, leading to structural disorganization.

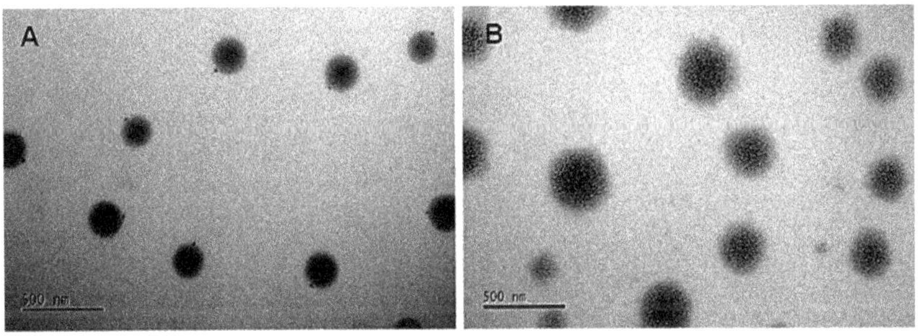

Figure 3. Photomicrograph obtained by transmission electron microscopy (TEM) for the taperebá pell extract encapsulated in NLCs. (**A**) NLC without NaDESs (NLC-TAP) and (**B**) NLC with NaDESs (NLC-TAP-NaDES).

These morphological differences provide critical insights into the impact of NaDESs on particle structure. Further evidence supporting this phenomenon, such as FTIR analyses showing reduced C-H band intensities in NaDES-containing formulations, will be discussed in detail later in this study.

3.1.4. Colloidal Stability

Colloidal stability is a critical parameter for the performance of nanostructured systems, and the results of this study emphasize the pivotal role of NaDESs in this context [32].

The polydispersity index (PDI), a key indicator of the homogeneity in particle size distribution, remained below 0.25 for most formulations under ambient and refrigerated conditions for up to 30 days (Figure 4). This indicates that the nanoparticles maintained high uniformity, essential for physical and functional stability.

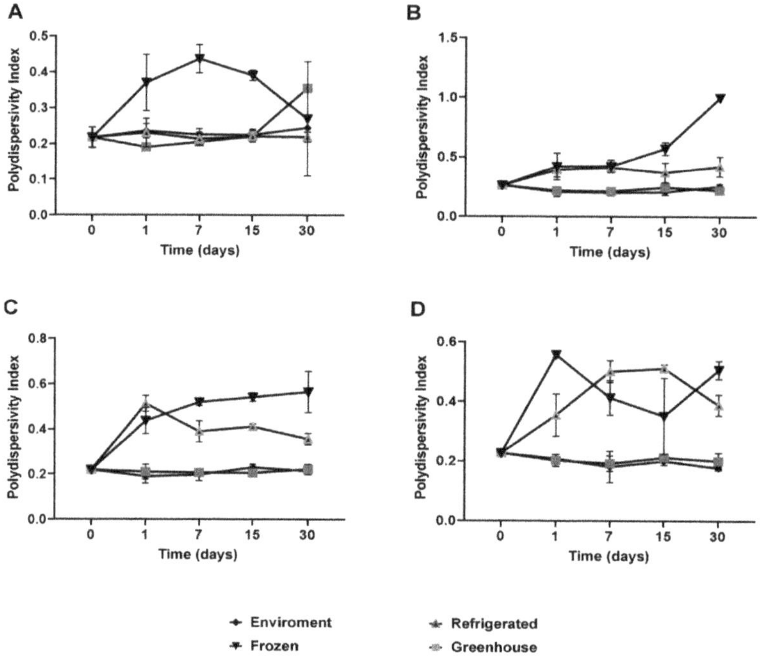

Figure 4. Polydispersity index (PDI) for each formulation stored at different temperature conditions over 30 days: NLC-Blank (**A**), NLC-NaDES (**B**), NLC-TAP-NaDESn (**C**), and NLC-TAP (**D**). Results are expressed as means of triplicates.

Colloidal stability assays over time showed that NaDES-containing formulations maintained consistent particle sizes and PDI values under ambient and refrigerated conditions for up to 30 days. Under thermal stress (~40 °C), NaDES formulations outperformed their non-NaDES counterparts, highlighting their efficacy in preserving nanoparticle integrity and bioactive retention.

In summary, the development of NLCs in this study demonstrates a high degree of innovation, from component selection to the application of advanced production and characterization methodologies. The combinations of lipids, surfactants, and NaDESs were optimized to maximize encapsulation efficiency, stability, and functionality of the nanoparticles. These advances pave the way for the application of NLCs in various fields, including nutraceuticals, pharmaceuticals, and cosmeceuticals, while representing a milestone in the sustainable utilization of agricultural byproducts in cutting-edge technologies.

Measurements of hydrodynamic diameter further reinforced the stabilizing effects of NaDESs. While formulations without NaDESs exhibited minimal size variations, NaDES-containing formulations demonstrated enhanced structural flexibility, observed through moderate size increases under thermal stress and freezing conditions (Figure 5). This behavior suggests that NaDESs modulate the lipid matrix, promoting greater thermal and functional stability.

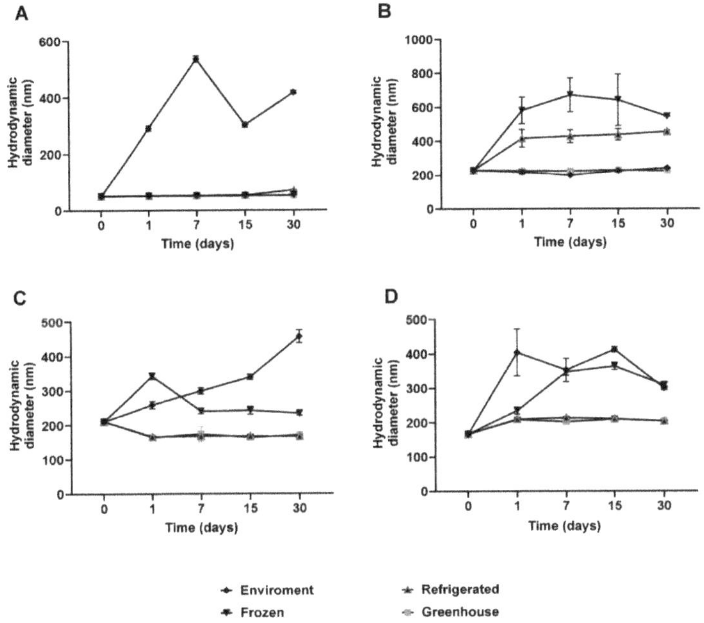

Figure 5. Hydrodynamic diameter (HD) size of the nanoparticle for each formulation stored at different temperature conditions over 30 days: NLC-Blank (**A**), NLC-NaDES (**B**), NLC-TAP-NaDES (**C**), and NLC-TAP (**D**). Results are expressed as means of triplicates.

3.1.5. Differential Thermal Analysis (DTA) and Thermogravimetric Analysis (TGA)

In the DTA curves shown in Figure 6A, it is possible to observe 3 endothermic events (127.27 °C, 260.70 °C, and 493.81 °C) and an exothermic event at 574.15 °C, which may be associated with the melting points of some components of the extract already quantified by this research group [7]. According to these quantification results, the taperebá peel extract contains several phenolic compounds, notably ellagic acid, quercetin, gallic acid and cis-Piceid [49].

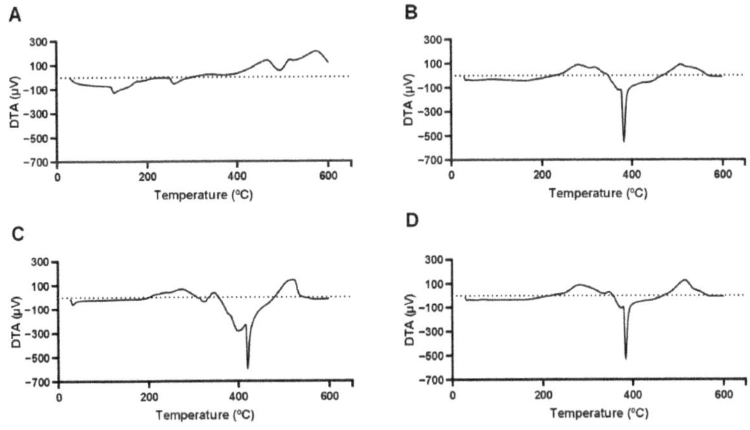

Figure 6. Differential thermal analysis (DTA) curves. (**A**) Tapereba extract; (**B**) NLC-NaDES; (**C**) NLC−TAP; (**D**) NLC−TAP−NaDES.

The other curves shown in Figure 6B,D represent an endothermic event around 380 °C, which shifts to higher values when NaDESs are not used. This result demonstrates that NaDESs enhance the dispersibility of the nanocarrier components, yielding a material with amorphous characteristics that are ideal for drug delivery systems [1]. This behavior is observed in the mass loss curves shown in Figure 7, indicating the influence of NaDESs on thermal stability.

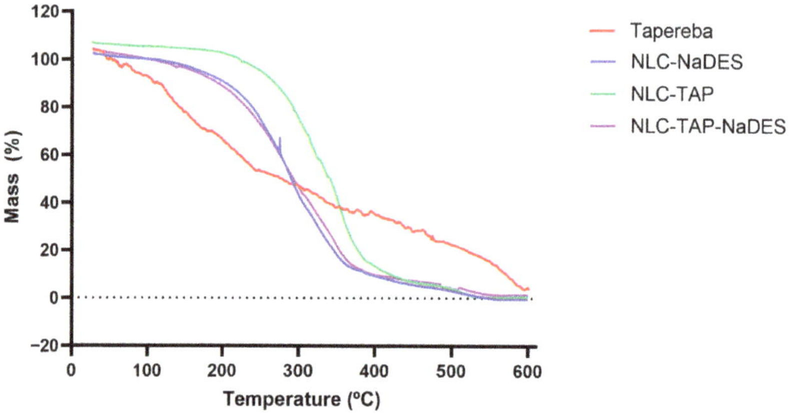

Figure 7. Thermogravimetric curves obtained for different materials and formulations: NLC-Blank, NLC−TAP, NLC−NaDES, and NLC−TAP−NaDES.

The thermogravimetric analysis (TGA) graph (Figure 7) illustrates the mass loss of different formulations of nanostructured lipid carriers (NLCs) and the pure taperebá extract as a function of temperature. The y-axis represents mass loss (%), indicating thermal degradation, while the x-axis represents temperature (°C), ranging from 0 to 600 °C. The curves correspond to different samples: Taperebá extract (red), NLC-NaDES (blue), NLC-TAP (green), and NLC-TAP-NaDES (purple).

The pure taperebá extract (red) exhibits the earliest degradation, with mass loss beginning at approximately 100–150 °C and a significant decomposition phase extending up to 400 °C. This indicates the volatilization and thermal breakdown of bioactive phenolic compounds present in the extract.

The formulations containing NaDESs (NLC-NaDES in blue and NLC-TAP-NaDES in purple) display higher thermal stability, with delayed mass loss compared to the pure extract. Degradation occurs primarily between 200 and 400 °C, suggesting that NaDESs play a protective role in reducing the volatility of bioactive molecules and stabilizing the lipid matrix at elevated temperatures.

The NLC-TAP formulation (green), which lacks NaDESs, shows a slightly delayed decomposition compared to the pure extract, initiating at around 150–200 °C. However, its degradation occurs more rapidly than in NaDES-containing formulations, reinforcing the hypothesis that NaDESs contribute to enhanced thermal stability.

The investigation into the thermal stability of various formulations reveals significant insights regarding the efficacy of nanostructured lipid carriers (NLCs) compared to pure extracts. Specifically, pure extracts exhibit lower thermal stability, which can be attributed to their unprotected nature against thermal degradation. In contrast, NLC formulations demonstrate improved thermal resistance, which is critical for maintaining the integrity of bioactive compounds during processing and storage [50]. Among the NLC formulations, those incorporating natural deep eutectic solvents (NaDESs) show enhanced thermal protection. This stability is likely due to favorable molecular interactions between NaDESs and the lipid matrix, which effectively minimize premature volatilization of the active ingredients. Such interactions are crucial as they protect the bioactive compounds from thermal degradation and enhance their retention within the lipid matrix [51]. The presence of NaDESs can alter the physicochemical properties of the lipid carriers, leading to improved encapsulation efficiency and stability under thermal stress [52]. The findings underscore the potential applications of NLC-NaDES systems across various fields, including pharmaceuticals, cosmetics, and nutraceuticals. The improved stability and bioactive retention offered by these formulations make them suitable for thermal processing, which is often a requisite in the production of food and cosmetic products [53]. The ability of NLCs to withstand thermal degradation while preserving bioactive compounds positions them as a promising delivery system, ensuring that the therapeutic efficacy of the encapsulated agents is maintained even under challenging conditions [52,54]. In conclusion, the integration of NaDESs into NLC formulations not only enhances thermal stability but also opens avenues for their application in diverse industries, ensuring that bioactive compounds are effectively preserved and delivered.

3.1.6. Retention and Stability of Phenolic Compounds

The integration of NaDESs into NLCs resulted in significantly higher retention of phenolic compounds, even under adverse conditions (Figure 8). After 30 days, the NLC-TAP-NaDES formulation retained approximately 85% of its phenolic content under ambient conditions and 95% under refrigeration, whereas the NLC-TAP formulation showed inferior retention, particularly under thermal stress (~40 °C) and freezing. These results reflect the stabilizing role of NaDESs, which reduce the exposure of phenolic compounds to environmental factors and prevent oxidative degradation.

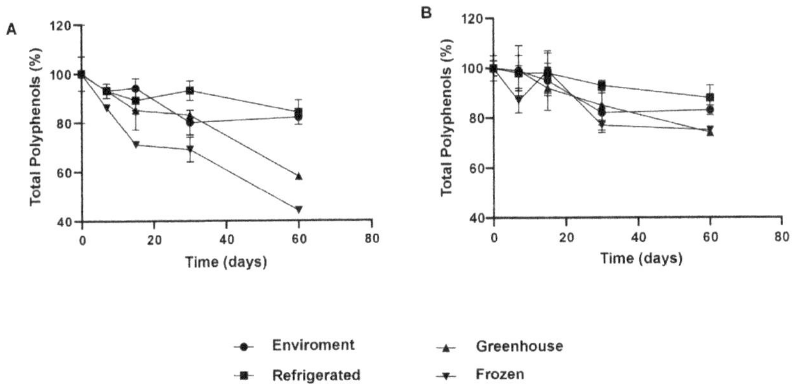

Figure 8. Representation of the concentration of total polyphenols (%) nanoencapsulated and stored at different temperature conditions. (**A**) NLC-TAP: formulation with murumuru butter, Brij® O10, buriti oil and extract and (**B**) NLC-TAP-NaDES: formulation with murumuru butter, Brij® O10, buriti oil and NaDES + extract.

The incorporation of natural deep eutectic solvents (NaDESs) into nanostructured lipid carriers (NLCs) has been demonstrated to significantly enhance the retention of phenolic compounds, even when subjected to adverse environmental conditions (Figure 8). After 30 days, the NLC-TAP-NaDES formulation retained approximately 85% of its phenolic content under ambient conditions and 95% under refrigeration, whereas the NLC-TAP formulation showed inferior retention, particularly under thermal stress (~40 °C) and freezing. These results reflect the stabilizing role of NaDESs, which reduce the exposure of phenolic compounds to environmental factors and prevent oxidative degradation.

About the results of the percentage of total polyphenol content (TP) retention of nanoparticles formulated with taperebá peel extract, NLC-TAP (without the addition of NaDESs) and NLC-TAP-NaDES (with the addition of NaDESs), it was verified that, between the beginning of the test and the 15th day, there was no significant difference between the temperatures studied ($p \geq 0.05$).

After 30 days of storage, it was found that refrigeration temperature showed the highest retention of TP in NLC-TAP (~95%), followed by ambient and stressful temperatures (~80%) ($p \geq 0.05$). Ambient (~80%) and refrigeration (~85%) temperatures were those that obtained the highest values of TP retention in the nanoparticles at the end of the 60 days of testing ($p \geq 0.05$).

NLCs without the addition of NaDESs (NLC-TAP) that were kept at freezing temperature were not able to protect the phenolic content (~40% TP retention) as effectively as under storage conditions at room temperature and refrigerated (~85%). This may be a consequence of the loss of colloidal stability of the nanoparticles due the phase separation during the freezing process. This separation leads to a high concentration of particles, which can generate irreversible aggregation and fusion of particulate material, in addition to the crystallization of ice, exerting mechanical stress on the system [41].

After 60 days of storage at stressful temperatures, NLCs without NaDESs (NLC-TAP) showed a significant decrease in TP retention (~50%). In theory, this type of entrapment of the active ingredient in nanostructures, which are made up of lipids in the solid and liquid phases (NLCs), has a lower melting point temperature than nanostructures made up only of lipids in the solid phase (SLN). This characteristic makes them unstable at stressful temperatures, but suitable for storage at room temperature [23]. Therefore, it is possible to suggest that there was instability of NLC-TAP when stored at ~40 °C, which promoted greater degradation of TP, as phenolic compounds are known to be thermolabile [6,37].

In general, at the end of this experiment, it was possible to verify that the NLCs with the addition of NaDESs obtained better results when compared to those without ($p \geq 0.05$). The best storage conditions were refrigeration and room temperatures (~85% TP retention), followed by stressful and freezing temperatures (~75% TP retention), demonstrating interesting results on the use of NaDESs in these formulations.

Transmission electron microscopy (TEM) results (Figure 3) complement these findings, showing that NLC-TAP-NaDES particles exhibited a more diffuse morphology compared to the organized structure of NLC-TAP particles. This structural disorganization in NaDES-containing particles, also evidenced by the reduction in C-H band intensity in FTIR, enhances thermal flexibility and stability, particularly under extreme storage conditions.

Under freezing conditions, the cryoprotective effect of NaDESs was evident. While the NLC-TAP-NaDES formulation retained approximately 75% of its phenolic compounds after 30 days, the NLC-TAP formulation showed a reduced retention of about 50% (Figure 8). This behavior can be attributed to the ability of NaDESs to mitigate ice crystal formation and phase separation, phenomena known to promote aggregation and degradation of bioactives.

3.1.7. FT-IR Spectroscopy

Samples containing NaDESs with extract (Figure 9C) and NaDESs without extract (Figure 9D) showed minimal variations in relation to the identified peaks positions. The largest shift observed was ± 5 cm^{-1}. Thus, since the NLCs were formulated with *Spondias mombin* L. extract, the reference values considered to this analysis will be given from the NaDESs with extract sample (C). The signatures (sig.) found are in consonance with the literature and correspond to the presence of glycerol, citric acid, and choline chloride. The broad band at 3321 cm^{-1} (sig. 1) is related to ν(OH), the narrow peaks at 2934 (sig. 2) and 2890 cm^{-1} (sig. 3) assign to $\nu_{as}(CH_2)$ and $\nu_s(CH_2)$, respectively. 1721 (sig. 4) and 1646 cm^{-1} (sig. 5) can be assigned to ν(C=O). In the fingerprint region (1500–500 cm^{-1}), the narrow and strong peak situated in 1035 cm^{-1} (sig. 9) refers to ν_{as}(C-C-O) assignment, and can be associated with glycerol, as well as choline chloride presence. The additional medium and weak peaks in this region at 1411 (sig. α), 1331 (sig. β), 1205 (sig. γ), 1107 (sig. 8), 991 (sig. π), 921 (sig. ω), 860 (sig. 10), and 780 cm^{-1} (sig. σ) may be accredited, correspondingly, to δ(C-O-H), ρ(C-O-H), ν(C-C-O), δ(OH), ν(CN), δ(OH), ν_s(C-C-O), and $\rho(CH_2)$. The taperebá extract did not indicate any influence regard to the molecular pattern in the IR spectra containing NaDESs.

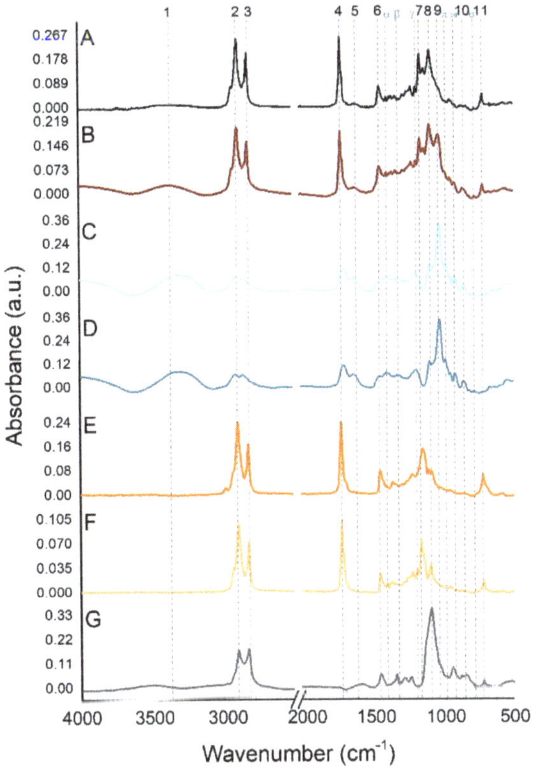

Figure 9. Fourier Transform Infrared (FT-IR) spectra. (**A**) NLC with extract and without NaDESs (NLC-TAP), (**B**) NLC with NaDESs and extract (NLC-TAP-NaDES), (**C**) NaDESs with extract, (**D**) NaDESs without extract, (**E**) Buriti oil, (**F**) Murumuru butter, and (**G**) Brij® O10. The numbered dashed lines correspond to the peak's positions, referring to sample B (nano extract with NaDESs). The dashed lines with Greek letters correspond to the peak's positions referring to sample D (NaDESs).

As occurs with NaDES samples, several functional groups with the same signature are present in the buriti oil, murumuru butter, and some in Brij® O10 IR spectra. What takes place with Brij® O10 signatures is that this surfactant comes from vegetable-based fatty ethers. Brij® O10 similar signatures to the lipid part used in the formulation (buriti and murumuru) correspond to $\nu_{as}(CH_2)$, $\nu_s(CH_2)$, $\delta(CH_2)$, ν(C-C-O), and $\rho(CH_2)$, respectively, 2920 (sig. 2), 2853 (sig. 3), 1463 (sig. 6), 1101 (sig. 8), and 723 cm^{-1} (sig. 11). The narrow medium peaks (absent in Brij® O10) around 1741 and 1744 cm^{-1} (sig. 4), and 1172 and

1161 cm^{-1} (sig. 7), for murumuru butter and buriti oil, correspond, subsequently, to ν(C=O) and ν(C=C-C-O).

Comparing the obtained NLCs IR spectra, it is observed, at ν(OH) (3367 and 3375 cm^{-1}, for NLC-TAP (Figure 9A) and NLC-TAP-NaDES (Figure 9B), respectively), the difference on the band shape between the samples. For NLC-TAP-NaDES this broad band (sig. 1) becomes defined, as well as presenting greater relative intensity, indicating that the amount/concentration of these (OH) groups is also higher. This contribution can be given due to the substantial availability of hydroxyl compounds related to glycerol, citric acid, and choline chloride, since water content used in the formulation is also smaller than NLC-TAP. The peaks corresponding to $\nu_{as}(CH_2)$ and $\nu_s(CH_2)$ (2914 and 2927 cm^{-1} (sig. 2), and 2855 and 2853 cm^{-1}(sig. 3)), for NLC-TAP-NaDES and NLC-TAP, resemble the same peaks present in the precursors (butter, oil and tensioactive). The shifts that occur in the spectral region between 4000 and 2500 cm^{-1} (vibrational modes ν(OH), ν(CH) or ν(NH)) may happen due to the overlapping of organic molecules involved in the reaction, as is the case of shifts (±10 cm^{-1}) situated in ν(OH) and $\nu_{as}(CH_2)$, when comparing the NLCs. The other signatures found (ν(C=O) (sig. 4), $\delta(CH_2)$ (sig. 6), ν(C=C-C-O) (sig. 7), and ρ (CH_2) (sig. 11)), in both samples, are in line with the buriti oil, and murumuru butter. The exclusive peaks found in the NLC-TAP-NaDES sample (1030 (sig. 9), 991 (sig. π), 923 (sig. ω), and 864 cm^{-1} (sig. 10), subsequently, ν_{as}(C-C-O), δ(OH), ν(CN), and ν_s(C-C-O), ascribed to NaDESs. Additionally, it should be evidenced that the presence of glycerol among the exclusive signatures mentioned for NLC-TAP-NaDES is relevant, since this compound, besides being coming from natural/vegetable bases, is related to several technological applications to the pharmaceutical (capsules, antibiotics, antiseptics), and cosmeceutical (moisturizers, deodorants, and makeup) industries.

3.2. Embryotoxicity, Cytotoxicity Testing and In Vitro ROS Production

Cytotoxicity assays in fibroblasts (L929) showed a higher IC50 for the NLC-TAP-NaDES formulation (56.48 μg/mL) compared to formulations without NaDESs (NLC–TAP), indicating reduced cytotoxicity in normal cells (Figure 10). These results align with the hypothesis that NaDESs enhance the encapsulation efficiency and stability of phenolic compounds, reducing their direct interaction with cellular targets and mitigating toxicity. The combined results of these bioassays suggest that while NaDESs-containing NLCs offer significant advantages in phenolic stabilization, further studies are needed to optimize their concentrations and evaluate their long-term effects in more complex biological systems. The cytotoxicity of NLCs was also tested on fibroblasts, and is represented in Figure 10. The IC50 values obtained were 39.95 μg/mL for NLC-Blank; 40.75 μg/mL for NLC-NaDES; 40.10 μg/mL for NLC-TAP; and 56.48 μg/mL for NLC-TAP-NaDES, the latter being the only one that showed a statistical difference ($p < 0.05$).

The embryotoxicity and cytotoxicity assays revealed important awareness into the biocompatibility and potential therapeutic window of NLC-TAP-NaDES. Zebrafish embryo tests showed a dose-dependent toxicity profile, with an LC50 of 5.05 μg/mL for the NLC-TAP-NaDES formulation. The results indicated significant mortality at higher concentrations, particularly at 37.63 μg/mL, where 100% lethality was observed within 24 h (Figure 11).

These findings underscore the importance of optimizing formulation concentrations for safe application in biological systems. Sublethal effects, such as delayed yolk sac absorption, yolk sac darkening, and pericardial edema, were observed predominantly at higher concentrations (Figure 12). Notably, the NLC-TAP-NaDES formulation demonstrated a less pronounced impact on embryonic development compared to formulations without NaDESs, suggesting a potential mitigating role of NaDESs in modulating the bioavailability and toxicity of phenolic compounds. It is also possible to observe the photodocumentation of organisms exposed to NLC-TAP in Figure 13.

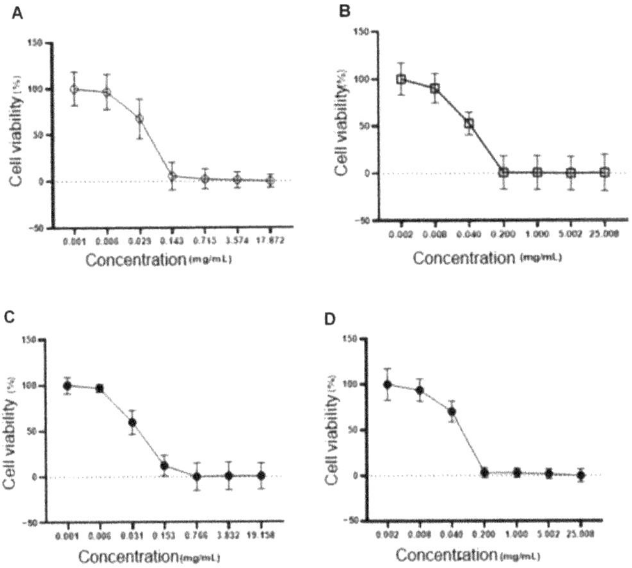

Figure 10. Cytotoxicity assays in fibroblasts (L929). The graphs illustrate the dose-dependent effect of different NLC formulations on cell viability (%), with IC50 values for each formulation. The IC50 values obtained were 39.95 µg/mL for NLC−Blank (**A**), 40.75 µg/mL for NLC−NaDES (**B**), 40.10 µg/mL for NLC−TAP (**C**), and 56.48 µg/mL for NLC−TAP−NaDES (**D**). The NLC−TAP−NaDES formulation exhibited significantly lower cytotoxicity compared to other formulations ($p < 0.05$), supporting the hypothesis that NaDESs reduce the direct interaction of phenolic compounds with cellular targets, thereby enhancing biocompatibility. These results highlight the potential of NaDES-containing NLCs in mitigating toxicity while maintaining phenolic stabilization.

The results of the embryotoxicity and cytotoxicity assays conducted on nanostructured lipid carriers (NLCs) containing natural deep eutectic solvents (NaDESs) provide compelling evidence for the viability of these formulations as a platform for the delivery of bioactive compounds. The findings indicate a significant reduction in cytotoxicity when these NLCs are administered to normal cells, suggesting a favorable biocompatibility profile [55]. This characteristic is particularly important in the context of drug delivery systems, where the safety of the carrier is paramount to ensure that therapeutic agents can be delivered effectively without causing undue harm to healthy tissues.

Moreover, the moderated impact on embryonic development observed at sublethal doses further supports the notion that NaDES-containing NLCs can be designed to minimize adverse effects during critical stages of development [56]. This is a crucial consideration, especially in applications involving reproductive health and developmental therapeutics. The ability to maintain a balance between efficacy and safety is a hallmark of successful drug delivery systems, and the data presented in this study suggest that NaDES-containing NLCs may achieve this balance effectively.

However, it is essential to note the dose-dependent toxicity observed at higher concentrations of these formulations. This finding underscores the necessity for meticulous optimization of the NLC formulations to ensure that they can be safely utilized across a range of concentrations [57]. The implications of this observation are significant; it highlights the importance of conducting thorough dose–response studies to establish safe dosage thresholds that maximize therapeutic benefits while minimizing potential risks.

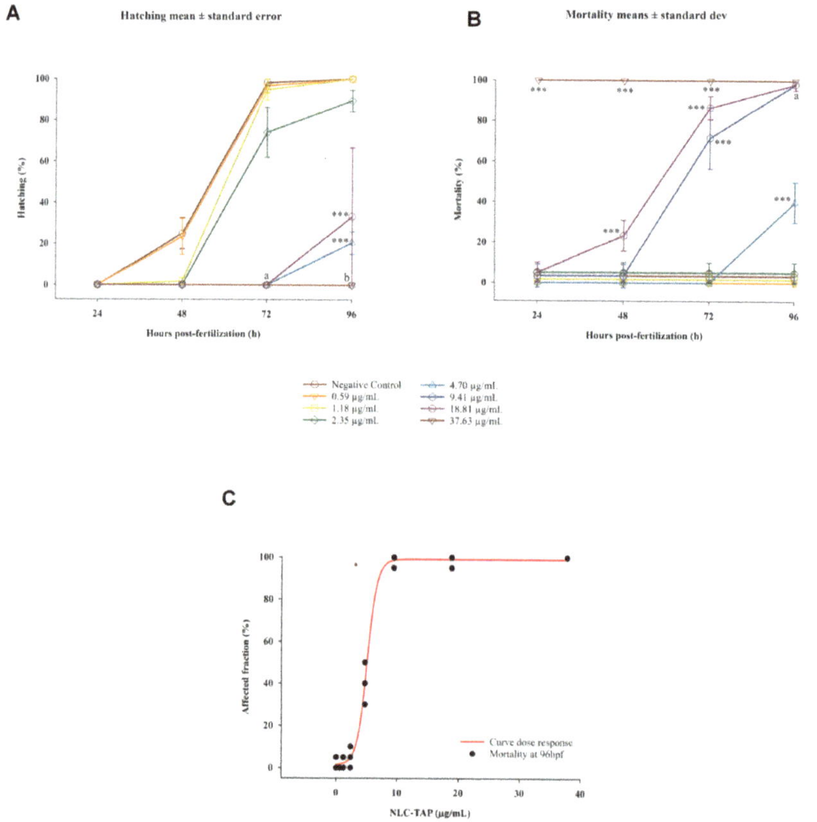

Figure 11. Graphics depicting the embryotoxicity test of NLC-TAP in zebrafish. (**A**). Chart illustrating the hatching rate over the 96 h exposure period. (**B**). Graph depicting the mortality rate throughout the 96 h exposure period. Significant differences compared to the negative control are indicated by *** $p < 0.001$, where both a and b also signify statistical differences of $p < 0.001$. In (**A**) concentrations of 4.70 µg/mL, 9.41 µg/mL, 18.81 µg/mL, and 37.63 µg/mL are associated, with data presented as mean ± standard error. In (**B**) concentrations of 9.41 µg/mL and 37.63 µg/mL are presented, with data shown as mean ± standard deviation. (**C**) Concentration-response curve (mortality) of organisms exposed to NLC-TAP for 96 h, revealing an LC50 of 5.05 µg/mL—Model: sigmoidal—4 parameters. $R^2 = 0.99$.

Figure 14 presents fluorescence images depicting the production of reactive oxygen species (ROS) in cells initially subjected to H_2O_2-induced oxidative stress, followed by treatment with the NLC-TAP-NaDES formulation in the treated group. Panel A represents the control group, where stressed cells were left untreated, while panel B shows the cellular response to the NLC-TAP-NaDES treatment.

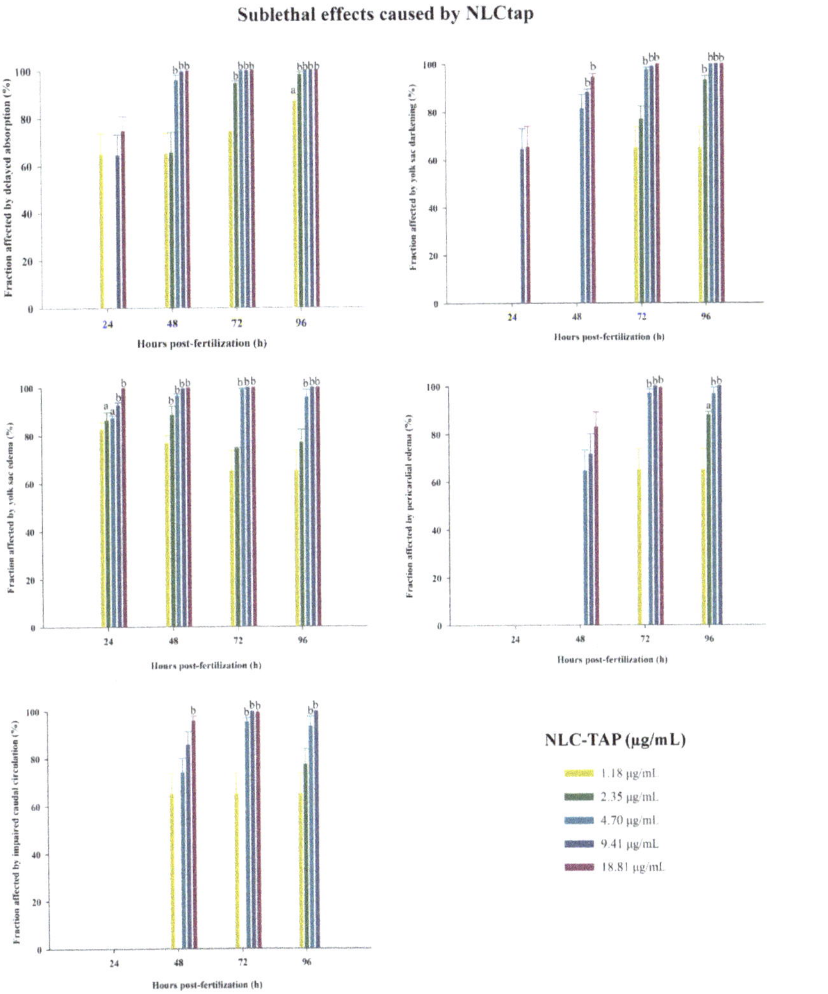

Figure 12. Graphics of sublethal effects caused by various concentrations of NLC-TAP during the embryo-toxicity test in zebrafish. Delayed absorption of the yolk sac, darkening of the yolk sac, edema in the yolk sac, edema in the pericardium, and alteration in caudal circulation. Significant differences are represented by letters (a and b), where a indicates $p < 0.005$ and b indicates $p < 0.001$. Data are presented as mean ± standard deviation.

The results highlight a markedly lower fluorescence signal in panel B, demonstrating the formulation's ability to mitigate the intracellular accumulation of ROS caused by H_2O_2. This antioxidant effect is attributed to the bioactive phenolic compounds derived from the peel extract of taperebá (*Spondias mombin*), which are rich in ellagic acid and quercetin—well-known radical scavengers. Previous studies by our group have shown that taperebá peel extract exhibits a high polyphenol content (2623 mg GAE/L) and strong antioxidant activity, as assessed by the DPPH (258 mM TEAC/100 mL) and ABTS (495 mM TEAC/100 mL) assays [7]. These properties make the extract a promising source for antioxidant applications.

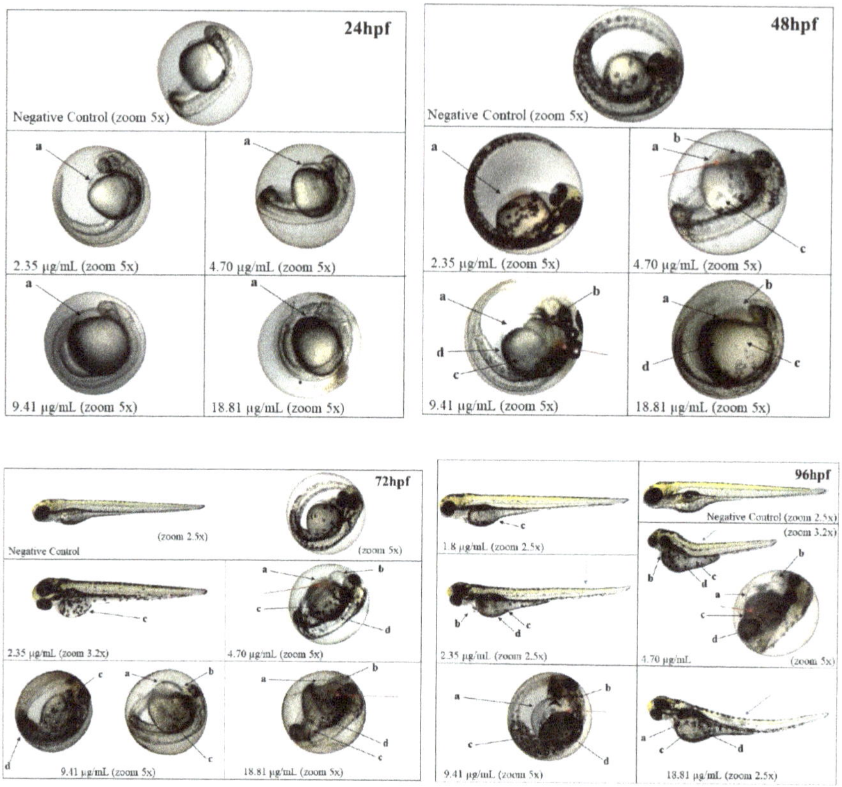

Figure 13. Photodocumentation of organisms exposed for 96 h to NLC-TAP. Black arrows—a: yolk sac edema; b: pericardial edema; c: delayed absorption; d: yolk sac darkening. Blue and red arrows indicate sublethal changes that did not show statistically significant differences. Blue arrows: alterations in the notochord. Red arrows: blood stasis.

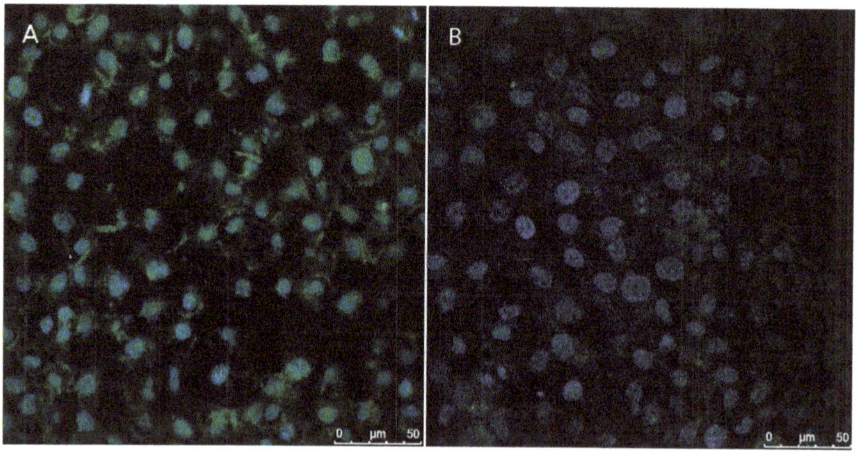

Figure 14. The fluorescence images of reactive oxygen species (ROS) production, assessed using the CellROX® Green Reagent assay after treatment with NLC-TAP-NaDES for 24 h, are shown. Panel (**A**) displays the control cells, while panel (**B**) depicts the cells treated with NLC-TAP-NaDES. ROS production is indicated in green, while DAPI staining, marking the cell nuclei, is shown in blue.

Moreover, the role of NaDESs combined with the NLC system was pivotal in enhancing the stability and bioavailability of the bioactive compounds. The NLC-NaDES system effectively protected polyphenols from oxidative degradation and enabled controlled release of antioxidants, targeting their action to mitigate the oxidative damage induced by H_2O_2. Consequently, treated cells exhibited a significantly reduced oxidative load compared to the control, as evidenced by the diminished fluorescence intensity associated with ROS production.

This study underscores the capability of NLC-NaDES-based formulations to alleviate oxidative damage under conditions of pre-induced stress, as demonstrated here with H_2O_2. The approach leverages underutilized by-products, such as taperebá peels, aligning with the principles of sustainability and circular bioeconomy. The proposed technology represents a substantial advancement in the development of innovative antioxidant therapies, with potential applications in addressing oxidative stress-related diseases, including cancer, neurodegenerative disorders, and chronic inflammation.

These findings also support the feasibility of employing this platform in preclinical studies to evaluate its efficacy under more complex conditions and, eventually, its application in pharmaceutical and nutraceutical formulations aimed at managing redox imbalance in living systems. The combination of bioactive natural extracts, NaDESs, and NLC exemplifies a modern paradigm of green nanotechnology with broad applications and global impact in the field of antioxidant science.

To further substantiate the therapeutic potential and safety of NaDES-containing NLCs, future research should prioritize in vivo assessments. These studies are critical for understanding the pharmacokinetics, biodistribution, and long-term effects of these formulations within a living organism [58]. In vivo models can provide insights that are not attainable through in vitro studies alone, particularly regarding the interactions between the NLCs and biological systems, including immune responses and metabolic pathways.

Additionally, long-term evaluations are necessary to assess the chronic effects of these formulations, particularly in relation to their cumulative exposure and potential for toxicity over extended periods [59]. Such studies will be instrumental in determining the feasibility of these NLCs for clinical applications, especially in health-related fields where sustained delivery of bioactive compounds is desired.

In conclusion, while the preliminary results are promising, the path forward requires a comprehensive approach that includes optimization of formulation parameters, rigorous in vivo testing, and long-term safety evaluations. By addressing these critical areas, researchers can pave the way for the successful application of NaDES-containing NLCs in various therapeutic contexts, ultimately contributing to advancements in drug delivery systems and improving patient outcomes.

3.3. *Sustainable Implications and Future Applications*

The integration of nanostructured lipid carriers (NLCs) with natural deep eutectic solvents (NaDESs) represents a significant advancement in the utilization of agricultural byproducts, particularly the peel of *Spondias mombin*. This innovative approach aligns with global sustainability trends and circular economy practices, emphasizing the efficient use of natural resources [60,61]. Agricultural and food industries produce substantial volumes of underutilized byproducts, which are often discarded as waste. The transformation of *S. mombin* peel, rich in bioactive phenolic compounds, into a valuable resource through advanced nanotechnology exemplifies the potential of co-product-based innovations to address critical environmental challenges, such as waste accumulation and resource inefficiency [62].

The application of NLCs and NaDESs not only enhances the bioavailability and stability of phenolic compounds but also reduces the environmental footprint associated with traditional manufacturing processes. By leveraging agricultural byproducts and eliminating the need for toxic solvents, this approach provides a sustainable model for industrial innovation [63]. This synergy between green solvents and nanostructured delivery systems illustrates how environmentally friendly and biocompatible technologies can support the production of scalable solutions that align with green chemistry principles [64,65].

From a neo-industrialization perspective, the valorization of *S. mombin* peel and similar co-products contributes to building resilient value chains that prioritize resource efficiency, reduced carbon emissions, and technological innovation. These efforts resonate with policies promoting green industrial development, particularly in emerging economies where agricultural byproducts represent an abundant yet untapped resource [66,67]. Furthermore, this study highlights the potential for such technologies to catalyze the development of next-generation materials that address global health challenges, integrating the principles of bioeconomy, circular economy, and technological innovation [68,69].

Future research should focus on scaling these technologies for industrial applications, exploring their potential in broader sectors such as environmental remediation, food preservation, and renewable energy systems. Collaborations between academia, industry, and policymakers will be essential to accelerate the adoption of co-product-based innovations, ensuring they contribute to global efforts towards a more sustainable and equitable industrial future [70,71].

4. Conclusions

The findings of this study demonstrate the successful development of nanostructured lipid carriers (NLCs) incorporating natural deep eutectic solvents (NaDESs) as a novel and sustainable platform for the encapsulation and stabilization of bioactive phenolic compounds extracted from *Spondias mombin* peel. The careful optimization of lipid ratios, surfactant concentrations, and the integration of NaDESs not only improved the physicochemical properties of the nanoparticles but also enhanced the retention and stability of the encapsulated bioactives under varying environmental conditions. The use of murumuru butter and buriti oil as lipid components, coupled with Brij® O10 (Sigma-Aldrich, St. Louis, MI, USA) as a surfactant, resulted in formulations with low polydispersity indices, stable zeta potentials, and hydrodynamic sizes suitable for advanced therapeutic and industrial applications.

The inclusion of NaDESs, comprising glycerol, choline chloride, and citric acid, played a pivotal role in solubilizing phenolic compounds, facilitating their incorporation into the lipid phase, and stabilizing the nanoparticles through robust molecular interactions. These interactions, evidenced by FTIR and corroborated by TEM analysis, underscored the protective microenvironment created by NaDESs, which mitigated oxidative and thermal degradation while providing flexibility to the lipid matrix. Moreover, the cryoprotective properties of the NaDESs contributed to improved nanoparticle stability under freezing conditions, further broadening the potential applications of these formulations.

The methodological advances in the production of NLCs, utilizing hot emulsification and rapid cooling, ensured consistent particle sizes and encapsulation efficiency, while the thorough characterization of colloidal properties validated the robustness and scalability of the formulations. The integration of NaDESs into NLCs represents a paradigm shift in the valorization of agricultural byproducts, aligning with global efforts towards sustainability, circular economy practices, and green industrial innovation. By transforming *S. mombin* peel—a byproduct often discarded as waste—into a high-value ingredient for health-related applications, this study highlights the potential for co-product-based technologies to address critical environmental and industrial challenges.

Future research should explore the scalability of these formulations to industrial levels, investigate their efficacy in diverse biological systems, and extend their application to other bioactive compounds. Additionally, fostering interdisciplinary collaborations between academia, industry, and policymakers will be essential to realize the full potential of these technologies, ensuring they contribute to a more sustainable and equitable future. This work not only sets a foundation for advanced delivery systems but also exemplifies how nanotechnology, coupled with sustainable practices, can drive innovation across health and industrial sectors.

Author Contributions: Conceptualization, V.C.M., S.N.B. and E.F.G.; data curation, E.A.F., S.N.B. and E.F.G.; formal analysis, C.K.G. and E.F.G.; funding acquisition, S.N.B. and E.F.G.; investigation, V.C.M., G.O.d.B., I.F., T.B.P., L.F.d.A.C. and A.P.S.; methodology, M.M.S., K.L.R.d.P., M.-K.M.S.S., G.O.d.B., M.A.R., I.F., E.A.F., N.S.A. and E.F.G.; project administration, V.C.M. and E.F.G.; resources, E.F.G.; supervision, C.K.G. and S.N.B.; validation, E.F.G.; visualization, E.A.F.; writing—original draft, V.C.M. and G.O.d.B.; writing—review and editing, M.M.S., K.L.R.d.P., M.-K.M.S.S., M.A.R., A.P.S., N.S.A., C.K.G. and S.N.B. All authors have read and agreed to the published version of the manuscript.

Funding: This research was funded by FAP-DF/Brazil (00193-00000165/2023-20; 0193.00002231/2022-15), the National Council for Scientific and Technological Development—CNPq (403033/2023-3), the Financier of Studies and Projects (01.08.0457.00), and the Higher Education Personnel Improvement Coordination—CAPES (0001).

Institutional Review Board Statement: Not applicable.

Informed Consent Statement: Not applicable.

Data Availability Statement: Data are contained within the article.

Conflicts of Interest: Victor Carlos Mello, Marina Arantes Radicchi, Isadora Florêncio, Leonardo Fróes de Azevedo Chang, Ariane Pandolfo Silveira, Marina Mesquita Simões, Karen Letycia Rodrigues de Paiva, and Nicole Santana Alves were employed by Cooil Cosmetics. The remaining authors declare that the research was conducted in the absence of any commercial or financial relationships that could be construed as a potential conflict of interest.

References

1. Carvalho, J.T.G.; Baldivia, D.S.; Leite, D.F.; de Araújo, L.C.A.; Espindola, P.P.; Toledo, F. Medicinal Plants from Brazilian Cerrado: Antioxidant and Anticancer Potential and Protection against Chemotherapy Toxicity. *Oxid. Med. Cell. Longev.* **2019**, *2019*, 3685264.
2. Sawyer, D.; Mesquita, B.; Coutinho, B.; Almeida, F.V.; Figueiredo, I.; Lamas, I. Perfil do Ecossistema Hotspot de Biodiversidade do Cerrado. Critical Ecosystem Partnership Fund. 2017, 506p. Available online: https://shs.hal.science/halshs-02870718/document (accessed on 20 March 2024).
3. Arruda, H.S.; Araújo, M.V.L.; Junior, M.R.M. Underexploited Brazilian Cerrado Fruits as Sources of Phenolic Compounds for Diseases Management: A Review. *Food Chem. Mol. Sci.* **2022**, *5*, 100148. [CrossRef] [PubMed]
4. Carvalho, P.E.R. Cajá-da-Mata: Spondias mombin. In *Coleção Espécies Arbóreas Brasileiras*; Embrapa: Brasília, Brazil, 2022; pp. 125–132.
5. Brito, S.A.; Barbosa, I.S.; de Almeida, C.L.F.; de Medeiros, J.W.; Silva Neto, J.C.; Rolim, L.A.; da Silva, T.G.; Ximenes, R.M.; de Menezes, I.R.A.; Caldas, G.F.R.; et al. Evaluation of Gastroprotective and Ulcer Healing Activities of Yellow Mombin Juice from *Spondias mombin* L. *PLoS ONE* **2018**, *13*, e0201561. [CrossRef] [PubMed]
6. Souza, V.R.; Brum, M.C.M.; Guimarães, I.D.S.; dos Santos, P.D.F.; do Amaral, T.O.; Abreu, J.P.; Passos, T.; Freitas-Silva, O.; Gimba ER, P.; Teodoro, A.J. Amazon Fruits Inhibit Growth and Promote Pro-Apoptotic Effects on Human Ovarian Carcinoma Cell Lines. *Biomolecules* **2019**, *9*, 707. [CrossRef] [PubMed]
7. de Brito, G.O.; Reis, B.C.; Ferreira, E.A.; Vilela Junqueira, N.T.; Sá-Barreto, L.C.L.; Mattivi, F.; Vrhovsek, U.; Gris, E.F. Phenolic Compound Profile by UPLC-MS/MS and Encapsulation with Chitosan of *Spondias mombin* L. Fruit Peel Extract from Cerrado Hotspot—Brazil. *Molecules* **2022**, *27*, 2382. [CrossRef] [PubMed]

8. Bataglion, G.A.; da Silva, F.M.A.; Eberlin, M.N.; Koolen, H.H.F. Determination of the Phenolic Composition from Brazilian Tropical Fruits by UHPLC–MS/MS. *Food Chem.* **2015**, *180*, 280–287. [CrossRef]
9. Eseberri, I.; Trepiana, J.; Léniz, A.; Gómez-García, I.; Carr-Ugarte, H.; González, M.; Portillo, M.P. Variability in the Beneficial Effects of Phenolic Compounds: A Review. *Nutrients* **2022**, *14*, 1925. [CrossRef]
10. Alara, O.R.; Abdurahman, N.H.; Ukaegbu, C.I. Extraction of phenolic compounds: A review. *Curr. Res. Food Sci.* **2021**, *4*, 200–214. [CrossRef]
11. Liu, C.; Ge, S.; Yang, J.; Xu, Y.; Zhao, M.; Xiong, L.; Sun, Q. Adsorption mechanism of polyphenols onto starch nanoparticles and enhanced antioxidant activity under adverse conditions. *J. Funct. Foods.* **2016**, *26*, 632–644. [CrossRef]
12. Lagoa, R.; Silva, J.; Rodrigues, J.R.; Bishayee, A. Advances in phytochemical delivery systems for improved anticancer activity. *Biotechnol. Adv.* **2020**, *38*, 107382. [CrossRef]
13. Gado, F.; Digiacomo, M.; Salsano, J.E.; Macchia, M.; Manera, C. Phenolic Compounds in Prevention and Treatment of Skin Cancers: A Review. *Curr. Med. Chem.* **2021**, *28*, 6730–6752. [CrossRef]
14. Yan, C.; Kim, S.R.; Ruiz, D.R.; Farmer, J.R. Microencapsulation for Food Applications: A Review. *ACS Appl. Bio Mater.* **2022**, *5*, 5497–5512. [CrossRef] [PubMed]
15. Ezhilarasi, P.N.; Muthukumar, S.P.; Anandharamakrishnan, C. Solid Lipid Nanoparticle Enhances Bioavailability of Hydroxycitric Acid Compared to a Microparticle Delivery System. *RSC Adv.* **2016**, *6*, 53784–53793. [CrossRef]
16. Gwinn, M.R.; Vallyathan, V. Nanoparticles: Health Effects—Pros and Cons. *Environ. Health Perspect.* **2006**, *114*, 1818–1825. [CrossRef]
17. Benvenutti, L.; Sanchez-Camargo, A.d.P.; Zielinski, A.A.F.; Ferreira, S.R.S. NADES as Potential Solvents for Anthocyanin and Pectin Extraction from *Myrciaria cauliflora* Fruit By-Product: In Silico and Experimental Approaches for Solvent Selection. *J. Mol. Liq.* **2020**, *315*, 113761. [CrossRef]
18. Mustafa, N.R.; de Winter, W.; van Iren, F.; Verpoorte, R. Initiation, Growth and Cryopreservation of Plant Cell Suspension Cultures. *Nat. Protoc.* **2011**, *6*, 715–742. [CrossRef] [PubMed]
19. Choi, Y.H.; van Spronsen, J.; Dai, Y.; Verberne, M.; Hollmann, F.; Arends, I.W.C.E.; Witkamp, G.-J.; Verpoorte, R. Are Natural Deep Eutectic Solvents the Missing Link in Understanding Cellular Metabolism and Physiology? *Plant Physiol.* **2011**, *156*, 1701–1705. [CrossRef] [PubMed]
20. Schuh, L.; Reginato, M.; Florêncio, I.; Falcao, L.; Boron, L.; Gris, E.F.; Mello, V.; Báo, S.N. From Nature to Innovation: The Uncharted Potential of Natural Deep Eutectic Solvents. *Molecules* **2023**, *28*, 7653. [CrossRef] [PubMed]
21. Schuh, L.; Salgado, L.A.; Piau, T.B.; Silveira, A.P.; Leal, C.; Romera, L.F.; Radicchi, M.A.; Santos, M.-K.M.S.; Falcao, L.; Grisolia, C.K.; et al. Integrating Natural Deep Eutectic Solvents into Nanostructured Lipid Carriers: An Industrial Look. *Pharmaceuticals* **2024**, *17*, 855. [CrossRef] [PubMed]
22. Vrhovsek, U.; Masuero, D.; Gasperotti, M.; Franceschi, P.; Caputi, L.; Viola, R.; Mattivi, F. A Versatile Targeted Metabolomics Method for the Rapid Quantification of Multiple Classes of Phenolics in Fruits and Beverages. *J. Agric. Food Chem.* **2012**, *60*, 8831–8840. [CrossRef]
23. Brand-Williams, W.; Cuvelier, M.E.; Berset, C. Use of a Free Radical Method to Evaluate Antioxidant Activity. *LWT-Food Sci. Technol.* **1995**, *28*, 25–30. [CrossRef]
24. Re, R.; Pellegrini, N.; Proteggente, A.; Pannala, A.; Yang, M.; Rice-Evans, C. Antioxidant Activity Applying an Improved ABTS Radical Cation Decolorization Assay. *Free Radic. Biol. Med.* **1999**, *26*, 1231–1237. [CrossRef]
25. da Silva, D.T.; Pauletto, R.; Cavalheiro, S.S.; Bochi, V.C.; Rodrigues, E.; Weber, J.; da Silva, C.d.B.; Morisso, F.D.P.; Barcia, M.T.; Emanuelli, T. Natural Deep Eutectic Solvents as a Biocompatible Tool for the Extraction of Blueberry Anthocyanins. *J. Food Compos. Anal.* **2020**, *89*, 103470. [CrossRef]
26. Mello, V. *Carreadores Lipídicos Nanoestruturados Contendo Alumínio-Ftalocianina para Terapia Fotodinâmica Contra Melanoma: Desenvolvimento, Caracterização e Teste de Eficácia In Vitro*; Universidade de Brasília: Brasília, Brazil, 2022.
27. Mello, V.; Araújo, V.H.S.; de Paiva, K.L.R.; Simões, M.M.; Marques, D.C.; da Silva Costa, N.R.; de Souza, I.F.; da Silva, P.B.; Santos, I.; Almeida, R.; et al. Development of New Natural Lipid-Based Nanoparticles Loaded with Aluminum-Phthalocyanine for Photodynamic Therapy Against Melanoma. *Nanomaterials* **2022**, *12*, 3547. [CrossRef] [PubMed]
28. Cabral, B.R.P.; Oliveira, P.M.; Gelfuso, G.M.; Quintão, T.S.C.; Chaker, J.A.; Margô Gomes, d.O.K.; Gris, E.F. Improving Stability of Antioxidant Compounds from *Plinia cauliflora* (Jabuticaba) Fruit Peel Extract by Encapsulation in Chitosan Microparticles. *J. Food Eng.* **2018**, *238*, 195–201. [CrossRef]
29. Mosmann, T. Rapid Colorimetric Assay for Cellular Growth and Survival: Application to Proliferation and Cytotoxicity Assays. *J. Immunol. Methods* **1983**, *65*, 55–63. [CrossRef] [PubMed]
30. OECD. *Test No. 236: Fish Embryo Acute Toxicity (FET) Test, OECD Guidelines for the Testing of Chemicals, Section 2*; OECD Publishing: Paris, France, 2013.

31. Danaei, M.; Dehghankhold, M.; Ataei, S.; Hasanzadeh Davarani, F.; Javanmard, R.; Dokhani, A.; Khorasani, S.; Mozafari, M.R. Impact of Particle Size and Polydispersity Index on the Clinical Applications of Lipidic Nanocarrier Systems. *Pharmaceutics* **2018**, *10*, 57. [CrossRef] [PubMed]
32. Viegas, C.M.; Patrício, A.B.; Prata, J.M.; Nadhman, A.; Chintamaneni, P.K.; Fonte, P. Solid Lipid Nanoparticles vs. Nanostructured Lipid Carriers: A Comparative Review. *Pharmaceutics* **2023**, *15*, 1593. [CrossRef] [PubMed]
33. Freire, R.; Hong, L.; Peterek, M.; Canarelli, S.; Rezzi, S.; Salentinig, S. Structure Formation in Tailor-Made Buriti Oil Emulsion During Simulated Digestion. *Adv. Funct. Mater.* **2023**, *33*, 2303854. [CrossRef]
34. Freitas, M.; Chisté, R.; Polachini, T.; Sardella, L.; Aranha, C.; Ribeiro, A.; Nicoletti, V.R. Quality Characteristics and Thermal Behavior of Buriti (*Mauritia flexuosa* L.) Oil. *Grasas Aceites* **2018**, *68*, 220. [CrossRef]
35. Bovi, G.; Petrus, R.; Pinho, S. Feasibility of Incorporating Buriti (*Mauritia flexuosa* L.) Oil Nanoemulsions in Isotonic Sports Drink. *Int. J. Food Sci. Technol.* **2017**, *52*, 2201–2209. [CrossRef]
36. Speranza, P.; Falcão, A.; Macedo, J.; Silva, L.; Rodrigues, A.; Macedo, G. Amazonian Buriti Oil: Chemical Characterization and Antioxidant Potential. *Grasas Aceites* **2016**, *67*, e135. [CrossRef]
37. Freitas, M.; Ribeiro, A.; Telis, V. Buriti Oil Emulsions as Affected by Soy Protein Isolate/High-Methoxyl Pectin Ratio, Oil Content and Homogenization Pressure. *Food Technol. Biotechnol.* **2020**, *58*, 159–172. [CrossRef] [PubMed]
38. Costa, P.; Ballus, C.; Filho, J.; Godoy, H. Fatty Acids Profile of Pulp and Nuts of Brazilian Fruits. *Food Sci. Technol.* **2011**, *31*, 950–954. [CrossRef]
39. Aquino, J.S.; Pessoa, D.C.N.d.P.; Araújo, K.d.L.G.V.; Epaminondas, P.S.; Schuler, A.R.P.; de Souza, A.G.; Stamford, T.L.M. Refining of Buriti Oil *(Mauritia flexuosa)* Originated from the Brazilian Cerrado: Physicochemical, Thermal-Oxidative and Nutritional Implications. *J. Braz. Chem. Soc.* **2012**, *23*, 212–219. [CrossRef]
40. Aquino, J.; Batista, K.; Araújo-Silva, G.; Santos, D.; Brito, N.; López, J.; da Silva, J.A.; das Graças Almeida, M.; Pincheira, C.G.; Magnani, M.; et al. Antioxidant and Lipid-Lowering Effects of Buriti Oil (*Mauritia flexuosa* L.) Administered to Iron-Overloaded Rats. *Molecules* **2023**, *28*, 2585. [CrossRef] [PubMed]
41. Paiva, A.; Craveiro, R.; Aroso, I.; Martins, M.; Reis, R.; Duarte, A. Natural Deep Eutectic Solvents—Solvents for the 21st Century. *ACS Sustainable Chem. Eng.* **2014**, *2*, 1063–1071. [CrossRef]
42. Sut, S.; Faggian, M.; Baldan, V.; Poloniato, G.; Castagliuolo, I.; Grabnar, I.; Perissutti, B.; Brun, P.; Maggi, F.; Voinovich, D.; et al. Natural Deep Eutectic Solvents (NADES) to Enhance Berberine Absorption: An In Vivo Pharmacokinetic Study. *Molecules* **2017**, *22*, 1921. [CrossRef] [PubMed]
43. Dai, Y.; Spronsen, J.; Witkamp, G.; Verpoorte, R.; Choi, Y. Ionic Liquids and Deep Eutectic Solvents in Natural Products Research: Mixtures of Solids as Extraction Solvents. *J. Nat. Prod.* **2013**, *76*, 2162–2173. [CrossRef]
44. Oomen, W.; Begines, P.; Mustafa, N.; Wilson, E.; Verpoorte, R.; Choi, Y. Natural Deep Eutectic Solvent Extraction of Flavonoids of *Scutellaria baicalensis* as a Replacement for Conventional Organic Solvents. *Molecules* **2020**, *25*, 617. [CrossRef]
45. Ma, Y.; Li, Y.; Ali, S.; Li, P.; Zhang, W.; Rauch, M.; Willot, S.J.-P.; Ribitsch, D.; Choi, Y.H.; Alcalde, M.; et al. Natural Deep Eutectic Solvents as Performance Additives for Peroxygenase Catalysis. *ChemCatChem* **2019**, *12*, 989–994. [CrossRef]
46. Coscarella, M. Alternative Assisted Extraction Methods of Phenolic Compounds Using NADES. *Antioxidants* **2023**, *13*, 62. [CrossRef] [PubMed]
47. Kolarević, L.; Horozić, E.; Ademović, Z.; Kundalić, B.; Husejnagić, D. Influence of Deep Eutectic Solvents (DESs) on Antioxidant and Antimicrobial Activity of Seed Extracts of Selected Citrus Species. *Int. Res. J. Pure Appl. Chem.* **2020**, *21*, 120–128. [CrossRef]
48. Stramarkou, M.; Oikonomopoulou, V.; Panagiotopoulou, M.; Papadaki, S.; Krokida, M. Sustainable Valorisation of Peach and Apricot Waste Using Green Extraction Technique with Conventional and Deep Eutectic Solvents. *Resources* **2023**, *12*, 72. [CrossRef]
49. Brito, G.O.; Reis, B.C.; Ferreira, E.A.; Junqueira, N.T.V.; Sá-Barreto, L.C.L.; Mattivi, F.; Vrhovsek, U.; Gris, E.F. Perfil de Compostos Fenólicos, Atividade Antioxidante e Microencapsulação com Quitosana do Extrato da Casca de Spondias mombin L. do Cerrado Brasileiro. *Molecules* **2020**, *25*, 9028924.
50. Tamjidi, F.; Shahedi, M.; Varshosaz, J.; Nasirpour, A. Stability of astaxanthin-loaded nanostructured lipid carriers in beverage systems. *J. Sci. Food Agric.* **2017**, *98*, 511–518. [CrossRef]
51. Varriale, S.; Delorme, A.; Andanson, J.; Devémy, J.; Malfreyt, P.; Verney, V.; Pezzella, C. Enhancing the thermostability of engineered laccases in aqueous betaine-based natural deep eutectic solvents. *ACS Sustain. Chem. Eng.* **2021**, *10*, 572–581. [CrossRef] [PubMed]
52. Aryani, N.; Siswandono, S.; Soeratri, W.; Putri, D.; Puspitasarini, P. Development, characterization in vitro and in silico of coenzyme q10 loaded myristic acid with different liquid lipids nanostructured lipid carriers. *J. Pharm. Pharmacogn. Res.* **2021**, *9*, 573–583. [CrossRef]
53. Shehata, M.; Ismail, A.; Kamel, M. Nose to brain delivery of astaxanthin–loaded nanostructured lipid carriers in rat model of alzheimer's disease: Preparation, in vitro and in vivo evaluation. *Int. J. Nanomed.* **2023**, *18*, 1631–1658. [CrossRef] [PubMed]

54. Kelidari, H.; Saeedi, M.; Âkbari, J.; Morteza-Semnani, K.; Valizadeh, H.; Maniruzzaman, M.; Nokhodchi, A. Development and optimisation of spironolactone nanoparticles for enhanced dissolution rates and stability. *Aaps Pharmscitech* **2016**, *18*, 1469–1474. [CrossRef] [PubMed]
55. Müller, R.H.; Mäder, K.; Gohla, S. Nanostructured Lipid Carriers (NLC) in Drug Delivery: A Review. *Eur. J. Pharm. Biopharm.* **2018**, *132*, 1–12.
56. Liu, Y.; Friesen, J.B.; McAlpine, J.B.; Lankin, D.C.; Chen, S.-N.; Pauli, G.F. Natural Deep Eutectic Solvents as a New Class of Solvents for the Extraction of Bioactive Compounds. *J. Nat. Prod.* **2017**, *80*, 2572–2581. [CrossRef]
57. Huang, M.M.; Yiin, C.L.; Lock, S.S.M.; Chin, B.L.F.; Othman, I.; Zauzi, N.S.A.; Chan, Y.H. Natural Deep Eutectic Solvents: A New Platform for Drug Delivery. *J. Control. Release* **2021**, *330*, 123–135.
58. Fonseca-Gomes, J.; Loureiro, J.A.; Tanqueiro, S.R.; Mouro, F.M.; Ruivo, P.; Carvalho, T.; Sebastião, A.M.; Diógenes, M.J.; Pereira, M.C. In Vivo Evaluation of Lipid-Based Nanocarriers for Drug Delivery. *Adv. Drug Deliv. Rev.* **2022**, *178*, 113–129. [CrossRef]
59. Mohammadpour, R.; Dobrovolskaia, M.A.; Cheney, D.L.; Greish, K.F.; Ghandehari, H. Subchronic and Chronic Toxicity Evaluation of Inorganic Nanoparticles for Delivery Applications. *Adv. Drug Deliv. Rev.* **2019**, *144*, 112–132. [CrossRef]
60. Długosz, O. Natural Deep Eutectic Solvents in the Synthesis of Inorganic Nanoparticles. *Materials* **2023**, *16*, 627. [CrossRef] [PubMed]
61. Madani, M.; Hosny, S.; Alshangiti, D.; Nady, N.; Alkhursani, S.; Alkhaldi, H.; Al-Gahtany, S.A.; Ghobashy, M.M.; Gaber, G.A. Green Synthesis of Nanoparticles for Varied Applications: Green Renewable Resources and Energy-Efficient Synthetic Routes. *Nanotechnol. Rev.* **2022**, *11*, 731–759. [CrossRef]
62. Fortunati, E.; Mazzaglia, A.; Balestra, G. Sustainable Control Strategies for Plant Protection and Food Packaging Sectors by Natural Substances and Novel Nanotechnological Approaches. *J. Sci. Food Agric.* **2018**, *99*, 986–1000. [CrossRef] [PubMed]
63. Bahadur, S. A Review on Current Prospective and Applications of Green Nanoparticles in Biomedical Applications. *Curr. Nanomed.* **2024**. [CrossRef]
64. Tsekhmistrenko, O.; Bityutskii, V.; Tsekhmistrenko, S.; Kharchyshyn, V.; Tymoshok, N.; Spivak, M. Efficiency of Application of Inorganic and Nanopreparations of Selenium and Probiotics for Growing Young Quails. *Theor. Appl. Vet. Med.* **2020**, 206–212. [CrossRef]
65. Özhava, D.; Duman, S. Solventless Dimethylamine Borane Dehydrogenation in the Presence of Transition Metal(0) Nanoparticles Loaded on Cellulose. *ChemCatChem* **2023**, *15*, e202201563. [CrossRef]
66. Bolade, O.; Williams, A.; Benson, N. Green Synthesis of Iron-Based Nanomaterials for Environmental Remediation: A Review. *Environ. Nanotechnol. Monit. Manag.* **2020**, *13*, 100279. [CrossRef]
67. Vorobyova, V. Plant Extract Based on Deep Eutectic Solvent-Mediated Biosynthesis of Silver Nanoparticles: Cytotoxicity and Antibacterial Effects. *Bioinorg. Chem. Appl.* **2023**, *2023*, 9672432. [CrossRef]
68. Apte, A.; Lubree, H.; Kapoor, M.; Juvekar, S.; Banerjee, R.; Bavdekar, A. Development and implementation of liposomal encapsulated micronutrient fortified body oil intervention for infant massage: An innovative concept to prevent micronutrient deficiencies in children. *Front Public Health.* **2021**, *8*, 567689. [CrossRef] [PubMed]
69. Zhou, Y.; Dou, F.; Alahmadi, T.; Alharbi, S.; Wainwright, M. Biosynthesis of Fe nanoparticles using *Alhagi sparsifolia* extract for the treatment of colorectal carcinoma in the in vitro condition: A pre-clinical trial study. *Arch Med. Sci.* **2021**. [CrossRef]
70. Kucuk, I. Green electrochemical nanosensor platform design for mexiletine detection based on *Citrus reticulata* peel-mediated iron nanoparticles and quantum dots and investigation of the adsorption mechanism by the DFT-D3 method. *New J. Chem.* **2024**, *48*, 3729–3740. [CrossRef]
71. Lamri, M.; Bhattacharya, T.; Boukid, F.; Chentir, I.; Dib, A.L.; Das, D.; Djenane, D.; Gagaoua, M. Nanotechnology as a processing and packaging tool to improve meat quality and safety. *Foods* **2021**, *10*, 2633. [CrossRef] [PubMed]

antioxidants

Article

Physical Properties of Cellulose Derivative-Based Edible Films Elaborated with Liposomes Encapsulating Grape Seed Tannins

Constanza Vidal [1], Johana Lopez-Polo [2] and Fernando A. Osorio [1,*]

1 Department of Food Science and Technology, Technological Faculty, University of Santiago-Chile—USACH, Av. El Belloto 3735, Estación Central, Santiago 9170022, Chile; constanza.vidala@usach.cl
2 Laboratorio de Biotecnología de los Alimentos, Instituto de Nutrición y Tecnología de los Alimentos, Universidad de Chile, El Líbano 5524, Macul, Santiago 783090, Chile; johana.lopez@inta.uchile.cl
* Correspondence: fernando.osorio@usach.cl; Tel.: +56-2-271-80550

Abstract: Combined use of edible films (EF) with nanoencapsulation systems could be an effective alternative for improving the films' physical properties and maintaining bioactive compounds' stability. This research work focuses on the combined use of EF of cellulose-derived biopolymers enriched with liposomes that encapsulate grape seed tannins and on the subsequent evaluation of the physical properties and wettability. Tannin-containing liposomal suspensions (TLS) showed 570.8 ± 6.0 nm particle size and 99% encapsulation efficiency. In vitro studies showed that the release of tannins from liposomes was slower than that of free tannins, reaching a maximum release of catechin of 0.13 ± 0.01%, epicatechin of 0.57 ± 0.01%, and gallic acid of 3.90 ± 0.001% over a 144 h period. Adding liposomes to biopolymer matrices resulted in significant decrease ($p < 0.05$) of density, surface tension, tensile strength, elongation percentage, and elastic modulus in comparison to the control, obtaining films with greater flexibility and lower breaking strength. Incorporating TLS into EF formulations resulted in partially wetting the hydrophobic surface, reducing adhesion and cohesion compared to EF without liposomes. Results indicate that the presence of liposomes improves films' physical and wettability properties, causing them to extend and not contract when applied to hydrophobic food surfaces.

Keywords: liposome; biopolymers; bioactive compounds; mechanical properties; wettability

1. Introduction

Condensed tannins from grape seeds, called proanthocyanidins, are monomeric, oligomeric, or polymeric flavonoids of flavan-3-ol units. The predominant components of these tannins are (+)—catechins (28.2%), (−)—epicatechins (8.8%), and gallic acid (1.3%) [1–3]. Grape seed tannins are natural phenolic compounds known for their potent antioxidant activity [4]. These tannins, found in abundance in grape seeds, have been the subject of increasing interest in scientific research due to their multiple health benefits. Among their most notable properties are the ability to neutralize free radicals, reduce oxidative stress, and prevent chronic diseases associated with oxidative damage, such as cardiovascular diseases and certain types of cancer [5,6]. Grape seed tannins are a rich source of proanthocyanidins, which are polymers of flavan-3-ols. These proanthocyanidins are highly effective in scavenging free radicals due to the presence of multiple hydroxyl groups in their molecular structures, which can donate electrons to neutralize free radicals. Studies have shown that grape seed tannins possess significantly higher antioxidant capacity than other natural antioxidant sources, such as vitamins C and E [7,8]. This potent antioxidant activity makes them promising candidates for applications in functional foods and nutraceutical products.

However, their oral administration and use as bioactive compounds in the food industry are limited due to their instability in the gastrointestinal tract, low water solubility, and poor bioavailability [9,10]. An innovative alternative to overcome these limitations of tannin instability is using liposomes as a nanoencapsulation technology, which allows them to be wrapped and protected from external conditions. Liposomes are nanometer-sized spherical vesicles composed of a phospholipid bilayer with hydrophilic heads and hydrophobic fatty acid tails surrounding an aqueous compartment [11]. These liposomes can be used to encapsulate hydrophilic, hydrophobic, and amphiphilic compounds [12]. Encapsulation in liposomes would stabilize and protect tannins against a series of chemical and environmental changes (temperature, pH, oxygen) typically used in the food industry, as well as improve their bioavailability and achieve a controlled release [13].

Recently, the combination of nanoliposomes with edible films (EF) has been studied as a novel strategy to improve and protect the physicochemical characteristics of bioactive compounds, prolong the shelf life of foods with edible films and achieve a gradual release of the compound [14,15]. EF are thin, flexible matrices that are made from natural biopolymers, applied directly to the surface of food [16]. EF are eco-friendly, non-toxic, biodegradable and can be consumed along with the food product [17,18]. Among the most commercially used biopolymers for EF production are polysaccharides derived from cellulose, such as Hydroxypropylmethylcellulose (HPMC) (CAS Number 9004-65-3) and Carboxymethylcellulose (CMC) (CAS Number 9004-32-4), which are generally recognized as safe (GRAS) biocompatible with other water-soluble materials, tasteless, colorless and transparent [19,20].

In the literature, some works have been published on the combined use of various biopolymers for edible coatings such as CMC with nanoliposomes that encapsulate antioxidants, i.e., sour tea extract (*Hibiscus sabdariffa* L.). The results showed that CMC and nanoliposomes from tea extracts reduce the oxidative deterioration process in fried chicken nuggets and generate a softer texture of the product [21]. Other works have also applied edible films and liposomes in meat products such as chicken fillets and cheese slices working with HPMC and κ-carrageenan edible films, which improved thermal stability, transparency and mechanical properties. Furthermore, it demonstrated strong antibacterial activity against food-borne Gram-positive and Gram-negative bacteria, which may have potential applications in extending the shelf life of these foods [22].

Although the research that has been developed in terms of the combination of films with liposomes is extensive, knowledge about polyphenols in edible films in the food industry is still in an incipient stage [23]. To the best of our knowledge, no work has been published that delves into the combination of an edible film containing liposomes encapsulating grape seed tannins. Therefore, this research aimed to evaluate the physical, mechanical, and wettability properties of edible films made from cellulose-derived biopolymers, specifically HPMC and CMC, enriched with liposomes encapsulating grape seed tannins. This analysis aims to determine the potential of these films for direct application in foods.

2. Materials and Methods

2.1. Materials

Grape seed tannins (TANIN VR GRAPE®; CAS Number:1401-55-4) were obtained from Laffort Chile (suitable for the products intended for direct human consumption in accordance with Regulation (EU) 2019/934). Soy lecithin was provided by Dimerco (Región Metropolitana, Chile). Citric acid anhydrous, tri-sodium citrate 2 hydrate, ethanol (99.9%), glycerol (>99%), ethyl acetate (99.8%), ethanol (99.9%) were obtained from Winkler (Región Metropolitana, Chile). Hydroxypropylmethylcellulose (HPMC) (Metrocel E19 Grade, Dow Wolff Cellulosics; CAS Number 9004-65-3), Carboxymethylcellulose (CMC) (CAS Number: 9004-32-4) (Sodium salt), (+)—Catequin hydrate, (−)—Epicatechin, Gallic acid (anhydrous), 2,2-diphenyl-1-picryhydrazyl ($DPPH^\bullet$), 2,2′-Azino-bis(3-ethylbenzothiazoline-6-sulfonic acid) diammonium salt ($ABTS^{\bullet+}$), Trolox ((±)—6-hydroxy-2,5,7,8-tetramethylchroman-2-carboxylic acid), Methanol (99.9%), Trifluoracetic acid (TFA) (>99%), Acetonitrile (ACN)

(99.9%), L-cysteine (98%) and dialysis bag (cellulose membrane of molecular weight 14,000 Da) were obtained from Sigma-Aldrich (St. Louis, MO, USA).

2.2. The Extraction of Partial Purified Phosphatidylcholine (PC)

The extraction of partial purified phosphatidylcholine (PC) was done from food-grade raw soy lecithin following the methodology described in our previous work with some modifications [24]. Soy lecithin (10 g) was dissolved in ethyl acetate (50 mL) at 20 °C. Then, distilled water (2 mL) was slowly added with manual stirring. The lower phase was separated by decantation and dispersed with acetone (30 mL), crushed with a glass rod, and the grinding process was repeated with a new aliquot of acetone. The precipitate was filtered under vacuum and dried in a desiccator at 20 °C for 48 h obtaining the partial purified PC. With this acetone extraction and washing method, a purification level of 95% of the lipids present is achieved. Taladrid et al. (2017) supports the effectiveness and reliability of the partial purified PC extraction methodology used in this study [24].

2.3. Preparation of Tannin-Containing Liposome Suspensions (TLS)

The condition for liposome preparation was determined based on previous studies conducted in our laboratory, which assessed stability over time and the formation of precipitates. During optimization, variations were made in the pH, partial purified PC, glycerol and bioactive compound concentrations. After evaluating various combinations of these factors, optimal concentrations were selected that provided the best stability and efficacy in tannin encapsulation. These concentrations were utilized in liposome preparation to ensure efficient encapsulation and controlled release of bioactive compounds. The tannin-containing liposome suspensions (TLS) were prepared using the heating/homogenization method with lamellarity reduction with some modifications [2]. Grape seed tannins (1 mg/mL) and partial purified PC (10 mg/mL) were dissolved in ethanol-citrate buffer (0.1 M at pH 3) at 80 °C for 1 h. Then, glycerol (0.76% w/v) [24] and a second heating period was carried out at 80 °C for 1 h. Then, 5 cycles of vortex and 20 cycles of ultrasound (HIELSCHER UP100H, Heidelberg, Germany, max. 100 W) were applied at 90% amplitude and 22.5 Hz. Two control samples were prepared: Free tannin suspension (FTS), prepared by dissolving tannins in ethanol-citrate buffer, and empty liposome suspension (LS), prepared by dissolving partial purified PC in ethanol-citrate buffer and following the same heating/homogenization procedure as the TLS sample.

2.4. Particle Size, Polydispersity Index and Zeta Potential

The analyzes of particle size, polydispersity index and z-potential were carried out via the dynamic light scattering (DLS) technique, using a refractive and phospholipid index of 1.330 and 1.334, respectively, and the measurement angle was 173° Backscatter (Zetasizer Nano ZS, Malvern Instruments Ltd., Malvern, UK). The samples were diluted 100 times in potassium phosphate buffer (PPB) (10 mM, pH 7.4) and vertical cuvettes of 2000 μL capacity were used at 25 °C.

2.5. Encapsulation Efficiency

The encapsulation efficiency (% EE) was determined with the centrifugation (Hanil Scientific Inc. Supra R22, Gimpo, Republic of Korea) method at 21,058× g for one hour [25]. The samples were quantified using Ultra High Performance Liquid Chromatography (UHPLC) (Thermo Fisher Scientific Ultimate 3000, Waltham, MA, USA) with the tannin standards: catechin, epicatechin and gallic acid, as detailed in the methodology Section "TLS Thiolysis and UHPLC Quantification". The EE % was determined with Equation (1).

$$EE\,\% = \frac{[T]_E - [T]_L}{[T]_E} \tag{1}$$

where: $[T]_E$ is the initial concentration of tannins in the liposomal suspension; $[T]_L$ is the concentration of free tannins in the medium.

2.6. Antioxidant Activity Analysis

2.6.1. ABTS$^{\bullet+}$ Radical Scavenging Assay of TLS

The TLS samples were analyzed by the 2,2′-azino-bis (3-ethylbenzothiazoline-6-sulfonic acid) (ABTS$^{\bullet+}$) radical scavenging method. To do this, 20 μL of TLS and 980 μL of ABTS$^{\bullet+}$ were mixed and left for 10 min at 25 °C in the dark [26]. The control sample was prepared with 20 μL of ethanol with 980 μL of ABTS$^{\bullet+}$. The percentage inhibition of ABTS$^{\bullet+}$ was determined at 734 nm using Equation (2).

$$\%\ \text{ABTS}^{\bullet+}{}_{\text{inhibition}} = \left[\frac{\text{Abs}_{\text{control}} - \text{Abs}_{\text{sample}}}{\text{Abs}_{\text{control}}}\right] \cdot 100 \quad (2)$$

where: $\text{Abs}_{\text{control}}$ is the absorbance of the control and $\text{Abs}_{\text{sample}}$ is the absorbance of the TLS sample.

2.6.2. DPPH$^{\bullet}$ Radical Scavenging Assay of TLS

TLS samples were analyzed by the 1,1–diphenyl-2 picrylhydrazyl (DPPH$^{\bullet}$) method. For this, 125 μL of TLS was mixed with 4875 μL of DPPH$^{\bullet}$ and allowed to rest for 30 min at 37 °C in the dark [27,28]. The control sample was prepared with 4875 μL of DPPH$^{\bullet}$ and 125 μL of absolute methanol. The absorbance value of the control solution used was 0.7 ± 0.02. The percentage inhibition of DPPH$^{\bullet}$ was determined at 514 nm using Equation (3).

$$\%\ \text{DPPH}^{\bullet}{}_{\text{inhibition}} = \left[\frac{\text{Abs}_{\text{control}} - \text{Abs}_{\text{sample}}}{\text{Abs}_{\text{control}}}\right] \cdot 100 \quad (3)$$

where: $\text{Abs}_{\text{control}}$ is the absorbance of the control and $\text{Abs}_{\text{sample}}$ is the absorbance of the TLS sample.

2.7. Detection of Total Phenolic Compounds (TPC) in TLS

One mL of TLS was added to a reaction mixture containing 1.6 mL of 7.5% sodium carbonate and 200 μL of Folin–Ciocalteu reagent. The reaction mixture was incubated at 25 °C for one hour in the absence of light and the absorbance at 760 nm was determined. The calibration curve was prepared with 5 to 25 (μg/mL) gallic acid.

2.8. Microstructure

The microstructure of the TLS was studied using transmission electron microscopy (TEM) with the Talos F200C G2 microscope (Thermo Scientific, Waltham, MA, USA). The samples were negatively stained to enhance contrast and then placed on a copper grid coated with Formvar/Carbon (300 mesh, 3 mm diameter HF 36). Subsequently, a 2% *w*/*v* uranyl acetate solution was added to the samples and allowed to rest for 1 min at 25 °C. Finally, the grids were air-dried in an oven (model LDO-150F, LabTech, Gwangju-si, Republic of Korea) at 25 °C for 30 min.

2.9. In Vitro Release of Tannins from Liposomes

The in vitro release of tannins was carried out following a methodology similar to that of Lopez-Polo et al. (2020), with some modifications, and using a simulated medium of ethanol–water fatty foods (50:50) according to EU Regulation No. 10/2011 [29]. The fatty food simulant was chosen for its accuracy in simulating contact conditions with fatty foods, aligning with our research on the future application of dairy derivatives and fatty foods. Additionally, this simulant has been used in other release studies to mimic fatty foods, thus endorsing its suitability for our purpose [30,31]. To do this, the TLS sample (2.5 mL) was incorporated into a dialysis bag (cellulose membrane with a molecular weight cut-off of 14,000 Da). The dialysis bag was immersed in the simulated medium (50 mL) and incubated at 37 °C, with constant shaking for 144 h [29,32]. Samples (2.5 mL) of the external medium were taken after 0, 0.08, 0.5, 1, 4, 8, 24, 48 and 144 h to quantify the concentration of released tannins by UHPLC and an equal volume of fresh medium was added to the system of dialysis. In this in vitro test, the FTS sample was used as a control. Subsequently, the in vitro release was determined through the percentage of cumulative release (%) calculated with Equation (4). Furthermore, during the in vitro release test, antioxidant activity was evaluated by $ABTS^{\bullet+}$ and $DPPH^{\bullet}$ assays, and TPC were quantified. In vitro release and antioxidant activity studies were performed in triplicate.

$$\text{Cumulative Release } (\%) = \left[\frac{[\text{T}] \cdot \text{factor dilution} \cdot \text{VR}}{[\text{T}] \text{ total}}\right] \cdot 100 \tag{4}$$

where: [T] is the initial concentration of tannins (μg/mL) in the liposomal suspension; VR is the volume of release medium (mL); T total is the total of tannins (μg).

TLS Thiolysis and UHPLC Quantification

To quantify the concentration of tannins from liposomes during in vitro release, they were depolymerized using acid thiolysis with cysteine, releasing their monomeric units of flavan-3-ol. Given that tannins are complex flavonoid polymers, analytical standards derived from grape seed tannins were employed, primarily composed of catechin (28.2%), epicatechin (8.8%), and gallic acid (1.3%) [2]. These predominant constituents allowed for the establishment of an indirect quantitative relationship regarding the tannin concentration present in the samples. To carry out thiolysis, the supernatant (200 μL) of the TLS sample was taken and mixed with the Cysteine-HCl-Methanol thiolysis medium (200 μL). Then, it was left to incubate for 1 h at 65 °C and the reaction was stopped with deionized water (1 mL). The analytical standards of catechin (5–100 μg/mL, R^2 = 0.999), epicatechin (10–100 μg/mL, R^2 = 0.999) and gallic acid (2.5–50 μg/mL, R^2 = 0.999) were quantified as measurement of tannins using UHPLC (Thermo Scientific Dionex UltiMate 3000). The UHPLC method conditions were based on the similar methodology by Bianchi et al. (2016), using a C18 column (5 μm, 250 × 4.6 mm, Perkin Elmer, Waltham, MA, USA) and a UV detector at 280 nm. The composition of Phase A was 0.1% trifluoroacetic acid (TFA) in deionized water and Phase B was 0.08% TFA in a 4/1 ratio of acetonitrile/deionized water at a mobile phase flow rate of 1 mL/min [33]. The FTS sample was used as a control during the test.

2.10. Preparation of Edible Films (EF)

Different biopolymer formulations were prepared using different concentrations of HPMC (2%, 3% and 4% *w*/*v*) and CMC (0.5, 1 and 2% *w*/*v*) according to preliminary tests carried out in our laboratory. The biopolymers were hydrated with deionized water and glycerol was added in different concentrations (20%, 30% and 40% *w*/*w* with respect to the biopolymer), for one hour with stirring at 90 °C until complete dissolution and cooled to 20 °C. Subsequently, one homogenization cycle with an Ultra-Turrax (IKA T18 digital, Guangzhou, China) was applied at 10,000 rpm for 5 min. The resulting mixture was degassed with an ultrasound bath (Elmasonic S30, Augsburg, Germany) for 15 min, applying three ultrasound cycles to remove air bubbles.

2.11. Physical Properties of EF

Density and Surface Tension

The density (ρ) of EF was measured at 20 °C using a pycnometer. The surface tension (γ) was determined using the pendant drop method according to Skurtys et al. (2011). Images of the drop shape were taken using a high-resolution optical system (Edmund Optics, NJ, USA) and the surface tension was determined from the fundamental Laplace equation. The solution of this equation was obtained with the Matlab 7.14 software (MathWorks, Inc., Natick, MA, USA) [34].

2.12. Preparation of Edible Films with Tannin-Containing Liposome Suspensions (EF/TLS)

According to the results obtained from density and surface tension measurements, the optimal concentrations of HPMC and CMC biopolymers for EF were selected, which were for HPMC (4% w/v HPMC with 33% w/w glycerol) and CMC (0.8% w/v CMC with 27% w/w glycerol). These optimal concentrations of EF formulations remained constant during the characterization of the edible films' physical, mechanical, and color properties. The optimal concentrations of HPMC and CMC were mixed with different concentrations of TLS to obtain edible films with tannin-containing suspensions (EF/TLS) with the following formulations (50:50), (60:40), (70:30), (80:20), and (90:10). These formulations were mixed using magnetic stirring for 15 min. Subsequently, one homogenization cycle with an Ultra-Turrax (IKA T18 digital, China) was applied at 10,000 rpm for 15 s. The resulting mixture was degassed with an ultrasound bath (Elmasonic S30, Germany) for 15 min, applying three cycles of ultrasound to remove air bubbles. The samples were stored and refrigerated (4 °C) until their measurements for four months.

2.13. Physical Properties of EF/TLS

Density and Surface Tension of EF/TLS

The density (ρ) and surface tension (γ) of EF/TLS were measured according to methodology described in Section "Density and Surface Tension".

2.14. EF/TLS Wettability Parameters

To determine the parameters associated with wettability, a smooth hydrophobic surface was used as a food simulant [35–37]. The hydrophobic surface was selected due to its high roughness and texture, as previously described by Monasterio et al. (2023), who reported surface roughness characteristics obtained through white light interferometry (WLI), utilizing a root mean square (RMS) roughness of 1.126 μm and a peak-to-valley difference of 6.933 μm [23]. This indicates that the hydrophobic surface exhibits high roughness and irregularities, providing relevant information on how films would behave in environments with similar surfaces. Subsequently, the contact angle (CA) was measured using the sessile drop method [38], on said hydrophobic surface, using a high-resolution optical system (Edmund Optics, Barrington, NJ, USA) and ImageJ software Version 1.8.0 (National Institutes of Health, Bethesda, MD, USA). A drop of the samples was deposited on the surface and photographs were taken in less than five seconds. The wettability parameters were calculated: work of adhesion (W_a), work of cohesion (W_c) and the spreading coefficient (S_{eq}), using Equations (5)–(7).

$$S_{eq} = W_a - W_c \tag{5}$$

$$W_a = \gamma_L \, (1 + Cos\,\theta) \tag{6}$$

$$W_C = 2\,\gamma \tag{7}$$

where: θ is the contact angle between the drop axis and the normal at the drop interface and γ is the surface tension of the liquid.

2.15. Mechanical Properties of EF/TLS

Tensile Test

For the measurement of mechanical properties, pieces of films were formed from the EF/TLS liquid formulations. To do this, the EF were placed on polystyrene plates and dried in an oven (Lab Tech LDO-150F, Republic of Korea) at 25 °C for 24 h and then placed in a desiccator at 58% relative humidity for 48 h. The solid films were cut into pieces of 80 × 25 mm^2 and the thickness (δ) was measured with a digital micrometer (Mitutoyo Co., Kawasaki shi, Japan). For the traction analysis, a texturometer (Zwick/Roell BDO-FBO.5T5, Ulm, Germany) was used with jaws separation of 60 mm (L_0) and a path speed of 10 mm/s. The tensile stress and strain were recorded, the slope of which corresponds to the elastic modulus (EM). These tensile parameters of tensile strength (TS) and percentage of elongation at break (EAB) were calculated with Equations (8) and (9).

$$TS = \frac{F_{max}}{A_t} \quad (8)$$

$$EAB\,(\%) = \frac{L_{max} - L_0}{L_{max}} \cdot 100 \quad (9)$$

where: F_{max} is the force at the elastic limit (N), A_t is the cross-sectional area of the sample (mm^2), L_{max} is the distance between the jaws at break (mm).

2.16. EF/TLS Color Parameters

The films were used to measure the color of the samples with a colorimeter (MiniScan XE Plus, Houston, TX, USA) that allows obtaining the parameters of L^*, a^* and b^*. Subsequently, the total color difference (ΔE) and the yellowness index (YI) were calculated using Equations (10) and (11).

$$\Delta E = \sqrt{(L* - L*_{ref})^2 + (a* - a*_{ref})^2 + (b* - b_{ref})^2} \quad (10)$$

$$YI = 142.86\left(\frac{b*}{L*}\right) \quad (11)$$

2.17. Statistical Analyzes

The experimental results were subjected to one-way analysis of variance (ANOVA) and Tukey's multiple comparison test using GraphPad Prism 8.01 statistical software (GraphPad software Inc. 8.01, San Diego, CA, USA). Statistical significance was statistically defined at a value of ($p < 0.05$). Microsoft Excel was used to calculate means and standard deviations. Figures were created using GraphPad Prism 8.01. To determine the optimal concentrations of EF, a multilevel factorial design was used, measuring the physical properties of density (ρ) and surface tension (γ) using the STATGRAPHICS Centurion XVI software (Version 16.2.03).

3. Results and Discussion

3.1. Particle Size, Polydispersity Index and Zeta Potential

The concentrations used and the heating/homogenization preparation method employed in this work allowed us to obtain liposome suspensions that encapsulate tannins, which were characterized by their physicochemical properties. Table 1 shows the results obtained for the particle size, polydispersity index and zeta potential of TLS, FTS and LS. It can be observed that the TLS presented an average size of 570.8 ± 6.0 nm, while for the LS a size of 126.8 ± 0.2 nm.

Table 1. Physicochemical properties of TLS, FTS and LS.

Analysis	TLS	FTS	LS
Mean particle size (nm)	570.8 ± 6.0 [a]		126.8 ± 0.2 [b]
Polydispersity index	0.56 ± 0.06 [a]		0.27 ± 0.01 [b]
Zeta potential (mV)	−37.9 ± 2.4 [a]		−30.1 ± 1.9 [b]
Encapsulation efficiency (% EE)			
(+)—Catechin	99.8 ± 0.01 [a]		
(−)—Epicatechin	99.7 ± 0.04 [a]		
Gallic acid	99.6 ± 0.06 [b]		
Antioxidant activity			
% ABTS$^{\bullet+}$ inhibition	60.0 ± 1.8 [a]	86.3 ± 0.4 [b]	7.1 ± 0.3 [c]
% DPPH$^{\bullet}$ inhibition	64.58 ± 0.6 [a]	74.28 ± 0.3 [b]	22.4 ± 0.5 [c]
TPC GAE (μg/mL)	185.6 ± 2.2 [a]	205.8 ± 3.7 [b]	48.4 ± 0.4 [c]

TLS: Suspension of liposomes containing tannins. FTS: Free tannin suspension. LS: Empty liposome suspension. Liposomes suspensions without tannins. ABTS$^{\bullet+}$: Percentage inhibition of 2,2′-azino-bis (3-ethylbenzothiazoline-6-sulfonic acid) radicals. DPPH$^{\bullet}$: Percentage inhibition of 1,1-diphenyl-2 picrylhydrazil. TPC: Total phenolic compounds. The mean of three replicates is shown. Letters a, b, c indicate significant differences between TLS, FTS, and LS.

These particle sizes are in the nanometer scale (30–1000 nm), which are favorable to achieve higher solubility, bioavailability and controlled release [39–41]. Other authors have reported sizes smaller than 309.9 ± 5.90 nm for liposomes prepared from soy phosphatidylcholine that encapsulate tannins from grape seed extracts, using the sonication heating/homogenization method. Sizes of 238.6 nm for liposomes prepared with phospholipids derived from soy and cholesterol, which encapsulate catechins from grape seed extracts using the reverse phase evaporation method were reported [2,42]. Furthermore, Chen et al. (2014) reported liposomes prepared with egg yolk phosphatidylcholine and cholesterol, which encapsulate catechins with larger size from 725.9 ± 23.9 to 1148.0 ± 87.9 nm using the reverse phase method [43]. These differences in particle size could be associated with the type of method and type of phospholipid used in the preparation of the liposomes, which can influence the stability and final size of the liposomes obtained [44]. In this way, the difference in particle size of the liposomes probably depends on the amount of mechanical force applied to the suspension, that is, when using a greater force, the particle size is reduced [45]. Furthermore, differences in liposome particle size have been observed when applying heating/homogenization and sonication, with some variations in the temperature [2], number of cycles and amplitude [23], as well as the buffer and bioactive used [29]. These methodological modifications could have significantly impacted the properties of the liposomes and consequently, the average particle sizes obtained [46]. Additionally, it has been demonstrated that prolonged ultrasound cycles can significantly affect the size of liposomes [47,48]; this could be attributed to the expansion effect of the lipid bilayer during prolonged sonication, thereby increasing the permeability of compounds encapsulated in the liposomes [48].

Significant differences ($p < 0.05$) were obtained between the polydispersity index values of TLS (0.56 ± 0.06) compared to LS (0.27 ± 0.01), indicating that TLS presented a more dispersed particle size distribution and less homogeneity. In previous studies, it has been suggested that this observation could be attributed to the ability of polyphenols to interact with the lipid membranes of liposomes, resulting in changes in their size and shape. These alterations may lead to more significant variability in particle size and contribute to a higher polydispersity index compared to empty liposomes [49].

Zeta potential is a key variable to evaluate the surface charge and determine the physical stability of liposomes. Table 1 shows the zeta potential value which was negatively charged, showing values of −37.9 ± 2.4 mV and −30.1 ± 1.9 mV for TLS and LS, respectively. These values indicate that the suspensions obtained can be considered stable, since there is a sufficient electrical charge to generate repulsion between the vesicles and avoid possible aggregation or fusion phenomena [50,51].

3.1.1. Encapsulation Efficiency (% EE)

The % EE was determined to quantify the ability to encapsulate tannins in liposomes using the heating and homogenization method employed in this work. The % EE values shown in Table 1 indicate that liposomes are efficient in encapsulating tannins (99.8 ± 0.01% for catechin; 99.7 ± 0.04% for epicatechin and 99.6 ± 0.06% for gallic acid); thus, they show a greater capacity to transport and protect these bioactive compounds inside. Other authors have reported % EE results that are much lower than those reported in this work [52–54]. The higher % EE values obtained in our work compared to the liposomes of other authors could be attributed to the liposome preparation technique used (heating and homogenization) with ultrasonication cycles, which has been shown to allow more stable liposomes with better encapsulation efficiency to be obtained [55]. Therefore, the application of ultrasound could be used to improve the % EE and the stability of a liposome loaded with the bioactive compound.

3.1.2. Antioxidant Activity and TPC

Table 1 shows the antioxidant activity of TLS, FTS and LS measured with the TPC, $ABTS^{\bullet+}$ and $DPPH^{\bullet}$ assays. The results demonstrated that FTS exhibited the highest total phenols and antioxidant activity, followed by TLS and LS. The TPC values were significantly ($p < 0.05$) higher for FTS (205.8 ± 3.7 GAE μg/mL) compared to TLS (185.6 ± 2.2 GAE μg/mL) and LS (48.4 ± 0.4 GAE μg/mL). The $ABTS^{\bullet+}$ and $DPPH^{\bullet}$ assay revealed significantly ($p < 0.05$) higher values for FTS ($ABTS^{\bullet+}$ = 86.3 ± 0.4% and $DPPH^{\bullet}$ = 74.28 ± 0.3%) compared to TLS ($ABTS^{\bullet+}$ = 60.0 ± 1.8% and $DPPH^{\bullet}$ = 64.58 ± 0.6%) and LS ($ABTS^{\bullet+}$ = 7.1 ± 0.3% and $DPPH^{\bullet}$ = 22.4 ± 0.5%). LS exhibited significantly lower values ($p < 0.05$) for TPC, $ABTS^{\bullet+}$ and $DPPH^{\bullet}$, and TPC parameters compared to TLS. These results of higher total phenols and antioxidant activity of FTS over TLS were anticipated because FTS (1 mg/mL) presents free tannins in suspension contrasting with TLS, which exhibited encapsulated tannins, as indicated by our % EE results, revealing a 99.8 ± 0.01% of catechin, 99.7 ± 0.04% of epicatechin, and 99.6 ± 0.06% of gallic acid. This is due to the fact that, in TLS, the tannins would be linked to active groups of the phospholipids of the liposomes, which reduces their availability to react with the free radicals present in the $ABTS^{\bullet+}$ and $DPPH^{\bullet}$ assay [2,56]. Olatunde et al. (2019) demonstrated that free extracts of ECHE (coconut shell extract), which contain the polyphenols tannic acid and catechin, exhibited higher antioxidant activity than liposomes encapsulating ECHE [57]. This is due to its greater availability to interact with $ABTS^{\bullet+}$ and $DPPH^{\bullet}$ radicals when ECHE is unencapsulated [53]. In addition to this interaction, it is crucial to consider possible losses caused by heating or exposure to light during the encapsulation process [58]. These factors can induce changes in the chemical structure of antioxidants, decreasing their capacity to neutralize free radicals. In contrast, LS (empty liposomes) had lower antioxidant activity than TLS. This decrease could be attributed to the presence of partially purified phosphatidylcholine (PC) used in the assembly of the liposomes, resulting in a limited intrinsic capacity of phospholipids to eliminate free radicals. These findings are consistent with those from previous studies on nanoliposomes loaded with catechin [59], quercetin [60], and curcumin [61].

3.2. Microstructure

The morphology of TLS and LS were analyzed using transmission electron microscopy (TEM). TEM images revealed that most prepared liposomes exhibited a semi-spherical vesicular and unilamellar structure (Figure 1). In Figure 1A, the TLS sample showed liposome vesicles with variations in their sizes, indicating a heterogeneous distribution. This finding aligns with the polydispersity index (PDI) presented in TLS (0.56 ± 0.06), indicating a broader size distribution. Additionally, the TLS sample (Figure 1B) displayed larger liposome sizes than LS (Figure 1C). These findings are consistent with the results obtained by mean particle size (MPS) analysis, where it was found that the MPS of TLS was larger than that of LS. These results are congruent with those reported for liposomes encapsulating soy protein hydrolysate [62] and liposomes encapsulating naringenin and trans-resveratrol [63], using a combined hydration and ultrasound method. Figure 1 allows for a comparison among treatments by means of their particle size.

3.3. *In Vitro* Release of Tannins from Liposomes

An in vitro tannin release study was carried out from TLS and FTS using dialysis bag methodology in a simulated fatty food medium for 144 h, with the primary purpose of investigating the stability of tannins and their release from the liposomes. Additionally, the aim was to understand how this release could be affected by environmental factors such as light, temperature, and antioxidant properties. Figure 2A shows that the percentages of cumulative release of catechins released from liposomes are significantly ($p < 0.05$) lower in TLS compared to FTS from the first hour of the in vitro test. The TLS sample reached a maximum release of 0.13 ± 0.01% of catechin after 24 h, maintaining that same release for 144 h, unlike FTS, which reached a maximum release of catechin of 0.41 ± 0.01% after 24 h and remained constant until 144 h. Regarding the releases of epicatechin (Figure 2B) and gallic acid (Figure 2C), they were significantly ($p < 0.05$) lower for TLS compared to FTS after the 24 h of study. It was observed that in TLS a maximum epicatechin release of 0.57 ± 0.01% was reached after 48 h of the study and remained constant for up to 144 h, unlike FTS which reached a maximum epicatechin release of 0.70 ± 0.02% after 144 h. In the case of gallic acid it was 3.90 ± 0.001% after 144 h, unlike FTS whose maximum release was 4.48 ± 0.02% after 144 h. These results indicate that the release rate of tannins encapsulated in liposomes was slower compared to the release rate of free tannins. This suggests that tannins encapsulated in liposomes have a lower release than non-encapsulated tannins. Because the encapsulated tannins would be contained in the liposome membrane, which generates a tortuous path for the passage of the active compound, they cannot be released quickly since they must pass through the entire liposomal bilayer before interacting with the medium abroad. Furthermore, this decrease in the release rate of tannins encapsulated in liposomes can also be attributed to the fact that polyphenol–phospholipid interactions would be occurring through hydrogen bonds [64,65]. The slower release of bioactive compounds, such as polyphenols, may improve their effectiveness as antioxidants by maintaining a constant release of bioactive compounds into the food over a longer period of time, which could extend the shelf life of the food [66]. This behavior is consistent with other studies that have found that liposomes offer greater affinity and protection to antioxidants, resulting in a slower release of these to the medium [67–70].

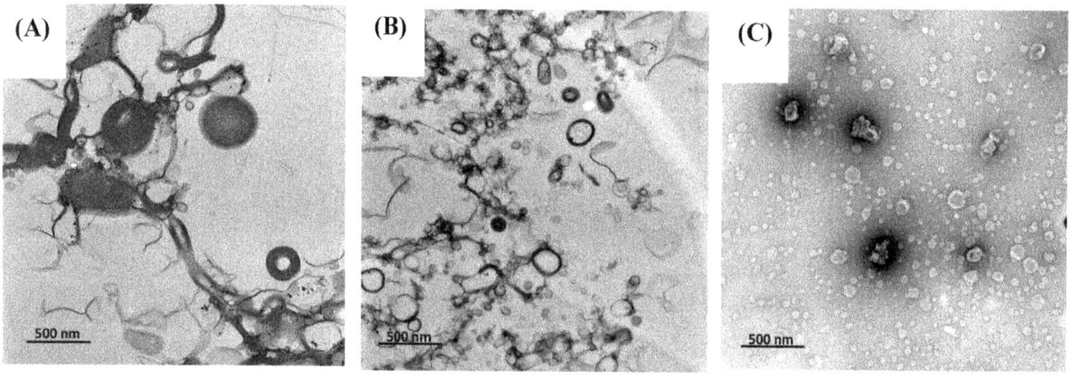

Figure 1. Transmission electron microscopy (TEM) microstructure (**A**,**B**) of TLS and (**C**) LS, magnified 17,500×.

During the in vitro release test, antioxidant activity ($ABTS^{\bullet+}$ and $DPPH^{\bullet}$) and TPC were measured in TLS compared to FTS. Figure 3A,B show that antioxidant activity values ($ABTS^{\bullet+}$ and $DPPH^{\bullet}$) were significantly ($p < 0.05$) higher in FTS compared to TLS from 24 h. Similarly, in Figure 3C, it was obtained that the quantification of TPC values is significantly ($p < 0.05$) higher in FTS compared to TLS from 8 h. These results suggest that encapsulation of tannins in liposomes could protect antioxidants and maintain their properties in the long term. Therefore, liposomes could be efficient as a protective vesicle against oxidative damage by creating a barrier that separates them from external conditions such as oxygen and/or pH changes [71,72]. Likewise, these results suggest that liposomes could be good nanovehicles for bioactive compounds during digestion since they could increase the bioavailability of antioxidants, by protecting them against the acids that are produced in the chemical digestive process, and therefore could ensure that these reached the absorption process in the intestine [73,74].

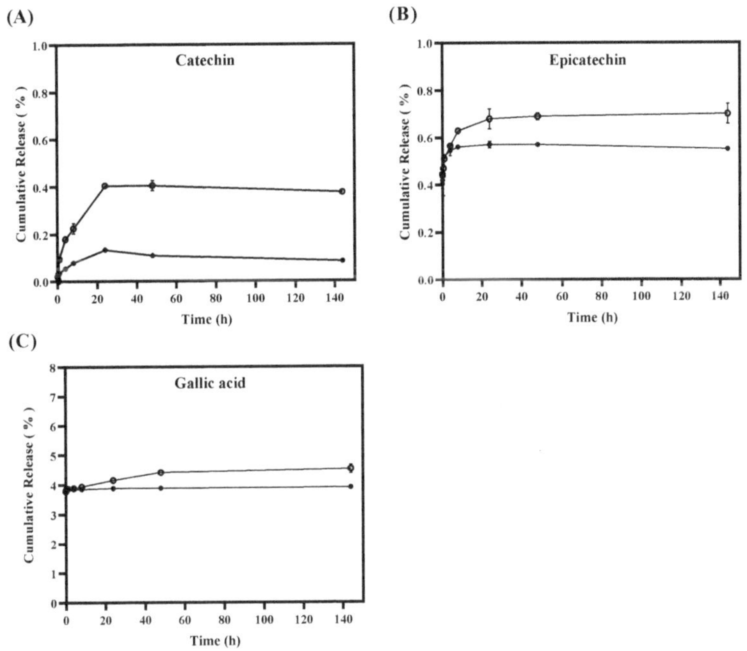

Figure 2. In vitro release of tannins from liposomes TLS (•) and tannins from free suspensions FTS (○) for 144 h by quantifying the cumulative release (%) of (**A**) catechin, (**B**) epicatechin and (**C**) gallic acid.

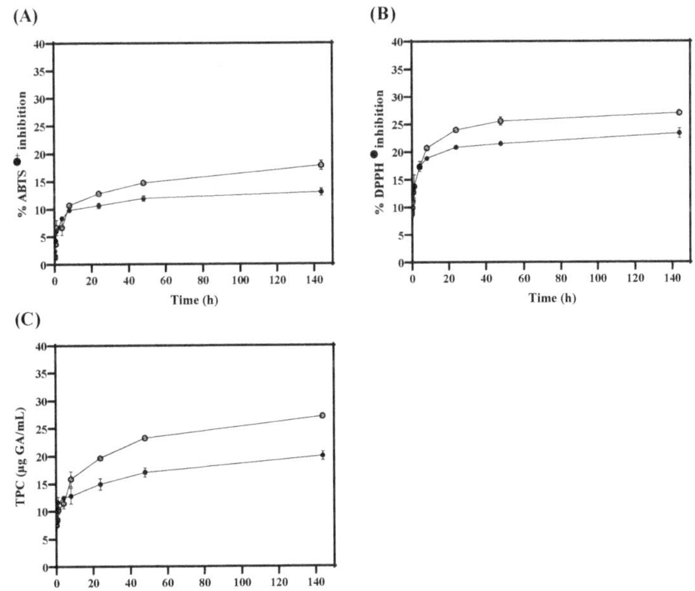

Figure 3. Antioxidant activity and total phenolic compounds of TLS (•) and FTS (○) obtained with the (**A**) $ABTS^{\bullet+}$, (**B**) $DPPH^{\bullet}$ and (**C**) TPC assays during in vitro tannin release.

Based on the characterization results of the physicochemical parameters of TLS, liposomes with semi-spherical vesicular morphology and nanometric size were observed, which were maintained after the encapsulation of grape seed tannins (% EE of 99.8 ± 0.01% for catechin, 99.7 ± 0.04% for epicatechin, and 99.6 ± 0.06% for gallic acid). Additionally, TLS exhibited lower antioxidant activity than FTS, suggesting greater protection and transport for the bioactive compound. Finally, it was found that TLS showed much slower release than FTS, maintaining its antioxidant properties for 144 h, which could protect the antioxidants and maintain their long-term properties during their food release compared to FTS. Therefore, we have chosen not to use FTS due to its low stability. Instead, we have chosen to work exclusively with TLS for the study of the physical and mechanical properties of the edible films in this study.

3.4. Physical Properties of EF/TLS

The TLS were mixed homogeneously with the formulation of the EF, which presented desirable characteristics for their subsequent application in food systems and did not present agglomerations or phase separation over 4 months, as can be observed in Figure 5B. The concentrations of biopolymers used in this study (HPMC and CMC) were selected using a multilevel factorial design that included 18 samples, for which 3 different combinations of biopolymer (2, 3 and 4% *w*/*v*) and glycerol (20, 30 and 40% *w*/*w*) (see Supplemental Table S1) using Statgraphics Centurion XVI software (V16.1.03). To select the optimal concentrations of EF, it was carried out by measuring the density and surface tension with a criterion of maximum values [23], since by increasing the density and surface tension the films could achieve a lower porosity [75] and, therefore, reduce the release values of the bioactive compound [76], which is desired in this work. The optimal concentrations of EF for HPMC were 4% *w*/*v* of HPMC with 33% *w*/*w* of glycerol in its formulation, and for CMC, they were 0.8% *w*/*v* of CMC with 27% *w*/*w* of glycerol. These two EF formulations remained constant, while liposome concentrations varied in different formulations (EF/TLS). Furthermore, to study EF physical properties, we chose to continue our study only with TLS due to the previously described results, which demonstrated better protection of the bioactive compound and slower release compared to FTS, as discussed in Section 3.3. The FTS sample was not used due to its low stability, which ruled it out for application in the physical and mechanical properties of EF/TLS.

3.5. Surface Tension and EF/TLS Density

EF/TLS were characterized by their physical properties. Table 2 shows the results obtained for the density and surface tension of the EF. It can be seen that, when incorporating liposomes into the EF formulation, the density values were significantly ($p < 0.05$) lower compared to the control film that did not have liposomes in its formulation. The formulation (70:30) of HPMC with tannin-containing liposome suspensions (HPMC/TLS) and 80:20 of CMC with tannin-containing liposome suspensions (CMC/TLS) reached the lowest density values being 1039.65 ± 1.3 kg/m^3, and 1014.4 ± 2.1 kg/m^3, respectively. Ghadermazi et al. (2019) reported that decreasing the density in EF increases the droplet size and apparent viscosity, which can affect the final thickness of the solid EF and reduce their stiffness. These authors suggest that the film density can be controlled and reduced using low-density essential oils to the HPMC suspension [77].

Table 2. Values of density and surface tension of EF/TLS.

Sample EF/TLS	ρ (kg/m³) at 20 °C		γ (mN/m)	
	HPMC/TLS	CMC/TLS	HPMC/TLS	CMC/TLS
Control (100:0)	1078.8 ± 0.7 ax	1042.1 ± 0.6 ay	47.9 ± 0.7 ax	74.5 ± 0.4 ay
(50:50)	1040.0 ± 1.4 bx	1019.4 ± 0.8 by	46.2 ± 0.5 abx	65.1 ± 1.4 bcy
(60:40)	1047.6 ± 1.3 bcx	1023.5 ± 0.7 bcy	42.4 ± 1.0 bcx	62.4 ± 1.2 by
(70:30)	1039.6 ± 1.3 bx	1027.5 ± 0.8 cy	39.2 ± 0.5 cx	64.5 ± 0.2 by
(80:20)	1052.0 ± 1.4 cx	1014.4 ± 2.1 dy	43.5 ± 1.9 bx	68.0 ± 1.5 cy
(90:10)	1049.2 ± 4.7 cx	1034.9 ± 4.7 ey	41.0 ± 0.7 bcx	68.1 ± 1.3 cy

EF: Edible films. EF/TLS: Edible films with tannin-containing liposome suspensions. HPMC/TLS: Hydroxypropylmethylcellulose (HPMC) with tannin-containing liposome suspensions. CMC/TLS: Carboxymethylcellulose (CMC) with tannin-containing liposome suspensions. ρ: density. γ: surface tension. The mean of three replicates is shown. Letters a, b, c, d, and e indicate significant concentration differences between EF/TLS. Letters x and y indicate significant differences between HPMC/TLS and CMC/TLS.

Therefore, lower density values with these EF formulations could reduce the stiffness of the films, allowing better adaptability of the film to the food surface.

Similarly, to the density, the presence of liposomes caused a significant decrease ($p < 0.05$) in surface tension, compared to the control. The 70:30 HPMC/TLS and 60:40 CMC/TLS formulations reached the lowest surface tension values of 39.2 ± 0.5 mN/m and 62.4 ± 0.5 mN/m, respectively. Other authors have shown that reducing surface tension increases wettability and improves the ability of films to adhere to food surfaces, favoring their protection and appearance [18,78,79]. These results are consistent in the literature, where it has been shown that liposomes made with soy lecithin decrease surface tension [80,81]. For example, Jiménez et al. (2014) incorporated soy lecithin nanoliposomes encapsulating orange essential oil and limonene to suspensions of 50:50 sodium caseinate and starch films and observed that the addition of nanoliposomes always decreased the surface tension compared to control [82]. Soy lecithin acts as an amphiphilic surfactant agent, meaning that it has a hydrophilic and a hydrophobic part [83]. When added to an aqueous solution, the lecithin molecules are oriented in such a way that the hydrophilic part is directed towards the water and the hydrophobic part is directed away from it, reducing the surface tension of the suspension, which translates into needing less energy to break the surface [17]. Furthermore, the presence of polyunsaturated fatty acids such as linoleic acid present in soy lecithin can also contribute to the reduction of surface tension [84,85]. Therefore, in this study, the decrease in surface tension could be explained because the liposomes were prepared from phosphatidylcholine that was partially purified from soy lecithin and still contains traces of soy lecithin components, such as polyunsaturated fatty acids in formulations.

3.6. EF/TLS Wettability Parameters

Wettability refers to the ability of a liquid to spread over a solid surface and is a key factor to consider in the formulation of EF, since it influences their ability to adhere and cover the surface of the food [86]. The wettability parameters of EF/TLS used in this study were measured by the contact angle method (θ), the work of adhesion (W_a), the work of cohesion (W_c) and the spreading coefficient (S_{eq}) on a hydrophobic surface. The hydrophobic surface selected for the study was utilized for its high roughness and irregular texture, aiming to simulate hydrophobic surfaces resembling those found in fatty dairy products [23]. Figure 4 shows that the contact angles (θ) formed between the droplets of the different EF/TLS formulations and the hydrophobic surface are less than 90°, indicating that the EF/TLS formulations moisturize partially the surface ($0 < \theta < 90$) [87]. Furthermore, it can be observed that, when incorporating TLS into the EF, the contact angle values are significantly ($p < 0.05$) lower compared to the control without liposomes. These results indicate that the addition of liposomes in the EF formulation causes a significant decrease in the contact angle with the surface, therefore, the liposomes could increase the affinity of the film with the food surface. Similar results were reported by Sapper et al. (2019), who studied soy lecithin liposomes encapsulating thyme essential oil (EO) in starch-gellan (80:20) coatings on the surfaces of apples and persimmons; their study demonstrated that the contact angle values (θ) decreased when incorporating the essential oils encapsulated in nanoliposomes in the coating, being lower than 90°, indicating surface wettability and greater extensibility of the coating on the surface of the fruits [88]. Furthermore, it has been reported that the contact angle is a property that also depends on the surface tension of the liquid and generally the contact angle decreases as the surface tension decreases, indicating better wettability of the solid surface by the liquid [17,89,90]. Considering the surface tension values obtained in this work for the EF/TLS formulations and discussed in Section 3.4, it would be reasonable to expect a decrease in the contact angle when incorporating liposomes in the EF, which could improve the adhesion of the films to the hydrophobic surface. These results are positive since they improve and favor the application of these films on different food surfaces.

The wettability of a film on the food surface is determined by an energy balance between Wa and Wc [91]. The Wa corresponds to the energy necessary for the liquid to spread over the surface of the food, while the Wc is a measure of the force of attraction between the molecules of a liquid, which causes contraction of the drop on the surface [38, 92]. These two factors are crucial to achieve proper adhesion and prevent film peeling. Table 3 shows that the values of Wa and Wc for EF/TLS decrease significantly ($p < 0.05$) compared to the control in both EF, which indicates that the presence of liposomes in the EF produces a decrease in the values of Wa and Wc on the hydrophobic surface. In the case of HPMC/TLS, the 70:30 formulation presented the lowest values of W_a (72.9 $\pm$ 1.1 mN/m) and W_c (78.3 $\pm$ 1.0 mN/m) in relation to the control. While in CMC/TLS, the 90:10 formulation showed the lowest values of W_a (105.8 $\pm$ 0.4 mN/m) and the 60:40 formulation presented the lowest values of W_c (126.1 $\pm$ 1.4 mN/m) on the surface.

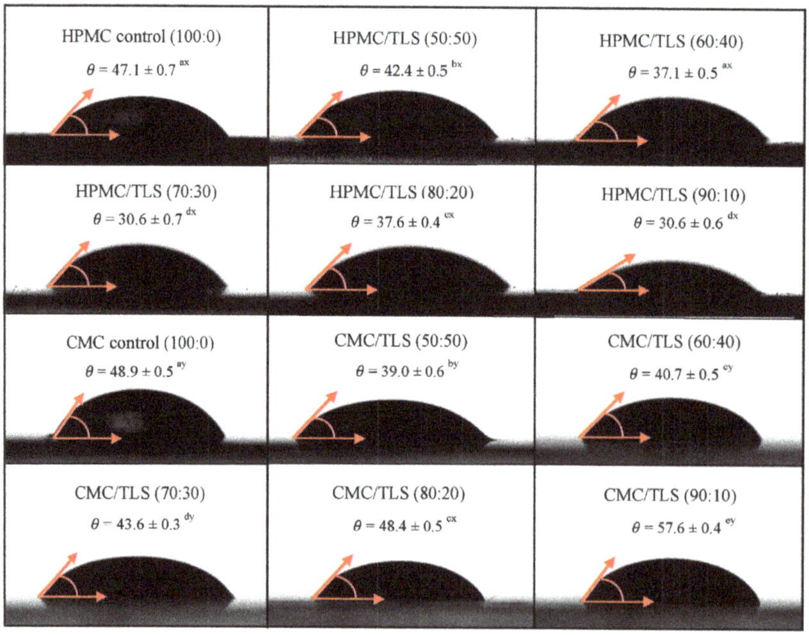

Figure 4. Contact angle between the hydrophobic surface and EF/TLS. (Letters a, b, c, d, and e indicate significant differences in concentrations between EF/TLS. Letters x and y indicate significant differences between HPMC/TLS and CMC/TLS).

Table 3. Wettability parameters on hydrophobic surface of EF/TLS.

Sample EF/TLS	Wa (mN/m)		Wc (mN/m)		Seq (mN/m)	
	HPMC/TLS	CMC/TLS	HPMC/TLS	CMC/TLS	HPMC/TLS	CMC/TLS
Control (100:0)	80.5 ± 0.3 ^{ax}	123.4 ± 0.7 ^{ay}	95.7 ± 0.7 ^{ax}	148.9 ± 0.9 ^{ay}	−15.3 ± 0.0 ^{ax}	−25.6 ± 0.3 ^{ay}
(50:50)	80.3 ± 0.8 ^{ax}	117.1 ± 0.8 ^{by}	92.4 ± 0.9 ^{ax}	131.9 ± 0.4 ^{by}	−12.1 ± 0.2 ^{bx}	−14.5 ± 0.4 ^{by}
(60:40)	76.2 ± 1.8 ^{abx}	110.8 ± 0.9 ^{cy}	84.8 ± 2.0 ^{bx}	126.1 ± 1.4 ^{cy}	−8.6 ± 0.3 ^{cx}	−15.1 ± 0.6 ^{by}
(70:30)	72.9 ± 1.1 ^{bx}	111.2 ± 0.2 ^{cy}	78.3 ± 1.0 ^{cx}	129.0 ± 0.5 ^{dy}	−5.4 ± 0.1 ^{dx}	−17.8± 0.2 ^{cy}
(80:20)	77.9 ± 3.6 ^{abx}	114.5 ± 0.9 ^{dy}	86.9 ± 3.9 ^{abx}	137.6 ± 0.7 ^{ey}	−9.0 ± 0.3 ^{cx}	−22.9 ± 0.4 ^{dy}
(90:10)	76.2 ± 0.1 ^{abx}	105.8 ± 0.4 ^{ey}	81.9 ± 1.4 ^{bcx}	137.8 ± 0.2 ^{ey}	−5.7 ± 0.1 ^{dx}	−31.6 ± 0.7 ^{ey}

Wa: Adhesion work. Wc: Cohesion work. Seq: Spreading coefficient. The mean of three replicates is shown. Letters a, b, c, d, and e indicate significant concentration differences between EF/TLS. Letters x and y indicate significant differences between HPMC/TLS and CMC/TLS.

These results could be favorable for the applications of fatty foods such as dairy derivatives, since they indicate that films with the addition of liposomes easily adhere to surfaces, allowing them to spread and not contract [38]. However, it is crucial to consider the variability among different types of fatty foods and the impact of surface roughness on adhesion [11]. In previous studies it has already been shown that, to obtain better films, a film formulation with low cohesive energy (W_c) should be selected to obtain better adhesion between the film suspension and the food surface [17,93]. Lopez-Polo et al. (2020) demonstrated that the presence of liposomes and cellulose nanofibers decrease the cohesive work (W_c) of HPMC, which partially hydrates the almond and chocolate surfaces, since they showed contact angles less than 90° [29]. Therefore, the incorporation of liposomes in the films could improve their adhesion and cohesion capacity and their effectiveness as a protective film, since it would have good adhesion on hydrophobic type surfaces without detaching or sliding. In this sense, our film could have a good application on foods such as dairy products (cheese) and fats in general.

In this study, wettability was also evaluated using the Seq, which indicates the ability of a liquid to spread over a solid surface, with the values closest to zero being the most suitable for coating the surface [94]. Table 3 presents the Seq values of the EF/TLS on the hydrophobic surface. It is observed that for the HPMC/TLS EF, the 70:30 formulation presented the best Seq values, (−5.4 ± 0.1 mN/m), followed by the 90:10 formulation (−5.7 ± 0.1 mN/m), which presented significant differences ($p < 0.05$) compared to the control. In the CMC/TLS case, it was observed that the 50:50 formulations on the food surface presented the best Seq values, (−14.5 ± 0.4 mN/m), followed by the 60:40 formulation (−15.1 ± 0.6 mN/m), which showed significant differences ($p < 0.05$) compared to the control. These results indicate that HPMC/TLS and CMC/TLS formulations have greater spreading and coverage capacity on the food surface compared to formulations that do not contain liposomes. This suggests that liposomes can improve the effectiveness and functionality of films by facilitating better wettability and uniform distribution over the food surface.

3.7. Mechanical Properties of EF/TLS

Tensile Test

Mechanical properties are used to evaluate the resistance of EFs to maintain and protect foods against physical and mechanical stress during transportation, storage and distribution [95]. In the mechanical properties of the EF/TLS, it is sought that they have adequate flexibility to adapt to the possible deformation of the food during storage without breaking, and, in addition, that they present a high tensile strength and adequate stretch to cover the food [96,97]. Table 4 shows the mechanical properties of the EF/TLS through tensile strength (TS), percentage of elongation at break (EAB) and elastic modulus (EM). The TS refers to the maximum stress supported by the solid films before breaking and EAB indicates the maximum elongation of the solid films before breaking [96]. EM is defined as the ability of a material to resist deformation under tensile stress [98]. In the case of

HPMC/TLS, the addition of liposomes caused the values of TS, EAB and EM to decrease significantly ($p < 0.05$) compared to the control.

Table 4. Mechanical properties and color of EF/TLS.

EF	Sample	TS (MPa)	EAB (%)	EM (MPa)	Δ *E*	YI
HPMC/TLS	Control (100:0)	22.0 ± 1.0 ^{ax}	8.4 ± 0.0 ^{ax}	1002.0 ± 0.5 ^{ax}	-	3.1 ± 0.5 ^{ax}
	(50:50)	6.3 ± 0.1 ^{bx}	2.9 ± 0.1 ^{bx}	261.4 ± 0.5 ^{bx}	22.4 ± 1.2 ^{ax}	36.6 ± 1.8 ^{bx}
	(60:40)	10.7 ± 0.2 ^{cx}	3.8 ± 0.1 ^{bx}	540.3 ± 0.9 ^{cx}	18.8 ± 0.9 ^{bx}	30.7 ± 1.2 ^{cx}
	(70:30)	17.1 ± 0.1 ^{ax}	6.2 ± 0.0 ^{cx}	692.6 ± 0.8 ^{dx}	13.1 ± 0.9 ^{cx}	22.0 ± 1.3 ^{dx}
	(80:20)	16.7 ± 0.6 ^{ax}	6.6 ± 0.3 ^{cx}	762.9 ± 0.9 ^{ex}	14.2 ± 0.3 ^{cx}	23.8 ± 0.4 ^{dx}
	(90:10)	26.7 ± 0.0 ^{dx}	8.7 ± 0.0 ^{ax}	953.7 ± 0.3 ^{fx}	9.5 ± 0.7 ^{dx}	17.0 ± 1.0 ^{ex}
CMC/TLS	Control (100:0)	19.0 ± 0.8 ^{ax}	2.1 ± 0.1 ^{ay}	891.3 ± 2.7 ^{ay}	-	2.5 ± 0.2 ^{ax}
	(50:50)	0.9 ± 0.5 ^{bx}	25.4 ± 1.1 ^{by}	0.10 ± 0.0 ^{by}	21.5 ± 0.4 ^{ax}	35.5 ± 0.8 ^{bx}
	(60:40)	1.6 ± 0.4 ^{by}	24.9 ± 0.7 ^{by}	0.12 ± 0.0 ^{by}	20.5 ± 0.9 ^{ay}	33.1 ± 1.0 ^{cy}
	(70:30)	14.9 ± 1.9 ^{abx}	16.5 ± 1.0 ^{cy}	24.2 ± 0.0 ^{cy}	11.3 ± 0.4 ^{by}	19.4 ± 0.5 ^{dy}
	(80:20)	7.6 ± 0.0 ^{by}	11.8 ± 0.2 ^{dy}	111.7 ± 0.3 ^{dy}	9.2 ± 0.5 ^{cy}	16.0 ± 0.7 ^{ey}
	(90:10)	19.4 ± 1.6 ^{bx}	3.8 ± 0.1 ^{ey}	774.2 ± 0.3 ^{ey}	4.5 ± 0.3 ^{dy}	8.9 ± 0.5 ^{fy}

TS: Tensile strength. EAB: Percentage elongation at break. EM: Modulus of elasticity. ΔE: Total color difference. YI: Yellowness index. The mean of three replicates is shown. Letters a, b, c, d, e, and f indicate significant differences between EF/TLS concentrations. Letters x and y indicate significant differences between HPMC/TLS and CMC/TLS.

Furthermore, it was observed that the TS and EAB values were similar for the 70:30 (TS = 17.1 ± 0.1 MPa, EAB = 6.2 ± 0.0%) and 80:20 (TS = 16.7 ± 0.6 MPa, EAB = 6.6) formulations. This indicates that the incorporation of liposomes into HPMC would lead to having lower tensile strength and lower stretch before breakage. Regarding the EM values, it was found that the 70:30 formulation presented significantly ($p < 0.05$) lower values (EM = 6.6 ± 0.3 MPa) compared to the 80:20 formulations (EM = 692.6 ± 0.8 MPa). These results would indicate that the 70:30 formulations would present more flexible characteristics, this being an important quality for the application of films on foods. Our results were in agreement with what was reported by Imran et al. (2012), who studied HPMC films containing nanoliposomes prepared from soy lecithin, which encapsulate nisin, and who observed that the addition of nanoliposomes produced a reduction in interchain links in polymer matrices, and as a result, a decrease in TS (37.0 ± 2.5 MPa) and EM (2228 ± 657 MPa) compared to the control (TS = 59.0 ± 6.8 MPa and EM = 2727 ± 361 MPa) [99]. These results attributed this to the fact that the incorporation of soy lecithin leads to more flexible and less resistant films to breakage [99]. Similarly, De Simone et al. (2020) reported that when adding soy L-α-phosphatidylcholine (PC) liposomes to a HPMC polymer matrix, they found similar TS values of 14.0–16.71 MPa and it was found that the different concentrations of liposomes (1% and 5%) do not significantly affect the particle size and fluidity, but they do present a lower rigidity of the biopolymer [100]. Therefore, the addition of liposomes to edible films could decrease the tensile strength due to their spherical structure and the surface charges of the liposomes that can interact with the functional groups present in the biopolymers of the films, which could affect intermolecular forces by increasing their deformation capacity [101].

Table 4 shows that in the case of CMC/TLS for most formulations, the addition of liposomes significantly decreased ($p < 0.05$) the TS and EM values and presented a significant increase ($p < 0.05$) in EAB values compared to the control. However, the 90:10 formulation presented a significant increase ($p < 0.05$) in the values of TS (19.4 ± 1.6 MPa) and EAB (3.8 ± 0.1%), and a significant decrease ($p < 0.05$) in the values of EM (774.2 ± 0.3 MPa) compared to the control, which would indicate that in this formulation the presence of liposomes showed a positive effect on mechanical resistance, flexibility and with greater rigidity compared to the control without liposomes. Mirzaei-Mohkam et al. (2020) reported that the addition of liposomes prepared with lecithin that encapsulate α-tocopherol (70%) in CMC films significantly decreased ($p < 0.05$) the values of TS (23.1 MPa) and EM (41.2 MPa) compared to the control (TS = 37.0 MPa, EM = 113.9 MPa). While the EAB (52.9%) increased significantly ($p < 0.05$) compared to the control (EAB = 32.3%) [102]. These results were mainly attributed to the structure of lecithin, which can affect the uniformity of the EF, and therefore cause a decrease in the TS and EM values, resulting in softer films [102]. Furthermore, Marín-Peñalver et al. (2019) prepared CMC films containing nanoliposomes loaded with a collagen hydrolysate, prepared with soy phosphatylcholine, and showed that TS (4.2 ± 0.8 MPa) decreases significantly ($p < 0.05$) in the presence of liposomes, when glycerol is added as a plasticizer, and they found an EAB of 50%, which contributes to increasing its elongation and flexibility [103]. Therefore, the behavior of different EF matrices with the addition of nanoliposomes may depend on the nature of the biopolymer, and the most appropriate one can be selected according to the need for protection, release or biological activity of the encapsulated compound.

Our tensile test results indicated that the TS and EM values in the CMC/TLS formulations were significantly ($p < 0.05$) lower compared to HPMC/TLS, indicating that CMC/TLS films are softer and have lower mechanical resistance. Furthermore, CMC/TLS formulations presented EAB values that are significantly ($p < 0.05$) higher compared to HPMC/TLS. Therefore, the results indicate that HPMC EF would have better tensile strength properties and greater stretchability without breaking, which could improve the quality and durability of the final product [104].

3.8. EF/TLS Color Parameters

Color is a fundamental characteristic in edible films for food, as it influences consumer perception and acceptability of the final food product. HPMC and CMC correspond to biopolymers that form transparent and colorless films; however, by incorporating specific materials into the formulation, such as glycerol, phospholipids, bioactive compounds, etc., the color properties of the resulting films can be affected [77]. Table 4 shows the results of the total color difference (ΔE) and yellowness index (YI) of EF/TLS. When TLS were incorporated into the EF, the ΔE and YI values increased significantly ($p < 0.05$) compared to the control that did not have liposomes in its formulation. The above indicates that there is a perceptible color difference and an increase in yellow color in the samples with liposomes compared to the control sample. However, as there is a lower concentration of TLS in the formulations, the values of ΔE and YI decrease significantly ($p < 0.05$). These results could indicate that, with a lower concentration of TLS, the perceptible color change in the films is reduced, which could be relevant for adjusting formulations according to desired color preferences. In HPMC/TLS, ranges of ΔE (9.5–22.4) and YI (17.0–36.6) values were presented and in the case of CMC/TLS, ranges of ΔE (4.5–21.5) and YI (8.9–35.5) were observed. These colors were in agreement with liposomes prepared with soy lecithin in chitosan/zein films (ΔE = 21.4–30.4) [105] and CMC (ΔE = 8.38 ± 0.54) [102], as well as the incorporation of sage leaf (SLE) and nettle (NLE) extracts at 15% with HPMC/chitosan films (ΔE SLE = 18.3 ± 1.1 and ΔE NLE = 22.2 ± 1.0) [106]. In Figure 5, the different formulations of HPMC/TLS and CMC/TLS can be observed, highlighting a more intense light brown or beige hue in the formulations with higher TLS concentration. Additionally, it is observed that as the concentration of TLS decreases, the coloration becomes more transparent and colorless. These differences in the color of liposome-containing films regarding the control (without liposomes), are due to the fact that the liposomes prepared in this work contain soy phosphatidylcholine which has a light-yellow color, in the same way the grape tannins that were used as encapsulated polyphenol also have a brown color. Therefore, when incorporating these into the EF, their color properties are modified. These findings underscore the importance of assessing how the use of liposomes affects the color properties in edible films; this could have significant implications in ingredient selection and formulation optimization to ensure the acceptability of the product.

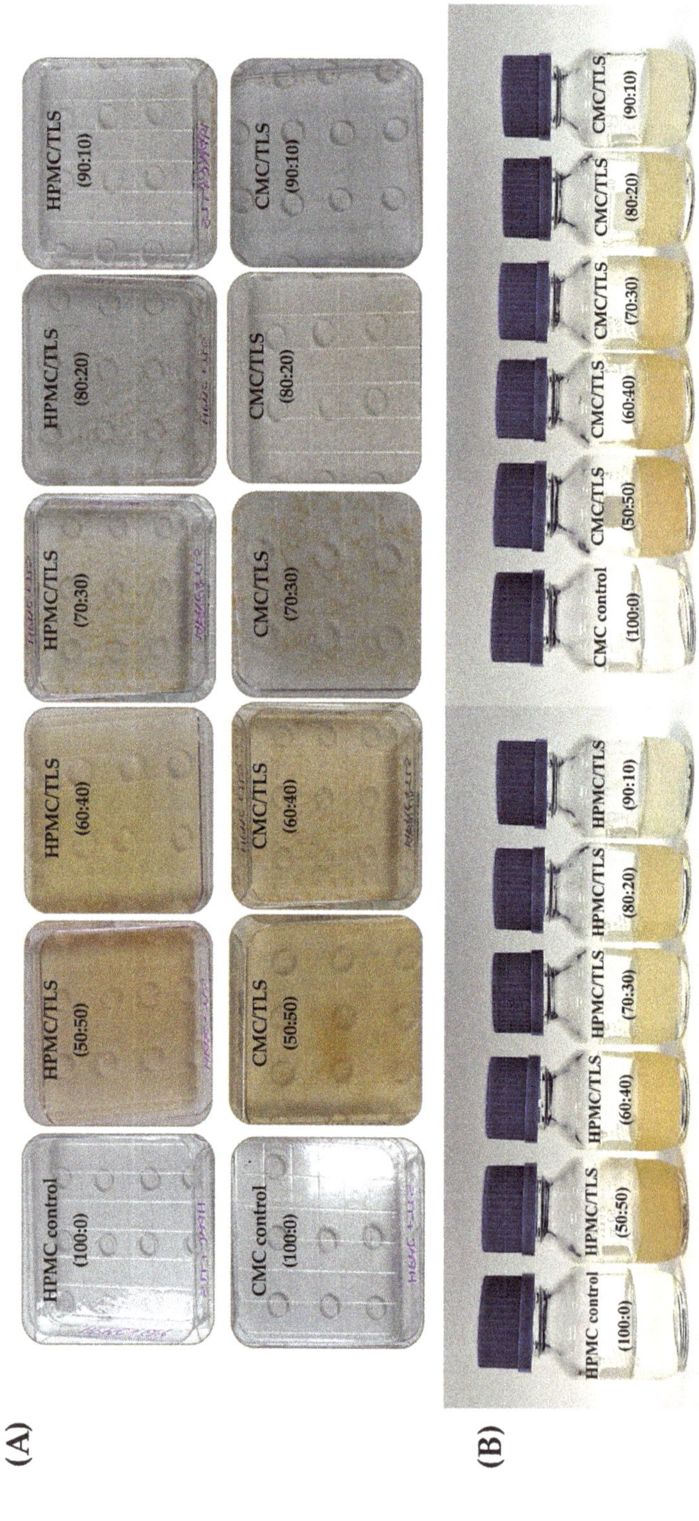

Figure 5. Images of the films produced from EF/TLS (**A**) and the preparation of EF/TLS formulations after 4 months (**B**).

4. Conclusions

In this research work, it was possible to obtain liposomes that are stable, encapsulate grape seed tannins with a nanometric size (570.8 ± 6.0 nm), and that demonstrate a high encapsulation efficiency of the active compound (99%), maintaining a semi-spherical structure. The values obtained for the analyses of antioxidant activity by $ABTS^{\bullet+}$ and $DPPH^{\bullet}$ were lower for tannins in liposomes, which suggests that encapsulation protects tannins and prevents them from reacting with free radicals; therefore, encapsulation in liposomes could protect antioxidants against external conditions (O_2, pH, temperature, etc.). Furthermore, we also found that the in vitro release rate of tannins from liposomes was slower than free tannins during the 144 h study, indicating that encapsulation in liposomes could improve the antioxidant efficacy of tannins for a longer period. This would help extend the shelf life of the foods on which the suspensions are applied. The suspensions of tannins encapsulated in liposomes were successfully added to the formulation of edible films, and no phase separation or agglomerations occurred for 4 months. Through studies of the wettability properties of the films, it was found that the addition of liposomes to the formulation caused a significant decrease in density, surface tension and contact angle values; this means that the liposome film partially moistens the hydrophobic surface studied, causing it to spread and not contract when applied, which could favor the protection and appearance of hydrophobic foods on which the film is applied.

Supplementary Materials: The following supporting information can be downloaded at: https://www.mdpi.com/article/10.3390/antiox13080989/s1, Table S1. Experimental design for density and surface tension of EF of HPMC/Gly and CMC/Gly at different concentration.

Author Contributions: Conceptualization, F.A.O.; methodology, F.A.O.; validation, J.L.-P. and C.V.; investigation, J.L.-P. and F.A.O.; project administration and resources, F.A.O.; supervision, F.A.O.; Final writing—review and editing, F.A.O. and J.L.-P.; data curation, C.V.; formal analysis, J.L.-P., F.A.O. and C.V.; writing—original draft, J.L.-P. and C.V.; funding acquisition, F.A.O. All authors have read and agreed to the published version of the manuscript.

Funding: F.A.O. and C.V.A. acknowledge Project AYUDANTE_DICYT, Código 082271OL, Vicerrectoría de Investigación, Innovación y Creación-USACH. F.A.O. would like to thank ANID-Fondecyt Chile (project 1241250) and DICYT-USACH. J.L.P. acknowledges the ANID grant for installation at the academy, calls for the year 2022, File 85220046 and Fondecyt Postdoctoral Project 3220441.

Institutional Review Board Statement: Not applicable.

Data Availability Statement: Data are available upon request.

Acknowledgments: F.A.O. and C.V.A. acknowledge Project AYUDANTE_DICYT, Código 082271OL, Vicerrectoría de Investigación, Innovación y Creación-USACH. F.A.O. would like to thank ANID-Fondecyt Chile (project 1241250) and DICYT-USACH.

Conflicts of Interest: The authors declare no conflicts of interest. The funders had no role in the design of the study; in the collection, analyses, or interpretation of data; in the writing of the manuscript; or in the decision to publish the results.

References

1. Costa, G.N.S.; Tonon, R.V.; Mellinger-Silva, C.; Galdeano, M.C.; Iacomini, M.; Santiago, M.C.P.A.; Almeida, E.L.; Freitas, S.P. Grape seed pomace as a valuable source of antioxidant fibers. *J. Sci. Food Agric.* **2019**, *99*, 4593–4601. [CrossRef] [PubMed]
2. Díaz, H.S.; Ríos-Gallardo, A.; Ortolani, D.; Díaz-Jara, E.; Flores, M.J.; Vera, I.; Monasterio, A.; Ortiz, F.C.; Brossard, N.; Osorio, F.; et al. Lipid-Encapsuled Grape Tannins Prevent Oxidative-Stress-Induced Neuronal Cell Death, Intracellular ROS Accumulation and Inflammation. *Antioxidants* **2022**, *11*, 1928. [CrossRef] [PubMed]
3. Shi, J.; Wang, Y.; Wei, H.; Hu, J.; Gao, M.T. Structure analysis of condensed tannin from rice straw and its inhibitory effect on Staphylococcus aureus. *Ind. Crops Prod.* **2020**, *145*, 112130. [CrossRef]
4. Li, W.; Yao, R.; Xie, L.; Liu, J.; Weng, X.; Yue, X.; Li, F. Dietary supplementation of grape seed tannin extract stimulated testis development, changed fatty acid profiles and increased testis antioxidant capacity in pre-puberty hu lambs. *Theriogenology* **2021**, *172*, 160–168. [CrossRef] [PubMed]
5. Soldado, D.; Bessa, R.J.; Jerónimo, E. Condensed tannins as antioxidants in ruminants—Effectiveness and action mechanisms to improve animal antioxidant status and oxidative stability of products. *Animals* **2021**, *11*, 3243. [CrossRef] [PubMed]

6. Peng, K.; Lv, X.; Zhao, H.; Chen, B.; Chen, X.; Huang, W. Antioxidant and intestinal recovery function of condensed tannins in Lateolabrax maculatus responded to in vivo and in vitro oxidative stress. *Aquaculture* **2022**, *547*, 737399. [CrossRef]
7. Ananga, A.; Obuya, J.; Ochieng, J.; Tsolova, V. Grape seed nutraceuticals for disease prevention: Current status and future prospects. In *Phenolic Compounds—Biological Activity*; InTech: Houston, TX, USA, 2017; pp. 119–137. [CrossRef]
8. Sochorova, L.; Prusova, B.; Jurikova, T.; Mlcek, J.; Adamkova, A.; Baron, M.; Sochor, J. The study of antioxidant components in grape seeds. *Molecules* **2020**, *25*, 3736. [CrossRef]
9. Jones, D.; Caballero, S.; Davidov-Pardo, G. Bioavailability of nanotechnology-based bioactives and nutraceuticals. In *Advances in Food and Nutrition Research*, 1st ed.; Elsevier Inc.: Amsterdam, The Netherlands, 2019; Volume 88. [CrossRef]
10. Peng, S.; Zou, L.; Zhou, W.; Liu, W.; Liu, C.; McClements, D.J. Encapsulation of Lipophilic Polyphenols into Nanoliposomes Using pH-Driven Method: Advantages and Disadvantages. *J. Agric. Food Chem.* **2019**, *67*, 7506–7511. [CrossRef] [PubMed]
11. Liu, W.; Hou, Y.; Jin, Y.; Wang, Y.; Xu, X.; Han, J. Research progress on liposomes: Application in food, digestion behavior and absorption mechanism. *Trends Food Sci. Technol.* **2020**, *104*, 177–189. [CrossRef]
12. Ben-Fadhel, Y.; Maherani, B.; Salmieri, S.; Lacroix, M. Preparation and characterization of natural extracts-loaded food grade nanoliposomes. *Lwt* **2022**, *154*, 112781. [CrossRef]
13. Pateiro, M.; Gómez, B.; Munekata, P.E.S.; Barba, F.J.; Putnik, P.; Kovačević, D.B.; Lorenzo, J.M. Nanoencapsulation of promising bioactive compounds to improve their absorption, stability, functionality and the appearance of the final food products. *Molecules* **2021**, *26*, 1547. [CrossRef] [PubMed]
14. Ballesteros, L.F.; Teixeira, J.A.; Cerqueira, M.A. Active Carboxymethyl Cellulose-Based Edible Coatings for the Extension of Fresh Goldenberries Shelf-Life[†]. *Horticulturae* **2022**, *8*, 936. [CrossRef]
15. Zambrano-Zaragoza, M.L.; González-Reza, R.; Mendoza-Muñoz, N.; Miranda-Linares, V.; Bernal-Couoh, T.F.; Mendoza-Elvira, S.; Quintanar-Guerrero, D. Nanosystems in edible coatings: A novel strategy for food preservation. *Int. J. Mol. Sci.* **2018**, *19*, 705. [CrossRef] [PubMed]
16. Bhagath, Y.B.; Manjula, K. Influence of composite edible coating systems on preservation of fresh meat cuts and products: A brief review on their trends and applications. *Int. Food Res. J.* **2019**, *26*, 377–392.
17. Parreidt, T.S.; Schott, M.; Schmid, M.; Müller, K. Effect of presence and concentration of plasticizers, vegetable oils, and surfactants on the properties of sodium-alginate-based edible coatings. *Int. J. Mol. Sci.* **2018**, *19*, 742. [CrossRef] [PubMed]
18. Yadav, A.; Kumar, N.; Upadhyay, A.; Sethi, S.; Singh, A. Edible coating as postharvest management strategy for shelf-life extension of fresh tomato (*Solanum lycopersicum* L.): An overview. *J. Food Sci.* **2022**, *87*, 2256–2290. [CrossRef]
19. Oztuna Taner, O.; Ekici, L.; Akyuz, L. CMC-based edible coating composite films from Brewer's spent grain waste: A novel approach for the fresh strawberry package. *Polym. Bull.* **2022**, *80*, 9033–9058. [CrossRef]
20. Wang, Y.; Jiang, S.; Chen, Y.; Qiu, D.; Weng, Y. Synthesis and Characterization of a Novel Composite Edible Film Based on Hydroxypropyl Methyl Cellulose Grafted with Gelatin. *Gels* **2023**, *9*, 332. [CrossRef] [PubMed]
21. Bahrami Feridoni, S.; Khademi Shurmasti, D. Effect of the nanoencapsulated sour tea (*Hibiscus sabdariffa* L.) extract with carboxymethylcellulose on quality and shelf life of chicken nugget. *Food Sci. Nutr.* **2020**, *8*, 3704–3715. [CrossRef] [PubMed]
22. Niaz, T.; Shabbir, S.; Noor, T.; Imran, M. Active Composite Packaging Reinforced with Nisin-Loaded Nano-Vesicles for Extended Shelf Life of Chicken Breast Filets and Cheese Slices. *Food Bioprocess Technol.* **2022**, *15*, 1284–1298. [CrossRef] [PubMed]
23. Monasterio, A.; Núñez, E.; Brossard, N.; Vega, R.; Osorio, F.A. Mechanical and Surface Properties of Edible Coatings Elaborated with Nanoliposomes Encapsulating Grape Seed Tannins and Polysaccharides. *Polymers* **2023**, *15*, 3774. [CrossRef] [PubMed]
24. Taladrid, D.; Marín, D.; Alemán, A.; Álvarez-Acero, I.; Montero, P.; Gómez-Guillén, M.C. Effect of chemical composition and sonication procedure on properties of food-grade soy lecithin liposomes with added glycerol. *Food Res. Int.* **2017**, *100*, 541–550. [CrossRef] [PubMed]
25. Babazadeh, A.; Ghanbarzadeh, B.; Hamishehkar, H. Phosphatidylcholine-rutin complex as a potential nanocarrier for food applications. *J. Funct. Foods* **2017**, *33*, 134–141. [CrossRef]
26. Re, R.; Pellegrini, N.; Proteggente, A.; Pannala, A.; Yang, M.; Rice-Evans, C. Antioxidant activity applying an improved ABTS radical cation decolorization assay. *Free Radic. Biol. Med.* **1999**, *26*, 1231–1237. [CrossRef] [PubMed]
27. Brand-Williams, W.; Cuvelier, M.E.; Berset, C. Use of a free radical method to evaluate antioxidant activity. *LWT -Food Sci. Technol.* **1995**, *28*, 25–30. [CrossRef]
28. Favarín, F.R.; Gündel, S.d.S.; Ledur, C.M.; Roggia, I.; Fagan, S.B.; Gündel, A.; Fogaça, A.d.O.; Ourique, A.F. Vitamin C as a shelf-life extender in liposomes. *Braz. J. Pharm. Sci.* **2022**, *58*, e20492. [CrossRef]
29. Lopez-Polo, J.; Silva-Weiss, A.; Zamorano, M.; Osorio, F.A. Humectability and physical properties of hydroxypropyl methylcellulose coatings with liposome-cellulose nanofibers: Food application. *Carbohydr. Polym.* **2020**, *231*, 115702. [CrossRef] [PubMed]
30. Estevez-Areco, S.; Guz, L.; Candal, R.; Goyanes, S. Release kinetics of rosemary (Rosmarinus officinalis) polyphenols from polyvinyl alcohol (PVA) electrospun nanofibers in several food simulants. *Food Packag. Shelf Life* **2018**, *18*, 42–50. [CrossRef]
31. Requena, R.; Vargas, M.; Chiralt, A. Release kinetics of carvacrol and eugenol from poly(hydroxybutyrate-co-hydroxyvalerate) (PHBV) films for food packaging applications. *Eur. Polym. J.* **2017**, *92*, 185–193. [CrossRef]
32. Guo, Y.; Shen, L.; Lu, Y.; Li, H.; Min, K.; Li, L.; Yu, C.; Zheng, X. Preparation of Rutin-liposome Drug Delivery Systems and Evaluation on Their in vitro Antioxidant Activity. *Chin. Herb. Med.* **2016**, *8*, 371–375. [CrossRef]

33. Bianchi, S.; Kroslakova, I.; Mayer, I. Determination of Molecular Structures of Condensed Tannins from Plant Tissues Using HPLC-UV Combined with Thiolysis and MALDI-TOF Mass Spectrometry. *Bio-Protocol* **2016**, *6*, e1975. [CrossRef]
34. Skurtys, O.; Velásquez, P.; Henriquez, O.; Matiacevich, S.; Enrione, J.; Osorio, F. Wetting behavior of chitosan solutions on blueberry epicarp with or without epicuticular waxes. *Lwt* **2011**, *44*, 1449–1457. [CrossRef]
35. Nguyen, P.T.M.; Nguyen, T.A.H.; Bhandari, B.; Prakash, S. Comparison of solid substrates to differentiate the lubrication property of dairy fluids by tribological measurement. *J. Food Eng.* **2016**, *185*, 1–8. [CrossRef]
36. Peter, A.; Cozmuta, L.M.; Nicula, C.; Cozmuta, A.M.; Apjok, R.; Talasman, C.M.; Drazic, G.; Peñas, A.; Calahorro, A.J.; Kamgang Nzekoue, F.; et al. Barrier properties, migration into the food simulants and antimicrobial activity of paper-based materials with functionalized surface. *Polym. Polym. Compos.* **2022**, *30*, 1–12. [CrossRef]
37. Zembyla, M.; Liamas, E.; Andablo-Reyes, E.; Gu, K.; Krop, E.M.; Kew, B.; Sarkar, A. Surface adsorption and lubrication properties of plant and dairy proteins: A comparative study. *Food Hydrocoll.* **2021**, *111*, 106364. [CrossRef] [PubMed]
38. Andrade, R.; Skurtys, O.; Osorio, F.; Zuluaga, R.; Gañán, P.; Castro, C. Wettability of gelatin coating formulations containing cellulose nanofibers on banana and eggplant epicarps. *Lwt* **2014**, *58*, 158–165. [CrossRef]
39. Danaei, M.; Dehghankhold, M.; Ataei, S.; Hasanzadeh Davarani, F.; Javanmard, R.; Dokhani, A.; Khorasani, S.; Mozafari, M.R. Impact of particle size and polydispersity index on the clinical applications of lipidic nanocarrier systems. *Pharmaceutics* **2018**, *10*, 57. [CrossRef] [PubMed]
40. Khorasani, S.; Danaei, M.; Mozafari, M.R. Nanoliposome technology for the food and nutraceutical industries. *Trends Food Sci. Technol.* **2018**, *79*, 106–115. [CrossRef]
41. Subramani, T.; Ganapathyswamy, H. An overview of liposomal nano-encapsulation techniques and its applications in food and nutraceutical. *J. Food Sci. Technol.* **2020**, *57*, 3545–3555. [CrossRef] [PubMed]
42. Montagner, G.E.; Ribeiro, M.F.; Cadoná, F.C.; Franco, C.; Gomes, P. Liposomes loading grape seed extract: A nanotechnological solution to reduce wine-making waste and obtain health-promoting products. *Future Foods* **2022**, *5*, 100144. [CrossRef]
43. Chen, G.; Li, D.; Jin, Y.; Zhang, W.; Teng, L.; Bunt, C.; Wen, J. Deformable liposomes by reverse-phase evaporation method for an enhanced skin delivery of (+)-catechin. *Drug Dev. Ind. Pharm.* **2014**, *40*, 260–265. [CrossRef] [PubMed]
44. Siyar, Z.; Motamedzadegan, A.; Mohammadzadeh Milani, J.; Rashidinejad, A. The effect of the liposomal encapsulated saffron extract on the physicochemical properties of a functional ricotta cheese. *Molecules* **2022**, *27*, 120. [CrossRef] [PubMed]
45. Eskandari, V.; Sadeghi, M.; Hadi, A. Physical and chemical properties of nano-liposome, application in nano medicine. *J. Comput. Appl. Mech.* **2021**, *52*, 751–767. [CrossRef]
46. Lombardo, D.; Kiselev, M.A. Methods of Liposomes Preparation: Formation and Control Factors of Versatile Nanocarriers for Biomedical and Nanomedicine Application. *Pharmaceutics* **2022**, *14*, 543. [CrossRef] [PubMed]
47. Chotphruethipong, L.; Hutamekalin, P.; Sukketsiri, W.; Benjakul, S. Effects of sonication and ultrasound on properties and bioactivities of liposomes loaded with hydrolyzed collagen from defatted sea bass skin conjugated with epigallocatechin gallate. *J. Food Biochem.* **2021**, *45*, e13809. [CrossRef] [PubMed]
48. Sun, L.; Wang, H.; Du, J.; Wang, T.; Yu, D. Ultrasonic-assisted extraction of grape seed procyanidins, preparation of liposomes, and evaluation of their antioxidant capacity. *Ultrason. Sonochemistry* **2024**, *105*, 106856. [CrossRef] [PubMed]
49. Yi, X.; Gao, S.; Gao, X.; Zhang, X.; Xia, G.; Liu, Z.; Shi, H.; Shen, X. Glycolipids improve the stability of liposomes: The perspective of bilayer membrane structure. *Food Chem.* **2023**, *412*, 135517. [CrossRef] [PubMed]
50. Faria, M.J.; Machado, R.; Ribeiro, A.; Gonçalves, H.; Real Oliveira, M.E.C.; Viseu, T.; das Neves, J.; Lúcio, M. Rational development of liposomal hydrogels: A strategy for topical vaginal antiretroviral drug delivery in the context of HIV prevention. *Pharmaceutics* **2019**, *11*, 485. [CrossRef] [PubMed]
51. Xu, J.; Jiang, S.; Liu, L.; Zhao, Y.; Zeng, M. Encapsulation of oyster protein hydrolysates in nanoliposomes: Vesicle characteristics, storage stability, in vitro release, and gastrointestinal digestion. *J. Food Sci.* **2021**, *86*, 960–968. [CrossRef] [PubMed]
52. Luo, X.; Guan, R.; Chen, X.; Liu, M.; Hao, Y.; Jiang, H. Optimized preparation of catechin nanoliposomes by orthogonal design and stability study. *Adv. J. Food Sci. Technol.* **2014**, *6*, 921–925. [CrossRef]
53. Wu, Z.; Guan, R.; Xiao, C.; Lyu, F.; Cao, G.; Liu, M.; Gao, J. Optimization of Catechin Nanoliposomes and Evaluation of Their Antioxidant Activity and Cytotoxicity. *Sci. Adv. Mater.* **2017**, *9*, 697–704. [CrossRef]
54. Ramili, N.A.; Ali, N.; Hamzah, S. Physicochemical Characterization of Quercetin-Loaded Liposomes Prepared by Sonication for Functional Food Application. *J. Sustain. Sci. Manag.* **2020**, *15*, 15–27. [CrossRef]
55. Gulzar, S.; Benjakul, S. Characteristics and storage stability of nanoliposomes loaded with shrimp oil as affected by ultrasonication and microfluidization. *Food Chem.* **2020**, *310*, 125916. [CrossRef]
56. Cheng, X.; Zang, M.; Wang, S.; Zhao, X.; Zhai, G.; Wang, L.; Li, X.; Zhao, Y.; Yue, Y. Physicochemical and Antioxidant Properties of Nanoliposomes Loaded with Rosemary Oleoresin and Their Oxidative Stability Application in Dried Oysters. *Bioengineering* **2022**, *9*, 818. [CrossRef] [PubMed]
57. Olatunde, O.O.; Benjakul, S.; Vongkamjan, K.; Amnuaikit, T. Liposomal Encapsulated Ethanolic Coconut Husk Extract: Antioxidant and Antibacterial Properties. *J. Food Sci.* **2019**, *84*, 3664–3673. [CrossRef] [PubMed]
58. Maqsoudlou, A.; Assadpour, E.; Mohebodini, H.; Jafari, S.M. The influence of nanodelivery systems on the antioxidant activity of natural bioactive compounds. *Crit. Rev. Food Sci. Nutr.* **2022**, *62*, 3208–3231. [CrossRef] [PubMed]
59. Rashidinejad, A.; Birch, E.J.; Sun-Waterhouse, D.; Everett, D.W. Delivery of green tea catechin and epigallocatechin gallate in liposomes incorporated into low-fat hard cheese. *Food Chem.* **2014**, *156*, 176–183. [CrossRef] [PubMed]

60. Caddeo, C.; Gabriele, M.; Fernàndez-Busquets, X.; Valenti, D.; Fadda, A.M.; Pucci, L.; Manconi, M. Antioxidant activity of quercetin in Eudragit-coated liposomes for intestinal delivery. *Int. J. Pharm.* **2019**, *565*, 64–69. [CrossRef] [PubMed]
61. De Leo, V.; Milano, F.; Mancini, E.; Comparelli, R.; Giotta, L.; Nacci, A.; Longobardi, F.; Garbetta, A.; Agostiano, A.; Catucci, L. Encapsulation of curcumin-loaded liposomes for colonic drug delivery in a pH-responsive polymer cluster using a pH-driven and organic solvent-free process. *Molecules* **2018**, *23*, 739. [CrossRef] [PubMed]
62. Pavlović, N.; Mijalković, J.; Đorđević, V.; Pecarski, D.; Bugarski, B.; Knežević-Jugović, Z. Ultrasonication for production of nanoliposomes with encapsulated soy protein concentrate hydrolysate: Process optimization, vesicle characteristics and in vitro digestion. *Food Chem. X* **2022**, *15*, 100370. [CrossRef]
63. Huang, M.; Wang, J.; Tan, C.; Ying, R.; Wu, X.; Chen, W.; Liu, J.; Ahmad, M. Liposomal co-delivery strategy to improve stability and antioxidant activity of trans-resveratrol and naringenin. *Int. J. Food Sci. Technol.* **2022**, *57*, 2701–2714. [CrossRef]
64. Ezzat, H.M.; Elnaggar, Y.S.R.; Abdallah, O.Y. Improved oral bioavailability of the anticancer drug catechin using chitosomes: Design, in-vitro appraisal and in-vivo studies. *Int. J. Pharm.* **2019**, *565*, 488–498. [CrossRef] [PubMed]
65. Gu, Y.; Zhao, Z.; Xue, F.; Zhang, Y. Alginate-Chitosan Coated Nanoliposomes as Effective Delivery Systems for Bamboo Leaf Flavonoids: Characterization, In Vitro Release, Skin Permeation and Anti-Senescence Activity. *Antioxidants* **2022**, *11*, 1024. [CrossRef] [PubMed]
66. Silva-Weiss, W.; Quilaqueo, M.; Venegas, O.; Ahumada, M.; Silva, W.; Osorio, F.; Giménez, B. Design of dipalmitoyl lecithin liposomes loaded with quercetin and rutin and their release kinetics from carboxymethyl cellulose edible films. *J. Food Eng.* **2018**, *224*, 165–173. [CrossRef]
67. Choudhary, P.; Dutta, S.; Moses, J.A.; Anandharamakrishnan, C. Nanoliposomal encapsulation of chia oil for sustained delivery of α-linolenic acid. *Int. J. Food Sci. Technol.* **2021**, *56*, 4206–4214. [CrossRef]
68. Jiao, Y.; Li, D.; Liu, C.; Chang, Y.; Song, J.; Xiao, Y. Polypeptide-decorated nanoliposomes as novel delivery systems for lutein. *RSC Adv.* **2018**, *8*, 31372–31381. [CrossRef] [PubMed]
69. Miao, Z.L.; Deng, Y.J.; Du, H.Y.; Suo, X.B.; Wang, X.Y.; Wang, X.; Wang, L.; Cui, L.J.; Duan, N. Preparation of a liposomal delivery system and its in vitro release of rapamycin. *Exp. Ther. Med.* **2015**, *9*, 941–946. [CrossRef] [PubMed]
70. Yarce, C.J.; Alhajj, M.J.; Sanchez, J.D.; Oñate-Garzón, J.; Salamanca, C.H. Development of Antioxidant-Loaded Nanoliposomes Employing Lecithins with Different Purity Grades. *Molecules* **2020**, *25*, 5344. [CrossRef] [PubMed]
71. Izadiyan, P.; Hemmateenejad, B. Multi-response optimization of factors affecting ultrasonic assisted extraction from Iranian basil using central composite design. *Food Chem.* **2016**, *190*, 864–870. [CrossRef] [PubMed]
72. Toro-Uribe, S.; López-Giraldo, L.J.; Alvarez-Rivera, G.; Ibánez, E.; Herrero, M. Insight of Stability of Procyanidins in Free and Liposomal Form under an in Vitro Digestion Model: Study of Bioaccessibility, Kinetic Release Profile, Degradation, and Antioxidant Activity. *J. Agric. Food Chem.* **2019**, *67*, 1990–2003. [CrossRef] [PubMed]
73. Ji, Y.; Wang, Z.; Ju, X.; Deng, F.; Yang, F.; He, R. Co-encapsulation of rutinoside and β-carotene in liposomes modified by rhamnolipid: Antioxidant activity, antibacterial activity, storage stability, and in vitro gastrointestinal digestion. *J. Food Sci.* **2023**, *88*, 2064–2077. [CrossRef] [PubMed]
74. Lisitsyn, A.; Semenova, A.; Nasonova, V.; Polishchuk, E.; Revutskaya, N.; Kozyrev, I.; Kotenkova, E. Approaches in animal proteins and natural polysaccharides application for food packaging: Edible film production and quality estimation. *Polymers* **2021**, *13*, 1592. [CrossRef] [PubMed]
75. Szulc, K.; Lenart, A. Surface modification of dairy powders: Effects of fluid-bed agglomeration and coating. *Int. Dairy J.* **2013**, *33*, 55–61. [CrossRef]
76. Huesca-Urióstegui, K.; García-Valderrama, E.J.; Gutierrez-Uribe, J.A.; Antunes-Ricardo, M.; Guajardo-Flores, D. Nanofiber Systems as Herbal Bioactive Compounds Carriers: Current Applications in Healthcare. *Pharmaceutics* **2022**, *14*, 191. [CrossRef] [PubMed]
77. Ghadermazi, R.; Hamdipour, S.; Sadeghi, K.; Ghadermazi, R.; Khosrowshahi Asl, A. Effect of various additives on the properties of the films and coatings derived from hydroxypropyl methylcellulose—A review. *Food Sci. Nutr.* **2019**, *7*, 3363–3377. [CrossRef] [PubMed]
78. Pavlath, A.E.; Orts, W. *Edible Films and Coatings for Food Applications*; Springer: New York, NY, USA, 2009; pp. 1–23. [CrossRef]
79. Xu, T.; Pan, M.; Chiou, Y.; Li, Z.; Wei, S.; Yin, X.; Ding, B. Improvement of emulsifying properties of potato starch via complexation with nanoliposomes for stabilizing Pickering emulsion. *Food Hydrocoll.* **2023**, *136*, 108271. [CrossRef]
80. Chen, M.; Li, R.; Lu, X.; Dai, Y.; Chen, T.; Xing, Y.; Xue, L.; Duan, Z.; Zhou, W.; Li, J. Fabrication and characterization of L-ascorbyl palmitate and phospholipid-based hybrid liposomes and their impacts on the stability of loaded hydrophobic polyphenols. *Food Chem.* **2023**, *398*, 133953. [CrossRef] [PubMed]
81. Topkanloo, S.P.; Tan, T.B.; Abas, F.; Azam, M.; Nehdi, I.A.; Tan, C.P. Improving Vesicular Integrity and Antioxidant Activity of Novel Mixed Soy Lecithin-Based Liposomes Containing Squalene and Their Stability against UV Light. *Molecules* **2020**, *25*, 5873. [CrossRef]
82. Jiménez, A.; Sánchez-González, L.; Desobry, S.; Chiralt, A.; Tehrany, E.A. Influence of nanoliposomes incorporation on properties of film forming dispersions and films based on corn starch and sodium caseinate. *Food Hydrocoll.* **2014**, *35*, 159–169. [CrossRef]
83. Yussof, N.S.; Tan, C.P.; Tan, T.B.; Utra, U.; Ramli Uhammad, E. Influence of Soy Lecithin and Sodium Caseinate on The Stability and in vitro Bioaccessibility of Lycopene Nanodispersion. *Food Technol. Biotechnol.* **2023**, *61*, 39–50. [CrossRef] [PubMed]

84. Fabra, M.J.; Jiménez, A.; Atarés, L.; Talens, P.; Chiralt, A. Effect of fatty acids and beeswax addition on properties of sodium caseinate dispersions and films. *Biomacromolecules* **2009**, *10*, 1500–1507. [CrossRef] [PubMed]
85. Le, N.T.T.; Cao, V.D.; Nguyen, T.N.Q.; Le, T.T.H.; Tran, T.T.; Hoang Thi, T.T. Soy lecithin-derived liposomal delivery systems: Surface modification and current applications. *Int. J. Mol. Sci.* **2019**, *20*, 4706. [CrossRef] [PubMed]
86. Pulla-Huillca, P.V.; Gomes, A.; Quinta Barbosa Bittante, A.M.; Lourenço, R.V.; Sobral, P.J.d.A. Wettability of gelatin-based films: The effects of hydrophilic or hydrophobic plasticizers and nanoparticle loads. *J. Food Eng.* **2021**, *297*, 110480. [CrossRef]
87. Avramescu, S.M.; Butean, C.; Popa, C.V.; Ortan, A.; Moraru, I.; Temocico, G. Edible and functionalized films/coatings-performances and perspectives. *Coatings* **2020**, *10*, 687. [CrossRef]
88. Sapper, M.; Palou, L.; Pérez-Gago, M.B.; Chiralt, A. Antifungal Starch-Gellan Edible coatings with thyme essential oil for the postharvest preservation of apple and persimmon. *Coatings* **2019**, *9*, 333. [CrossRef]
89. Falcó, I.; Randazzo, W.; Sánchez, G.; López-Rubio, A.; Fabra, M.J. On the use of carrageenan matrices for the development of antiviral edible coatings of interest in berries. *Food Hydrocoll.* **2019**, *92*, 74–85. [CrossRef]
90. Kalin, M.; Polajnar, M. The wetting of steel, DLC coatings, ceramics and polymers with oils and water: The importance and correlations of surface energy, surface tension, contact angle and spreading. *Appl. Surf. Sci.* **2014**, *293*, 97–108. [CrossRef]
91. Osorio, F.; Valdés, G.; Skurtys, O.; Andrade, R.; Villalobos-Carvajal, R.; Silva-Weiss, A.; Silva-Vera, W.; Giménez, B.; Zamorano, M.; Lopez, J. Surface free energy utilization to evaluate wettability of hydrocolloid suspension on different vegetable epicarps. *Coatings* **2018**, *8*, 16. [CrossRef]
92. Ribeiro, C.; Vicente, A.A.; Teixeira, J.A.; Miranda, C. Optimization of edible coating composition to retard strawberry fruit senescence. *Postharvest Biol. Technol.* **2007**, *44*, 63–70. [CrossRef]
93. Pirozzi, A.; Del Grosso, V.; Ferrari, G.; Donsì, F. Edible Coatings Containing Oregano Essential Oil Nanoemulsion for Improving Postharvest Quality and Shelf Life of Tomatoes. *Foods* **2020**, *9*, 1605. [CrossRef] [PubMed]
94. Mohd Yusof, N.; Jai, J.; Sharif, Z.I.M.; Mustapha, F.A.; Pinijsuwan, S. Effect of different amount chitosan, starch and glycerol in composite edible coating. *J. Phys. Conf. Ser.* **2019**, *1349*, 012077. [CrossRef]
95. Jafarzadeh, S.; Mohammadi Nafchi, A.; Salehabadi, A.; Oladzad-abbasabadi, N.; Jafari, S.M. Application of bio-nanocomposite films and edible coatings for extending the shelf life of fresh fruits and vegetables. *Adv. Colloid Interface Sci.* **2021**, *291*, 102405. [CrossRef] [PubMed]
96. Cazón, P.; Velazquez, G.; Ramírez, J.A.; Vázquez, M. Polysaccharide-based films and coatings for food packaging: A review. *Food Hydrocoll.* **2017**, *68*, 136–148. [CrossRef]
97. Pirozzi, A.; Ferrari, G.; Donsì, F. The use of nanocellulose in edible coatings for the preservation of perishable fruits and vegetables. *Coatings* **2021**, *11*, 990. [CrossRef]
98. Sinha, A.; Bhargav, A. Young's modulus estimation in food samples: Effect of experimental parameters. *Mech. Ind.* **2020**, *21*, 404. [CrossRef]
99. Imran, M.; René, N.; Jamshidian, M.; Akhtar, M.J.; Arab-tehrany, E.; Jacquot, M.; Desobry, S. Food Hydrocolloids Microstructure and physico-chemical evaluation of nano-emulsion-based antimicrobial peptides embedded in bioactive packaging films. *Food Hydrocoll.* **2012**, *29*, 407–419. [CrossRef]
100. De Simone, V.; Dalmoro, A.; Bochicchio, S.; Caccavo, D.; Lamberti, G.; Bertoncin, P.; Barba, A.A. Nanoliposomes in polymeric granules: Novel process strategy to produce stable and versatile delivery systems. *J. Drug Deliv. Sci. Technol.* **2020**, *59*, 101878. [CrossRef]
101. Kamkar, A.; Molaee-Aghaee, E.; Khanjari, A.; Akhondzadeh-Basti, A.; Noudoost, B.; Shariatifar, N.; Sani, M.A.; Soleimani, M. Nanocomposite active packaging based on chitosan biopolymer loaded with nano-liposomal essential oil: Its characterizations and effects on microbial, and chemical properties of refrigerated chicken breast fillet. *Int. J. Food Microbiol.* **2021**, *342*, 109071. [CrossRef] [PubMed]
102. Mirzaei-Mohkam, A.; Garavand, F.; Dehnad, D.; Keramat, J.; Nasirpour, A. Physical, mechanical, thermal and structural characteristics of nanoencapsulated vitamin E loaded carboxymethyl cellulose films. *Prog. Org. Coat.* **2020**, *138*, 105383. [CrossRef]
103. Marín-Peñalver, D.; Alemán, A.; Gómez-Guillén, M.; Montero, P. Carboxymethyl cellulose films containing nanoliposomes loaded with an angiotensin-converting enzyme inhibitory collagen hydrolysate. *Food Hydrocoll.* **2019**, *94*, 553–560. [CrossRef]
104. Zhou, X.; Liu, X.; Liao, W.; Wang, Q.; Xia, W. Chitosan/bacterial cellulose films incorporated with tea polyphenol nanoliposomes for silver carp preservation. *Carbohydr. Polym.* **2022**, *297*, 120048. [CrossRef] [PubMed]
105. Mehdizadeh, A.; Shahidi, S.A.; Shariatifar, N.; Shiran, M.; Ghorbani-HasanSaraei, A. Physicochemical characteristics and antioxidant activity of the chitosan/zein films incorporated with *Pulicaria gnaphalodes* L. extract-loaded nanoliposomes. *J. Food Meas. Charact.* **2022**, *16*, 1252–1262. [CrossRef]
106. Bigi, F.; Haghighi, H.; Siesler, H.W.; Licciardello, F.; Pulvirenti, A. Characterization of chitosan-hydroxypropyl methylcellulose blend films enriched with nettle or sage leaf extract for active food packaging applications. *Food Hydrocoll.* **2021**, *120*, 106979. [CrossRef]

antioxidants

MDPI

Article

Valorization of *Citrus reticulata* Blanco Peels to Produce Enriched Wheat Bread: Phenolic Bioaccessibility and Antioxidant Potential

Esther Gómez-Mejía *, Iván Sacristán , Noelia Rosales-Conrado *, María Eugenia León-González and Yolanda Madrid

Department of Analytical Chemistry, Faculty of Chemistry, Complutense University of Madrid, 28040 Madrid, Spain; ivasacri@ucm.es (I.S.); leongon@ucm.es (M.E.L.-G.); ymadrid@ucm.es (Y.M.)
* Correspondence: egomez03@ucm.es (E.G.-M.); nrosales@ucm.es (N.R.-C.)

Abstract: The fortification of foods with bioactive polyphenols aims to improve their functional properties and to provide health benefits. Yet, to exert their benefits, phenolic compounds must be released from the food matrix and absorbed by the small intestine after digestion, so assessing their bioaccessibility is crucial to determine their potential role. This work aims to incorporate *Citrus reticulata* Blanco peel extracts into wheat bread as a promising opportunity to increase their bioactive potential, along with supporting the sustainable management of citrus-industry waste. A control and a wheat bread enriched at 2% and 4% (w/v) with a phenolic extract from mandarin peels were prepared and analyzed for antioxidant activity and phenolic composition using LC-MS and UV-Vis spectrophotometry. In addition, in vitro digestion was performed, and the digested extracts were analyzed with HPLC-MS/MS. The results showed a significant increase in total flavonoid content (TFC, 2.2 ± 0.1 mg·g^{-1}), antioxidant activity (IC_{50} = 37 ± 4 mg·g^{-1}), and contents of quercetin, caffeic acid, and hesperidin in the 4% (w/v) enriched bread. Yet, most polyphenols were completely degraded after the in vitro digestion process, barring hesperidin (159 ± 36 μg·g^{-1}), highlighting the contribution of citrus enrichment in the development of an enriched bread with antioxidant potential.

Keywords: mandarin peels; polyphenols; enriched wheat bread; waste valorization; in vitro bioaccessibility; antioxidant activity

1. Introduction

Over the last decade, consumers' nutritional awareness has increased considerably around the world, leading to the search for healthier and more nutritious foods that ensure greater safety and promote well-being [1]. As a result, a growing interest is now being shown in foods that, in addition to providing basic nutrients, contain a high antioxidant potential [2]. According to scientific reports, the deficiency of antioxidants in the daily diet is not only the cause of the organism aging, but also of the appearance of numerous diseases of affluence derived from oxidative stress [2], including cancer, Alzheimer's disease, obesity, and osteoporosis, among others [3,4]. For this reason, both industries and researchers are engaged in optimizing food production technology to develop enriched foodstuffs with functional components, which improve the quality, taste, performance, and bioavailability of food products, whilst also reducing the burden on health services [1,3].

One of the most abundant families of natural antioxidants are phenolic compounds. Polyphenols are secondary metabolites synthesized by plants as essential physiological compounds, comprising a large family of molecules with one or more phenolic rings [4]. In addition to being potent antioxidants, they are also known to exhibit anti-allergic, antiviral, anti-inflammatory, and antimutagenic properties [3,4]. These compounds are present in many plant foods, such as citrus fruits. *Citrus* (Rutaceae) is the most widely produced tree fruit crop in the world, with more than 130 million tons per year. About 33% of citrus fruits are processed industrially for juice production, resulting in the generation of over 15 million tons of citrus waste per year, namely peels, membranes, and seeds, the management of which is a major economic and environmental concern [5]. These citrus by-products, and in particular the peel, are rich in bioactive polyphenols such as hesperidin, coumaric acid, ferulic acid, rutin, and luteolin, among others [6,7]. Therefore, based on their composition, their low cost, and their easy availability, citrus waste peels should be considered a potential nutraceutical source of antioxidant and value-added ingredients for the elaboration of functional foods. Therefore, this approach allows one to follow a circular economy strategy that offers alternative and green opportunities for the disposal of citrus waste, allowing for more sustainable production and consumption within the agri-food sector [5,6]. In general, cereal-based foods, such as bread and bakery products, play an important role in human nutrition, given that they are considered a good source of energy and irreplaceable nutrients. In fact, they represent up to 50% of dietary intake in some communities [2,3]. Thus, given their widespread consumption, bread and bakery products are considered to be the foremost appropriate carriers of functional supplements. Previously, Taglieri et al. studied the preparation of a bread enriched with 8% (*w*/*w*) purple potato flour and 0.75% (*w*/*w*) sour orange (*Citrus* × *aurantium*) albedo, drawing a significant rise in phenolic compounds such as apigenin 7-*O*-ruthinoside and neohesperidin, as well as a higher antioxidant activity and a longer shelf life of the enhanced bread [8]. On the other hand, Yaqoob et al. prepared cookies enriched with kinnow (*Citrus reticulate* L.) pomace and peel powder at 5–20% (*w*/*w*) and citrus peel phenolic extract at 1–4% (*w*/*w*). As a result, a significant improvement in the DPPH antioxidant capacity as well as in the total contents of phenolic compounds, flavonoids, and carotenoids was detected when the cookies were enriched with the phenolic extracts. In addition, a greater oxidative stability of the citrus-residue-enriched cookies was noted compared with those with the artificial antioxidant butylated hydroxyanisole [9]. And Laganà et al. substituted 2.5% to 15% (*w*/*w*) wheat flour with bergamot (*Citrus bergamia*) pomace to obtain improved cookies, showing a proportional increase in total phenolic content and total flavonoid content in the enriched cookies, especially at the highest level of enrichment (3.64 mg GAE·g^{-1} and 3.90 mg CE·g^{-1}, respectively) [10]. Although, in the aforementioned studies, the preparation of fortified foods was carried out by adding the bioactive residue or extract in a solid state [8–10], a number of advantages regarding diffusion, dosage, and application are well-known when ready-to-use nutraceutical ingredients are available in a liquid state. Furthermore, solvents can provide synergistic activity not only in the overall extraction of polyphenolic compounds, but also in their underlying bioactivity [11]. Therefore, both facts seem to indicate that the formulation of natural additives in liquid form for the preparation of fortified foods is becoming increasingly attractive.

Ultimately, an issue to be taken into consideration when designing an enriched food is the stability of the bioactive compounds involved in the digestion process, which may influence not only their bioaccessibility but also their potential activity [12]. Since phenolic compounds are usually degraded by oxidation during digestion, it is essential to evaluate their digestive stability, generally using in vitro gastrointestinal procedures, in which the mechanical and physiological conditions of each stage of the gastrointestinal digestion process are mimicked [13].

In view of the above, this study focuses on exploring the feasibility of preparing wheat bread enriched with different ratios of hydroalcoholic phenolic extract derived from mandarin peels. The resulting breads were compared in terms of total phenolic and flavonoid content and DPPH antioxidant activity using spectrophotometric methods. Furthermore, the individual phenolic composition was studied and the in vitro digestive stability of low-molecular-weight polyphenols, i.e., phenolic acids, flavonoids, and stilbenes, in the prepared breads was evaluated using liquid chromatography-mass spectrometry.

2. Materials and Methods

2.1. Raw Citrus Material

'Orri' hybrid mandarins (*Citrus reticulata* Blanco) were purchased at a local market in Madrid (Spain). The peels were manually separated from the fruit, cleaned with Milli-Q water, and cut into equally sized portions (1 × 0.5 cm) using stainless-steel scissors. Finally, they were stored in hermetically sealed glass containers at −20 °C until processing.

2.2. Reagent, Solvent, and Polyphenol Standards

Analytical-grade reagents and purified water from a Milli-Q system (Merck, Madrid, Spain) were used. Absolute ethanol HPLC gradient quality (EtOH), acetonitrile (ACN), methanol (MeOH), and formic acid (FA) of MS quality were provided by Scharlab (Barcelona, Spain). Dimethyl sulfoxide (DMSO, ≥99.9%), 2N Folin–Ciocalteu reagent, 2,2-diphenyl-1-picrylhydrazyl (DPPH), urea (≥99.5%), α-amylase from Bacillus subtilis (powder, 50 U/mg), bile salts, pepsin from porcine gastric mucosa, and pancreatin from porcine pancreas were all supplied by Sigma-Aldrich (St. Louis, MO, USA). Ammonium molybdate tetrahydrate, aluminum chloride 6-hydrate, sulfuric acid (95–98%), sodium carbonate anhydrous, tri-sodium phosphate 12-hydrate, monosodium phosphate monohydrate (≥98.0%), anhydrous sodium sulphate (≥99.9%), potassium chloride (99.5%), potassium thiocyanate (98.0%), sodium bicarbonate (99.5%), hydrochloric acid (37%), sodium hydroxide, and sodium nitrite were obtained from Panreac (Barcelona, Spain).

Phenolic-standard gallic acid monohydrate (≥98.0%), dihydroxybenzoic acid (≥97.0%), chlorogenic acid (≥95.0%), catechin (≥98.0%), caffeic acid (≥98.0%), *p*-coumaric acid (≥98.0%), epicacatechin (≥98.0%), *trans*-ferulic acid (98%), rutin trihydrate (≥95.0%), myricetin (≥96.0%), resveratrol (≥99.0%), quercetin (≥95.0%), kaempferol (≥97.0%), and naringin (≥95.0%) were obtained from Sigma-Aldrich (St. Louis, MO, USA). Hesperidin (≥98.0%) was provided by European Pharmacopoeia. Phenolic stock solutions (200 $mg \cdot L^{-1}$) were prepared in MeOH, ethanol–water mixture 80:20 (v/v) (quercetin), or 5% (v/v) DMSO aqueous solution (hesperidin). They were stored in the dark at 4 °C or at −80 °C (myricetin, hesperidin, *trans*-ferulic, and caffeic acid) for up to one month. Fresh working standard solutions were prepared daily by diluting stock solutions as needed.

2.3. Moisture Determination

The moisture content of mandarin peel and bread samples was obtained according to AOAC method 20.013 [14]. Briefly, 1.0000 g of sample, previously ground, was weighed in triplicate and dried to constant weight at 105 °C (±0.1 °C) (P-Selecta oven, Panreac, Barcelona, Spain). The free-water content was calculated gravimetrically and expressed as a percentage (mean ± standard deviation, n = 3).

2.4. *Citrus reticulata* Blanco Peel Extract Preparation

Polyphenols from mandarin peels were extracted using a procedure previously optimized elsewhere [15], with slight modifications. Heat-assisted solid–liquid extraction (SLE) was performed at 90 °C under magnetic stirring (3 rpm) for 15 min (VELP Scientifica, Us-mate, MB, Italy) using 1.5000 g (2%, w/v) or 3.0000 g (4%, w/v) of citrus peel waste and 75 mL of 20:80 (v/v) ethanol–water. The obtained extracts were cooled to room temperature and centrifuged at 1528× *g* (centrifuge 5804, Eppendorf, Sigma Aldrich, Madrid, Spain). Finally, the supernatants were collected for further use and analysis. Extracts were prepared in triplicate.

2.5. Production of Enriched Wheat Bread

The enriched bread was prepared by mixing 125 g of T65-strength wheat flour, 1.7500 g of dry yeast, 0.2500 g of salt, and 3.7500 g of extra virgin olive oil (Picual variety) with 75 mL of 2% (w/v) or 4% (w/v) mandarin peel extract. Additionally, a control bread was prepared using a 20:80 (v/v) ethanol–water mixture. All ingredients were manually kneaded for 10 min until a homogeneous dough was formed, which subsequently fermented for 2 h at

27 °C. The dough was then divided into three portions of approximately 60 g and put into baking pans lined with parchment paper. Finally, control and enriched breads were baked at 200 °C for 20 min in a P-Selecta oven (Panreac).

2.6. Phenolic Extraction of Enriched Wheat Bread

An amount of 1.000 g of ground wheat bread was added to 20 mL of 70:30 (v/v) ethanol–water mixture and held at 60 °C under magnetic stirring (3 rpm) for 30 min. The phenolic extract was cooled to room temperature and centrifuged at 11,000 rpm for 10 min. Ultimately, the supernatant was collected for further analysis. Samples were prepared in triplicate.

The selection of the aforementioned procedure was based on a study in which the effect of the extraction technique on the extraction efficiency was evaluated using total phenolic content (TPC), total flavonoid content (TFC), and antioxidant activity determinations, using the control bread as a matrix model, while maintaining the extraction solvent (70:30 (v/v) ethanol-water) and the sample-to-solvent ratio (1/20). The extraction techniques assessed were SLE assisted by mechanical stirring (29.5 kHz, 25 °C, P-Selecta, Barcelona, Spain), SLE assisted by magnetic stirring and heating (3 rpm, 60 °C, VELP Scientifica, Us-mate, Italy) for 30 min, and ultrasound-assisted extraction (UAE) working at 40% of amplitude and 25 °C for 20 min. The UAE was performed using two different instruments, an ultrasonic homogenizer (HD 3200, Sonopuls, Bandelin, Berlin, Germany) equipped with a titanium probe (25 × 15.5 × 25.7, mm) fitted with a 200 W high-frequency generator at 20 kHz frequency, and a Vibra-Cell ultrasound probe (Sonic, Newton, CT, USA) equipped with a 2 mm diameter titanium microtip fitted with a 130 W high-frequency generator at 20 kHz frequency.

2.7. Spectrophotometric Analysis of Phenolic Extracts: Total Polyphenol Content, Total Flavonoid Content, and Antioxidant Activity

The total phenolic content (TPC) of mandarin peel and wheat bread extracts were assessed using the Folin–Ciocalteu method [16]. The phenolic extracts (1 mL for wheat bread or 400 µL for mandarin peel) were mixed with 70 µL of the Folin–Ciocalteu reagent and 60 µL of 7.5% (w/v) Na_2CO_3 to a final volume of 10 mL. Gallic acid was used as standard for external calibration (0–40 µM, n = 5). The absorbance of the solutions was measured at 720 nm (UV-Vis spectrophotometer Cary 60, Agilent Technologies, Madrid, Spain) and the results were expressed as mg of gallic acid equivalent per g of dry sample (mg GAE$\cdot$g^{-1}). The assay was performed in triplicate.

The total flavonoid content (TFC) was determined according to the aluminum complexation colorimetry assay [16]. Sample aliquots (1 mL for wheat bread or 500 µL for mandarin peel) were added to 2 mL of water, 150 µL of 5% (w/v) $NaNO_2$, and 150 µL of 10/(w/v) $AlCl_3$. After two incubation periods of 5 min, 1 mL of 1 M NaOH was mixed with the reaction solution and stored for 15 min; finally, the solution was diluted to 10 mL with water. The absorbance of the solutions was measured at 450 nm using a UV-Vis spectrophotometer. Quercetin was used, as is standard, to obtain a calibration curve (0–45 µM, n = 6) and the results were expressed as mg of quercetin equivalent per g of dry sample (mg QE$\cdot$g^{-1}). Samples were analyzed three times.

The antioxidant activity of wheat bread and mandarin peel samples was assessed based on the ability of the extracts to scavenge the DPPH radical [17]; thus, they were assessed in terms of their antiradical activity. Working solutions were prepared combining 500 µL of 0.28 mM DPPH (MeOH) and 100–500 µL of sample aliquots. In addition, a DPPH control and a blind control (sample aliquot plus pure MeOH) were prepared. After a 30 min incubation in the dark, the absorbance was measured at 515 nm. Antioxidant activity was tested in triplicate and denoted as IC_{50} value in mg of extract per g of dry sample.

2.8. Chromatographic Analysis of Phenolic Extracts Using cLC-ESI-MS and HPLC-ESI-QTOF

Individual polyphenol determination of mandarin and wheat bread extracts was carried out using capillary liquid chromatography coupled to a mass simple quadrupole analyzer (cLC-ESI-MS), following the procedure previously described by Gómez-Mejía et al. [17] with minor adjustments. The extracts were analyzed using an Agilent liquid chromatography system (Mod. 1100 Series), outfitted with a G1376A binary capillary pump, a G1379A degasser, a simple quadrupole mass analyzer (6120), and a micro electrospray ionization source (ESI). Agilent Chemstation B.04.01 software was utilized to gather and process data, while an external stainless-steel loop (10 μL) was positioned into a Rheodyne® injection valve. A Synergi™ Fusion C18 capillary analytical column (150 × 0.3 mm i.d., 4 μm, Phenomenex, Torrance, CA, USA) and a mobile phase consisting of 0.05% (*v*/*v*) formic acid aqueous solution at pH 2.9 (A) and acetonitrile (B), operating in gradient elution mode at 10 $\mu L \cdot min^{-1}$, were used to separate the phenolic compounds. The gradient was run as follows: 8% B for 0 to 3 min, 8% to 34% B for 3 to 17 min, 8% to 34% B for 17 to 21 min, and 8% to 34% B for 21 to 24 min. Prior to analysis, each mobile phase was filtered with nylon membrane filters (0.22 m, Teknokroma, Barcelona, Spain). The molecular ion $[M-H]^-$ was chosen for online identification of polyphenols using mass detection in negative ion mode, where ESI capillary voltage was fixed at 3.5 kV. The drying gas temperature was set to 325 °C and a flowrate of 8.0 L min^{-1}. The nebulizer pressure was fixed at 17 psi. Identification of phenolic compounds was carried out by comparing the retention times and molecular ions acquired from the standards with those of the sample extracts. External calibration curves were obtained for quantifying purposes. For on-column focusing purposes, injection solutions were prepared by adding to sample aliquots 50 μL of ACN, 800 μL of MeOH, 0.05% (*v*/*v*) aqueous formic acid solution at pH 2.9, and Milli-Q water to a final volume of 5 mL.

For a more thorough and wider determination of the bioactive compounds present in the mandarin residues and in the samples subjected to the in vitro digestion process, high-performance liquid chromatography coupled to a quadrupole time-of-flight mass spectrometer (HPLC-ESI-QTOF) was employed. The phenolic analysis was performed in an Agilent liquid chromatography system (Mod. 1200), a quaternary pump (G1311A), a coupled degasser (G1322A), a thermostated automatic injector (G1367B), a thermostated column module (G1316A), and a QTOF mass spectrometer (Agilent G6530A) with atmospheric-pressure electrospray ionization source (ESI) and JetStream technology, operating in negative mode and scanning mode (SCAN) in the m/z range 100–1000, using a capillary voltage of 4 kV and a 45 psi pressure. Data processing was performed with Masshunter Data Acquisition B.05.00 and Masshunter Qualitative Analysis B.07.00. Nitrogen was used as both nebulizing and drying gas (10.0 $L \cdot min^{-1}$, 325 °C).

HPLC-QTOF separation was performed on a Synergi™ C18 Fusion-RP 80 Å analytical column (150 mm × 3 mm I.D., 4 μm, Phenomenex, USA), maintained at 30 °C and using a mobile phase gradient based on a mixture of 0.1% (*v*/*v*) FA in ACN (solvent A) and 0.1% (*v*/*v*) FA aqueous solution (solvent B) as follows: 10% solvent B holding for 0.1 min, linear increase to 35% B within 30 min, and to 70% B within another 5 min. This condition was held for 2 min, then a final linear increase to 90% B was attained within 3 and was held for 5 min, subsequently followed by a re-equilibration of the column. The flow rate was set at 0.50 $mL \cdot min^{-1}$ and the injection volume was fixed at 20 μL.

The identification of phenolic compounds was carried out by comparing the retention times and the m/z of the molecular ions $[M-H]^-$ acquired from the standards with those of the sample extracts. For quantification purposes, external calibration curves were obtained. Nevertheless, the effect of the matrix on the suppression/enhancement of the ESI/MS signal was studied by comparing the peak areas of the 2 $mg \cdot L^{-1}$ standard solutions with those obtained for the samples spiked in the former standard mixture. The matrix effect was then calculated using the modified version of the equation described by Matuszewki [11] (Equation (1)).

$$\text{matrix effect, \%} = \left(\frac{A_{\text{sample}}}{A_{\text{standard}}}\right)\cdot 100 \quad (1)$$

The performance of both LC-MS methods was evaluated for the standard solutions under optimal chromatographic conditions in terms of linear range and limits of detection (LOD) and quantification (LOQ) [18,19]. Linear ranges ($n \geq 4$) were set at concentrations between 0.002 $\mu g \cdot L^{-1}$ and 2000 $mg \cdot L^{-1}$. Chromatographic peak areas were analyzed using linear least squares regression, and linearity was assessed as determination coefficients (R^2). LOD and LOQ were calculated for analyte concentration as 3 signal-to-noise (*S/N*) at height and 10 *S/N*, respectively. Finally, the precision was estimated at 80 $\mu g \cdot L^{-1}$ for gallic acid, dihydroxybenzoic acid, *p*-coumaric acid, resveratrol, quercetin, and kaempferol; 44 $\mu g \cdot L^{-1}$ for caffeic acid; 40 $\mu g \cdot L^{-1}$ for *trans*-ferulic acid; and 480 $\mu g \cdot L^{-1}$ for catechin. Intraday variation (n = 3) was assessed by injecting three standard solutions at the target concentration for each analyte on the same day, while inter-day precision was similarly obtained from three successive days (n = 9, three injections per day). The relative standard deviation (RSD, %) was calculated for both the retention factor (k) and peak areas of each analyte.

2.9. *In Vitro Gastrointestinal Digestion of Phenolic Compounds from Bread*

The 4% (w/v) fortified and control wheat bread were subjected to an in vitro digestion process, according to the procedure described by Minekus et al. [20], slightly modified. The salivary phase was initiated by mixing 0.2500 g of minced bread with 40 mg of α-amylase and 4 mL of simulated salivary fluid (KCl (179.2 $g \cdot L^{-1}$), KSCN (40 $g \cdot L^{-1}$), NaH_2PO_4 (177.6 $g \cdot L^{-1}$), Na_2SO_4 (114.0 $g \cdot L^{-1}$), NaCl (350.6 $g \cdot L^{-1}$), $NaHCO_3$ (169.4 $g \cdot L^{-1}$), and urea (50.0 $g \cdot L^{-1}$). The pH was set to 6.8 with 0.1 M HCl and incubated at 37 °C for 15 min. Subsequently, 5 mL of pepsin dissolved in 0.1 M HCl was combined, the pH was adjusted to 1.8 with 6 M HCl, and the gastric mixture was maintained at 37 °C for 2 h. The duodenal phase was then initiated by adjusting the pH to 6.8 with saturated aqueous $NaHCO_3$ solution. Lastly, 3 mL of 1.5% (w/v) pancreatin and 0.15% (w/v) bile salts, both dissolved in 0.15 M NaCl, were added and the mixture was incubated at 37 °C for 2 h. Gastrointestinal digestion blanks were prepared in parallel. The procedure was performed in triplicate with constant shaking (100 rpm) and digested samples were analyzed fresh to prevent phenolic degradation, following the procedure described in Section 2.8.

Finally, the in vitro bioaccessibility index (IVBA), i.e., the percentage content of a polyphenol at the duodenal stage following the in vitro gastrointestinal step [12], was determined, when possible, by applying Equation (2).

$$\text{IVBA, \%} = \left(\frac{[\text{Polyphenol}]_{\text{duodenal stage}}}{[\text{Polyphenol}]_{\text{initial}}}\right)\cdot 100 \quad (2)$$

2.10. *Statistical Analysis*

Data were statistically analyzed using two-tailed paired *t*-Student test, one-way analysis of variance (ANOVA), and the least-significant difference (LSD) multiple comparison test using the software package Statgraphics 19 (Statgraphics Technologies Inc., Rockville, MD, USA).

3. Results and Discussion

3.1. *Performance of the Chromatographic Methods*

A cLC-ESI-MS analytical method was developed, optimized, and validated for the determination of gallic acid, dihydroxybenzoic acid (DHB), catechin, caffeic acid, *p*-coumaric acid, *trans*-ferulic acid, resveratrol, quercetin, and kaempferol, seeking the optimal chromatographic resolution in the minimum analysis time. Based on the LC separation proposed by Gómez-Mejía et al. [21], the former nine compounds were determined in less than 25 min (Table S1). Calibration was performed using analyte standard solutions, where linearity and correlation coefficients were determined via external calibration using peak area values as responses. As shown in Table S1, wide linear ranges were found, namely for kaempferol, quercetin, resveratrol, and *p*-coumaric acid (0.5–180 $\mu g \cdot L^{-1}$), with R^2 values above 0.9900. Further, acceptable LODs and LOQs were estimated in the range 0.1–6.0 $\mu g \cdot L^{-1}$ and 0.3–20 $\mu g \cdot L^{-1}$, respectively, apart from catechin (LOD = 100 $\mu g \cdot L^{-1}$), for which a lower sensitivity was observed, possibly associated with the negative ionization mode [22]. In addition, the repeatability and intermediate precision of the cLC-ESI-MS method were assessed for each polyphenol using the retention factor and peak area. Satisfactory RSD values were observed for all polyphenols analyzed, with RSD values below 7.8%.

To complement this analysis, an HPLC-ESI-QTOF method was also developed and validated to determine a larger number of phenolic compounds, including those reported to be abundant in citrus peels, i.e., hesperidin, naringin, and rutin [15,23]. Exact-mass analysis offered the advantage of unequivocally identifying those bioactive compounds present in the extracts, as well as enhancing selectivity, which is particularly relevant when analyzing complex matrices, such as digested samples. Analyte standard solutions allowed for performing calibration curves (n = 4) by using peak area values, showing wide linear ranges (2–2000 $\mu g \cdot L^{-1}$) and suitable R^2 ($\geq$0.9990) (Table S2). On the other hand, appropriate LODs and LOQs were estimated, under 8.9 $\mu g \cdot L^{-1}$ and 28.7 $\mu g \cdot L^{-1}$ (Table S2), respectively, evidencing an adequate performance of the method. The matrix effect was evaluated by comparing the peak areas of pure standard with those of spiked samples (undigested and digested samples), as described Equation (1). A marked matrix effect was observed for all the polyphenols studied in the undigested and digested bread samples. In bread extract, this effect was less than 61%, apart from *trans*-ferulic acid, which showed a signal inhibition of 91%. As for the digested samples, the highest matrix effect was observed in the salivary stage given the high salinity of this digestive fluid (above 90% except for quercetin and kaempferol, both of which had 76% inhibition). Furthermore, the gastric phase showed a matrix inhibition below 70% by most of the phenolic compounds, while in the duodenal phase this effect was enhanced, especially for gallic acid, DHB, caffeic acid, and *p*-coumaric acid (>91%). Therefore, the quantification of the samples was carried out considering the inhibition percentages determined with Equation (1).

3.2. Determination of the Extraction Conditions of Polyphenols from Wheat Bread

Prior to the evaluation of the functionality of the enriched bread, an initial extraction step of phenolic compounds is required. Thus, to select the most suitable extraction method, different techniques were evaluated, namely, conventional SLE extraction (assisted by mechanical stirring or magnetic stirring with heating) and UAE, using different equipment: an HD ultrasonic homogenizer with a 15.5 mm diameter probe and a Vibra-Cell homogenizer with a 2 mm tip. Conventional solvent extraction was selected because of its widespread use for phenolic extraction in a variety of agri-food matrices, including wheat bread [2]. Furthermore, UAE, a non-conventional technique employed in phenolic extraction from bakery products [24,25], was proposed based on its potential to shorten extraction times, promote matrix tissue breakdown, and increase the mass transfer surface area of the phenolic compounds [26]. On the other hand, all extractions were based on the use of ethanol–water 70:30 (*v*/*v*) mixtures, since they are considered efficient, GRAS, and environmentally friendly [17].

The extraction efficiency of each tested condition was expressed in terms of the TPC, TFC, and DPPH antioxidant activity and compared using ANOVA and LSD tests, showing significant differences (*p*-value < 0.05) in all determinations. As can be observed in Figure 1a,c, the SLE assisted by magnetic stirring and heating showed the highest TPC

(0.14 mg GAE·g^{-1}) and antioxidant activity, i.e., the lowest IC_{50} (28 mg·g^{-1}), followed by the UAE performed with the 15.5 mm probe. Positive correlations have been found between the TPC and the antioxidant activity of phenolic extracts [2,3,12]. Particularly, gallic acid, dihydroxybenzoic acid, and ferulic acid have been described to be potent antiradical agents present in wheat, flour, and bakery samples [3,21]. Moreover, in line with the obtained results, other authors have described the better efficiency of conventional solid–liquid extraction versus ultrasound-assisted extraction, mainly aimed at the recovery of hydroxycinnamic acids [27], which can be due to the oxidation of the phenolic compounds by the formation of free radicals [28].

For the TFC, shown in Figure 1b, the SLE assisted by magnetic stirring and heating was significantly lower than the UAE performed with the 2 mm probe (0.9 mg QE·g^{-1} and 1.46 mg QE·g^{-1}, respectively). The better results of the probe in this respect could be due to the more efficient release of the matrix-bound flavonoids present in the wheat, such as rutin [29], associated with the massive energy released by the ultrasound probe [28]. Furthermore, this compound is not very efficient against DPPH radicals [21], which in turn would account for the higher IC_{50} value compared with the SLE (Figure 1c).

Overall, given the importance of antioxidant activity in the functionality of bakery products and its good correlation with TPC [3,16], as well as the easiness of handling, SLE assisted by stirring and heating was selected as the most favorable technique for extracting bread polyphenols. These results agree with previous studies reporting a higher efficiency of SLE in the recovery of phenolic compounds compared with UAE [30], which could be related to the lower potential to extract other non-phenolic compounds, such as polysaccharides, which not only impair the selectivity but also increase the viscosity of the extract [31].

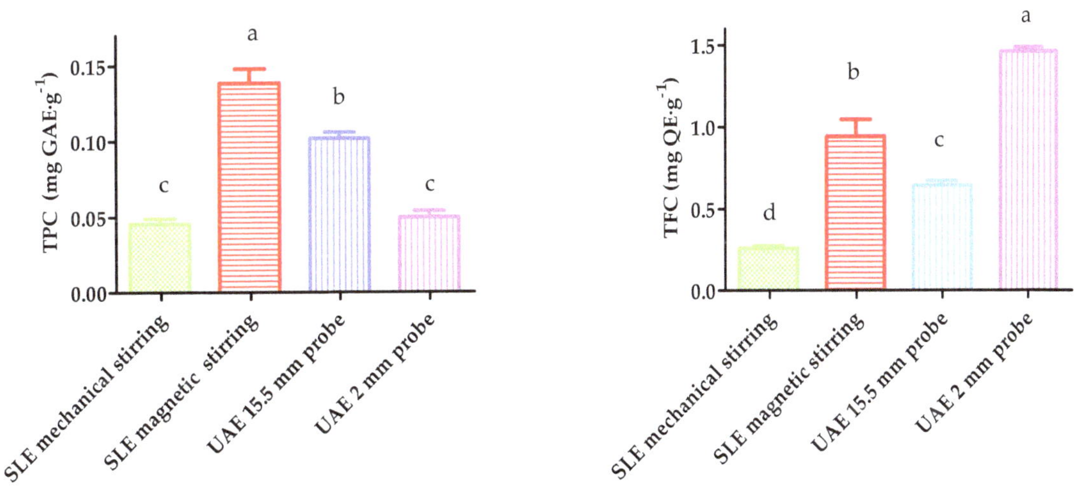

(**a**) (**b**)

Figure 1. *Cont.*

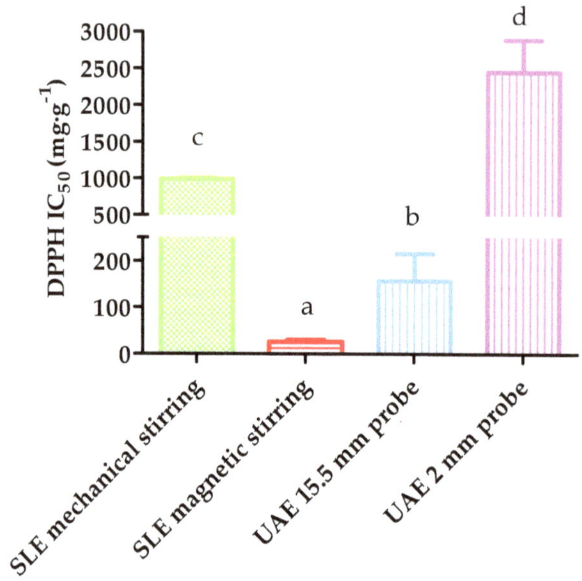

(c)

Figure 1. Comparison of the different extraction techniques used in the recovery of phenolic compounds from bread, according to (**a**) total phenolic content; (**b**) total flavonoid content; and (**c**) DPPH antioxidant activity. Data with different letters are significantly different at $p-$value < 0.05, according to one-way ANOVA and Fisher's LSD test.

3.3. Total Contents and Antioxidant Characterization of Mandarin Peel and Enriched Bread

Citrus extracts were obtained following the SLE procedure described in Section 2.4, given its simplicity, improved efficiency, and easy application on an industrial scale. In this method, a 20:80 (v/v) ethanol–water mixture was used, due to its greater effectiveness compared with extraction with water alone [15]. In addition, ethanol is a Generally Recognized as Safe solvent according to the American Food and Drug Administration [32], so its use avoids the disposal of the solvent, moving towards zero-waste processes, and harmonizes the applicability of ready-to-use phenolic extract with enhanced functionality in the food industry [11,32]. Analogously, the phenolic extracts of the control and enriched breads were obtained according to the SLE method described in Section 2.6, due to its greater effectiveness in the extraction of compounds with DPPH-radical-inhibition capacity, as previously established. The phenolic extracts obtained were characterized in terms of TPC, TFC, and DPPH antiradical activity (Figure 2), which provided rapid and practical information on the variability of phenolic composition in foods and extracts [12,15], and they were then compared with ANOVA and LSD tests, showing significant differences (p-value < 0.05) in all determinations. According to the data included in Figure 2, both total content and antioxidant activity were significantly higher in the mandarin peel extract than in the control and functionalized breads. This is due not only to the fact that citrus peels are particularly abundant in antioxidants [6], but also to the loss of the grain polyphenols in the processing of refined flour and during bread baking [3].

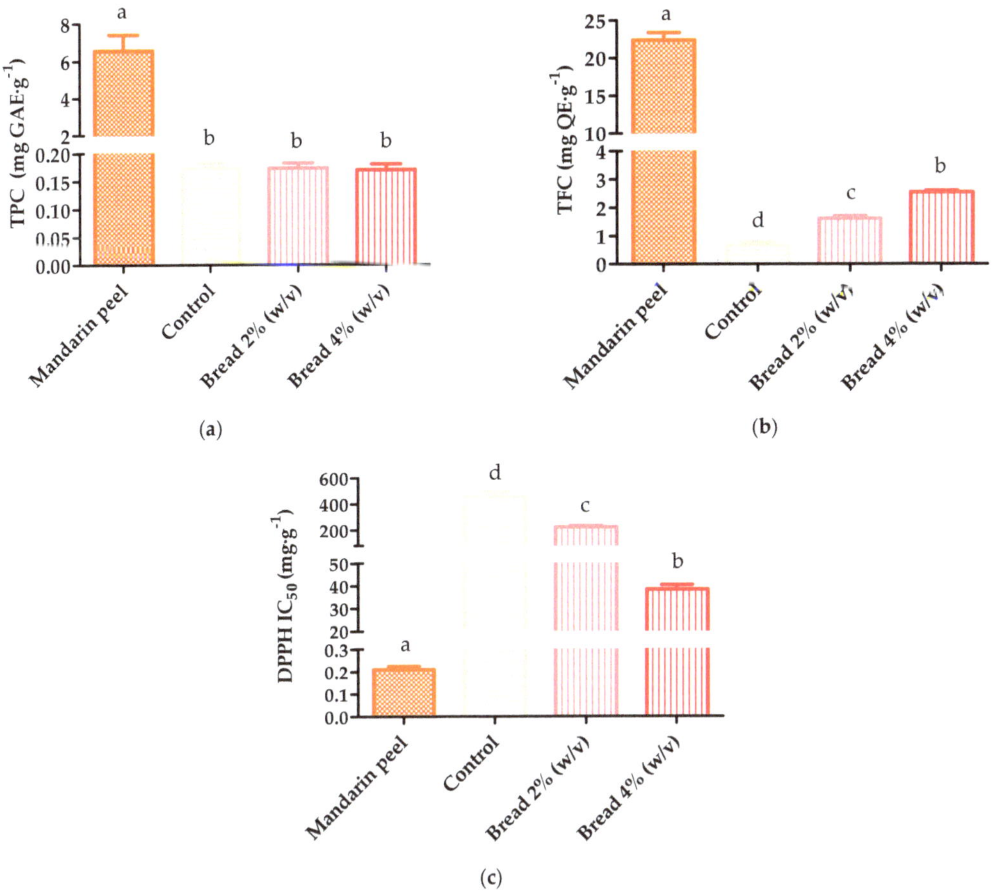

Figure 2. Spectrophotometric determinations of phenolic extracts of mandarin peel, control bread, and enriched bread at 2% (w/v) and 4%(w/v): (**a**) total phenolic content; (**b**) total flavonoid content; (**c**) DPPH antioxidant activity. Data with different letters are significantly different at $p-$value < 0.05, according to one-way ANOVA and Fisher's LSD test.

As a basis for comparison, Anticona et al. determined a TPC ranging from 6 to 9 mg GAE$\cdot$g^{-1} and a TFC varying between 4 and 6 mg CE$\cdot$g^{-1} when analyzing mandarin peel extracts (*C. reticulata* Blanco × *C. Sinensis* Osbeck) with EAU [33], with the values reported in this study being comparable or even higher (TPC = 7 ± 1 mg$\cdot$g^{-1} and TFC 22 ± 1 mg$\cdot$g^{-1}), demonstrating their potential as a source of high value-added compounds. Similarly, the antioxidant activity determined in this study was over 63 mg/100 g, exceeding the value reported herein (IC_{50} = 0.95 mg$\cdot$g^{-1}) for a mandarin peel citrus residue. The higher antioxidant activity of the present extract may be related to a greater content in phenolic compounds with significant free-radical-inhibition activity, such as gallic acid and quercetin [21]. Thus, the promising results of this mandarin peel extract could be attributed to both the efficiency of the extraction method and the polyphenolic potential of the residue evaluated, suggesting its prospective for the fortification and functionalization of white bread.

As for the total indices and antioxidant activity of the fortified breads, a significant dependence on the percentage of fortification was observed for both TFC and DPPH, in contrast to TPC, where all values were roughly comparable (Figure 2). The lack of effect of bread fortification on the TPC could be caused by the presence of sugars, especially abundant in white bread [3], in the extract obtained using SLE with an ethanol–water 70:30 (*v*/*v*) mixture. These sugars also react with the Folin–Ciocalteu reagent and may interfere with the determination and thereby alter the outcome, as previously stated [21]. Conversely, Cedola et al. observed that the TFC of *taralli* (Italian baked bread) quadrupled from 0.09 mg QE$\cdot$g^{-1} to 0.36 mg QE$\cdot$g^{-1} when the dough was enriched with 17% (*w*/*w*) olive leaf extract [34]. A similar trend was reported by Laganà et al. when they studied cookies enriched with bergamot (*Citrus bergamia*) pomace. In particular, a significant proportional increase in TFC was recorded when the citrus residue replaced from 2.5% to 15% (*w*/*w*) of the wheat flour in the formulation [10]. On the other hand, the improvement in the antioxidant activity of the 4% (*w*/*v*) enriched bread was quite substantial, with an IC_{50} reduction of more than tenfold (IC_{50} = 38 $\pm$ 2 mg$\cdot$g^{-1}) compared with the control bread (IC_{50} = 451 $\pm$ 40 mg$\cdot$g^{-1}), while the 2% (*w*/*v*) enriched bread halved its IC_{50} over the control (Figure 2c). Accordingly, the antioxidant potency of citrus fortification in baked goods has been observed in other studies [8,9], highlighting that supplementation with extracts is much more profitable due to the higher purity of phytochemicals compared with whole-residue fortifiers [9].

3.4. Individual Phenolic Composition of Mandarin Peel and Enriched Bread

While spectrophotometric methods are very useful for estimating total phenolic content and antioxidant activity, their lack of selectivity and information regarding the identity of the polyphenols present in the extracts make it necessary to complement the characterization of phenolic extracts using chromatographic methods [12]. As such, the phenolic extract obtained from mandarin peel, control, and fortified breads were analyzed with cLC-ESI-MS and LC-ESI-MS/MS. In total, ten phenolic compounds were identified and quantified, when possible, in the mandarin peel extract (Table 1). The use of HPLC-ESI-MS/MS enabled the unequivocal identification of those bioactive compounds present in the extract, as well as a selectivity improvement, particularly relevant in the analysis of complex samples, such as bread. Thus, HPLC-ESI-MS/MS analysis confirmed the presence of dihydroxybenzoic acid, *p*-coumaric acid, *trans*-ferulic acid, and quercetin, at concentration levels consistent with those obtained using cLC-ESI-MS. Moreover, it allowed the determination of caffeic acid and kaempferol, given a higher sensitivity and selectivity (Tables S1 and S2). However, gallic acid was not detected at the LOD levels of the HPLC-ESI-MS/MS method, although still quantified using cLC-ESI-MS, possibly due to the enhanced LOD of the latter, as it combines the use of the capillary LC column and the on-column focusing technique, thus increasing the sensitivity for these phenolic acid determinations [12]. As a novelty, naringin, hesperidin, rutin, and myricetin were identified and quantified by means of the HPLC-ESI-MS/MS method in the control and 4% (*w*/*v*) fortified bread (Table 1). These phenolic compounds could not be included in the cLC-ESI-MS method, since, as described before, they present a limited ionization, impairing their MS sensitivity against UV-Vis detectors [16,21]. Therefore, for comparative and unequivocal identification purposes, only the phenolic extracts from mandarin peel, the control bread, and the 4% enriched bread were analyzed using HPLC-MS/MS.

Table 1 summarizes the phenolic compounds determined in the phenolic extracts of mandarin peels and the studied breads. The mandarin peel extract was found to be significantly most abundant in the flavonoid family, mainly due to the richness of hesperidin (6.2 mg$\cdot$g^{-1}). Several studies have reported the mentioned flavanone as the predominant phenolic compound in citrus peels, as such hesperidin has been determined in concentrations ranging from 1 to 15 mg$\cdot$g^{-1} in *Citrus reticulata* Blanco [35,36] and *Citrus* $\times$ *clementina* peels [5,16]. These results agree with our data, pointing out that variability in concentration is most likely attributable to the extraction method, the genotype, and variety of the mandarin fruit or the environmental conditions in which it grew [4]. Moreover, the flavone myricetin was found at a significant concentration, 138 µg$\cdot$g^{-1}, followed by quercetin and kaempferol, which were quantified at levels around 60 µg$\cdot$g^{-1}, and, lastly, by rutin and naringin, which were minor components (Table 1). Closely, other authors have found myricetin as a rich compound in *Citrus sinensis* peels [37], while quercetin, kaempferol, and naringin were determined at low concentrations in *Citrus reticulate* L. [36] and *Citrus × clementina* peel extracts [15], respectively. As for rutin, a great variability in its concentration was observed, fluctuating from not detected to 13 $mg \cdot g^{-1}$, in different mandarin peel extracts [36], again probably due to the extraction condition and the environmental and genetic factors [4]. As regards phenolic acids, these accounted for 7% of the total phenolic composition, with gallic acid standing out with a concentration of 280 $\mu g \cdot g^{-1}$, followed by *trans*-ferulic, *p*-coumaric, and caffeic acid, which were present at levels between 96 and 38 $\mu g \cdot g^{-1}$ (Table 1). Consistent with the results obtained, a low amount of caffeic acid (0.32–1.6 mg/g) was also found by Safdar et al. [36]; in contrast, gallic, *p*-coumaric, and *trans*-ferulic acids have been described as the leading acids in peel extracts of *Citrus reticulata* Blanco [38] and *Citrus × clementina* [16]. As for the control bread, more than 70% of the total polyphenol content corresponded to phenolic acids, specifically hydroxycinnamic acids, namely *trans*-ferulic acid (2.01 ± 0.03 $\mu g \cdot g^{-1}$) and *p*-coumaric acid (3.50 ± 0.07 $\mu g \cdot g^{-1}$); followed by the hydroxybenzoic acids; gallic acid (3.52 ± 0.01 $\mu g \cdot g^{-1}$); and dihydroxybenzoic acid, whose concentration did not exceed 1 $\mu g \cdot g^{-1}$ (Table 1). Hesperidin, rutin, and resveratrol appeared in a concentration range between 0.5 and 2 $\mu g \cdot g^{-1}$. Coherent with the above results, phenolic acids have been reported to be more abundant than flavonoids in wheat, flour, and bakery products [3], as well as in extra virgin olive oil [39]. Ferulic acid accounted for more than 59% of the total phenolic acids in refined bread and whole bread, observing *p*-coumaric acid concentrations of 4.5 $\mu g \cdot g^{-1}$ [40]. On the other hand, Sharma et al. [29], reported that different wheat varieties contained concentrations of hesperidin and rutin (3 $\mu g \cdot 100\ g^{-1}$) comparable to those in this study (Table 1). It is also interesting to consider the contribution of extra virgin olive oil to the phenolic composition of prepared bread, although to a lesser extent than wheat, since it accounts for 3% of the bread dough. In this sense, the presence of 3,4-dihydroxybenzoic acid, *p*-coumaric acid, *trans*-ferulic acid, and quercetin has been described in extra virgin olive oil marketed at concentrations lower than 0.46 $\mu g \cdot g^{-1}$, while kaempferol was not detected [39], consistent with the results reported in Table 1. Overall, mandarin peel extracts were found to be more plentiful in phenolic compounds, with a total amount of 7 $mg \cdot g^{-1}$ of the polyphenols screened vs. 12.9 ± 0.3 $\mu g \cdot g^{-1}$ in the control bread, demonstrating their potential as a source of bioactive polyphenols to be used as functional ingredients in the development of enriched bread.

Table 1. Phenolic compounds determined in mandarin peel, control, and fortified wheat bread extracts. Data are expressed as mean ± standard deviation (n = 3).

Compound ($\mu g \cdot g^{-1}$ DW)	Mandarin Peel	Control Bread	2% (*w/v*) Fortified Bread	4% (*w/v*) Fortified Bread
Gallic acid	280 ± 6 [a]	3.52 ± 0.01 [c]	5.3 ± 0.5 [b]	5.6 ± 0.5 [b]
Dihydroxybenzoic acid	*n.d.*	0.29 ± 0.02 [b]	0.42 ± 0.03 [a]	0.44 ± 0.02 [a]
Caffeic acid	38 ± 1 [a]	*n.d.*	*n.d.*	0.75 ± 0.02 [b]
p-Coumaric acid	72.4 ± 0.2 [a]	3.50 ± 0.07 [b]	2.28 ± 0.07 [c]	2.34 ± 0.09 [c]
trans-Ferulic acid	96.2 ± 0.5 [a]	2.01 ± 0.03 [c]	2.4 ± 0.2 [bc]	2.57 ± 0.08 [b]
Rutin	45 ± 4 [a]	2.06 ± 0.01 [c]	*n.a.*	7.3 ± 0.5 [b]
Naringin	13 ± 1 [a]	*n.d.*	*n.a.*	3.0 ± 0.2 [b]
Hesperidin	(6.2 ± 0.9) × 10^3 [a]	1.1 ± 0.4 [c]	*n.a.*	83 ± 3 [b]
Myricetin	138 ± 20 [a]	*n.d.*	*n.a.*	16.6 ± 0.9 [b]
Resveratrol	*n.d.*	0.502 ± 0.001 [a]	0.501 ± 0.001 [a]	0.502 ± 0.002 [a]
Quercetin	63 ± 3 [a]	*n.d.*	22.8 ± 0.6 [c]	33.3 ± 0.6 [b]
Kaempferol	56 ± 8	*n.d.*	*n.d.*	*n.d.*

Table 1. *Cont.*

Compound (μg·g^{-1} DW)	Mandarin Peel	Control Bread	2% (*w*/*v*) Fortified Bread	4% (*w*/*v*) Fortified Bread
Total Phenolic Acids	489 ± 8 ^{a}	9.3 ± 0.1 ^{b}	10.7 ± 0.03 ^{b}	12.4 ± 0.3 ^{b}
Total Flavonoids	6400 ± 900 ^{a}/ *119 ± 10 ^{a}*	3.1 ± 0.4 ^{d}/ *0.502 ± 0.01 ^{c}*	*22.7 ± 0.2^c*	141 ± 3 ^{b}/ *33.8 ± 0.2 ^{b}*
Total Polyphenols	6900 ± 940 ^{a}/ *607 ± 18 ^{a}*	12.9 ± 0.3 ^{d}/ *9.8 ± 0.1 ^{c}*	*33.8 ± 0.2 ^{c}*	154 ± 3 ^{b}/ *46.3 ± 0.9 ^{b}*

Mean values with different letters in the same column indicate significant differences (p-value < 0.05) according to ANOVA and Fisher LSD test. *n.d.* = not detected; *n.a.* = not analyzed. Total values in italics exclude hesperidin, myricetin, rutin, and naringin. DW: dry weight (moisture content of: mandarin peels (38.8 ± 0.6)%, control bread (33.8 ± 0.3)%, 2% (*w*/*v*) enriched bread (29.4 ± 0.5)%, and 4% (*w*/*v*) enriched bread (28.8 ± 0.4)%).

As for the effect of bread enrichment, Table 1 shows significant differences in the profile and content of the fortified breads, both with the control bread and with the crude mandarin peel extract. As for the sum of individual polyphenols, it was three times higher in the bread enriched at 2% (*w*/*v*) compared with the control bread, while in the bread enriched at 4% (*w*/*v*), it was twelvefold higher (Table 1). These results clearly indicate the potential of the 4% (*w*/*v*) enriched bread to improve the total polyphenol content of wheat-based baking products. Specifically, the main effect of mandarin peel phenolic extract fortification was a significant increase in the flavonoid fraction, mainly focused on quercetin, myricetin, and naringin, which were not previously found in the control bread (Table 1), but also on hesperidin, whose concentration reached 83 μg·g^{-1} in the 4% (*w*/*v*) enriched bread and was the main phenolic compound in mandarin peel (Table 1). Likewise, the addition of mandarin peel extract to the dough had a positive effect on the content of *trans*-ferulic acid and gallic acid, with comparable concentrations at both levels of enrichment (p-value > 0.05), probably due to the bonding of their free forms to the matrix components because of the baking process [3]. On the contrary, no effect was observed for kaempferol, which was not detected in either of the two enriched breads, nor when it came to p-coumaric acid, where a lower concentration (p-value < 0.05) was observed for the enriched bread compared with the control. Likewise, Xiao et al. reported the loss of free kaempferol aglycone in a fermented buckwheat bread dough after steaming [41]. These forfeits could be attributed to the oxidation of kaempferol to the benzofuranone form, favored not only by the temperature and heat used during baking, but also by the presence of oxidative enzymes such as polyphenol oxidase, which also leads to the development of the characteristic brown color of the bread [42]. On the other hand, the lower presence of free p-coumaric acid in the enriched breads compared with the control could be attributed to the role of this polyphenol in the inhibition of acrylamide, according to the well-known Millard reaction, which is favored in the presence of reducing sugars, which are possibly co-extruded in the mandarin extract [15,42,43]. Xu and An revealed that p-coumaric acid most likely reacted with a precursor of acrylamide (3-oxopropanamide), giving rise to 2-(propenamide)coumaric acid [42]. Resveratrol, which was not identified in the mandarin peel extract, showed no significant differences between the breads (Table 1), while dihydroxybenzoic acid was significantly increased in the 2%(*w*/*v*) and 4%(*w*/*v*) enriched bread, with a concentration around 40 μg·g^{-1} in each. This could be related to the hydrolysis of the higher-molecular-weight dihydroxybenzoic acid derivatives, since the phenolic extract would have a lower pH than the EtOH–water mixture used in the control bread preparation, thus supporting their breakdown [44]. Similarly, Taglieri et al., concluded that some phenolic compounds, such as feruloyl acid, diosmetin, and glucosidase eriocitrin, were lost during the preparation of bread enriched with 0.75% (*w*/*w*) sour orange albedo, compared with the control [9]. Therefore, the addition of phenolic compounds in food matrices does not always translate to a final enrichment, whereby the effect of the cooking and the matrix plays a pivotal role in the final composition [3].

3.5. In Vitro Gastrointestinal Digestion Study of Phenolic Compounds in Bread

Determining the content of phenolic compounds in foodstuff is not sufficient to predict their potential bioactivity. Indeed, it is well-known that the most widespread polyphenols in foods and beverages are not necessarily the most accessible, nor the most active, given that to perform their function, polyphenols must be released from the matrix, transferred into the bloodstream, and reach up to the target tissue or organ while undergoing mechanical, enzymatic, and metabolic transformations [13]. Hence, a first approach to investigate the effect of the digestive environment on the phenolic stability is to submit the foodstuff to an in vitro gastrointestinal assay [13,34]. In this study, fifteen monomeric and low-molecular-weight phenolic compounds were carefully selected, including phenolic acids, flavonoids, and stilbenes, since these properties would favor their bioaccessibility and eventual bioavailability [12]. In addition, the in vitro digestive stability study of the polyphenols evaluated was performed using the bread itself (control and enriched) and not the derived extracts, since the presence of other phytochemicals and the matrix is essential to representatively assess the bioaccessibility of phenolic compounds in any food [12,13]. As can be seen in Table 2, seven phenolic compounds were identified and quantified, when possible, in all or some of the digestive stages, namely the phenolic acids dihydroxybenzoic, caffeic, *p*-coumaric, and *trans*-ferulic acids and the flavonoids rutin, hesperidin, and quercetin.

Table 2. Phenolic compounds determined during the in vitro digestion process using HPLC-ESI-MS/MS in control and 4% (*w*/*v*) enriched bread (mean ± SD, n = 3).

Compound ($\mu g \cdot g^{-1}$ DW)	Control Bread			4% (*w*/*v*) Fortified Bread		
	Salivary Phase	**Gastric Phase**	**Duodenal Phase**	**Salivary Phase**	**Gastric Phase**	**Duodenal Phase**
Dihydroxybenzoic acid	*n.d.*	0.062 ± 0.009	*n.d.*	*n.d.*	0.09 ± 0.01	*n.d.*
Caffeic acid	*n.d.*	*n.d.*	*n.d.*	0.63 ± 0.02	*n.d.*	*n.d.*
p-Coumaric acid	1.06 ± 0.07	*n.d.*	*n.d.*	0.979 ± 0.002	*n.d.*	*n.d.*
trans-Ferulic acid	0.31 ± 0.06 **	*n.d.*	*n.d.*	0.03 ± 0.01	*n.d.*	*n.d.*
Rutin	0.34 ± 0.03 [b]	1.57 ± 0.04 [a]	*n.d.*	0.41 ± 0.02 [b]	2.6 ± 0.1 [a]	*n.d.*
Hesperidin	*n.d.*	*n.d.*	77 ± 5 **	3.8 ± 0.2 [c]	28.7 ± 0.2 [b]	159 ± 36 [a]
Quercetin	*n.d.*	*n.d.*	*n.d.*	1.25 ± 0.02	*n.d.*	*n.d.*
Total Phenolic Acids	1.37 ± 0.01 [a]	0.062 ± 0.009 [b]	-	2.26 ± 0.06 [a]	0.09 ± 0.01 [b]	-
Total Flavonoids	0.34 ± 0.03 [c]	1.57 ± 0.04 [b]	77 ± 5 [a]	5.48 ± 0.20 [c]	31.3 ± 0.2 [b]	159 ± 36 [a]
Total Polyphenols	1.71 ± 0.05 [b]	1.64 ± 0.03 [b]	77 ± 5 [a]	7.1 ± 0.3 [c]	31.4 ± 0.1 [b]	159 ± 36 [a]

Mean values with different letters in the same column indicate significant differences (*p*-value < 0.05), according to ANOVA and Fisher LSD test. ** Statistical differences < 0.05 by applying a two-tailed paired *t*-Student test to different bread samples at the same digestive stage. *n.d.* = not detected. DW: dry weight (moisture content of: mandarin peels (38.8 ± 0.6)%, control bread (33.8 ± 0.3)%, 2% (*w*/*v*) enriched bread (29.4 ± 0.5)%, and 4% (*w*/*v*) enriched bread (28.8 ± 0.4)%).

Considering the salivary stage, the total polyphenol content was significantly higher in the 4% (*w*/*v*) enriched bread (7.1 ± 0.3 $\mu g \cdot g^{-1}$) compared with the control (1.71 ± 0.05 $\mu g \cdot g^{-1}$), demonstrating the effectiveness of fortification. *p*-Coumaric acid and rutin were determined in comparable concentrations in the salivary phases of both breads (Table 2), while *trans*-ferulic acid was higher in the control bread, and hesperidin, quercetin, and caffeic acid were only determined in the salivary extract of the 4% (*w*/*v*) enriched bread, as these compounds came directly from the mandarin extract (Table 1). Several authors have described good stability of polyphenols such as quercetin, caffeic acid, and *trans*-ferulic acid under oral biochemical conditions [12,45,46].

However, this condition is greatly altered under gastric environments, observing a general shift in both the content and distribution of polyphenols in the bread (Table 2). In this context, a total loss of the previously determined phenolic acids (*p*-coumaric, *trans*-ferulic, and caffeic), as well as of the flavonol quercetin, occurs in both bread samples, either due to acid hydrolysis caused by the low pH of the gastric medium or by their interaction with pepsin via non-covalent bonds [12,46]. On the contrary, dihydroxybenzoic acid appears for the first time at this stage in both samples and at a similar concentration (around 0.08 $\mu g \cdot g^{-1}$) (Table 2). This fact could be due to the release of dihydroxybenzoic acid bound to the baking matrices in acidic media. Previously, Arranz et al. described this behavior when studying the extraction of dihydroxybenzoic acid in wheat flour, inferring that an appreciable number of polyphenols bound to cell-wall constituents or trapped within the food matrix may remain insoluble after aqueous–organic extraction and/or alkaline treatment [44]. Rutin and hesperidin were also released in the gastric phase, with a significantly higher concentration in the 4% (w/v) enriched bread (Table 2). In agreement with current findings, some authors have noted a rather remarkable gastric stability of flavonoid glycosides, such as rutin and hesperidin, even reporting increases in their concentration. As such, it has been suggested that the cleavage of polyphenols with a higher degree of glycosylation in the gastric environment could lead to those disaccharide flavonoids of lower molecular mass [12,47].

After the duodenal phase, complete depletion of phenolic compounds occurs, except for hesperidin (Table 2). A similar observation was previously made by Cedola et al. when studying the digestive stability of oleuropein, hydroxytyrosol, and verbascoside in Italian breads enriched with 17% (w/w) olive leaf extract, reporting such a significant decrease that the enrichment effect was suppressed [34]. Consequently, it can be safely stated that the degradation of bioactive compounds occurs mainly in the intestine, where a mild alkaline pH facilitates the epimerization and auto-oxidation of these compounds in addition to the interaction of phenolic compounds with pancreatin, which reduces the phenolic free form [34,45,46]. As regards hesperidin, it highlights the progressive enrichment of this flavonoid over the different digestive stages (Table 2), which could be explained by the release of matrix-bound hesperidin and/or deglycosylation of high-molecular-weight glycoside derivatives, particularly favored at the mild alkaline pH of the duodenum, as previously reported during the digestion of white tea and whole grapes [12,48]. Hesperidin presented in vitro bioaccessibility indexes above 100% in both cases, reaching (220 ± 6)% in the 4% (w/v) enriched bread, with double the duodenal concentration in the aforementioned case ((159 ± 36) $\mu g \cdot g^{-1}$ vs. (77 ± 5) $\mu g \cdot g^{-1}$ in the control). This fact is noteworthy, not only because it demonstrates the relevance and potential of mandarin-peel-enriched bakery products, but also because different models have shown that hesperidin consumption prevents lung damage, modulates antioxidant enzymes that induce apoptosis and cancer cell proliferation, and prevents cognitive deficits in cell lines, mice, and even in humans [49]. This suggests that consumption of the fortified bread proposed in this study could have beneficial health impacts in consumers, although further in vivo and clinical studies should be conducted.

4. Conclusions

This study has proposed the valorization of citrus peel wastes by obtaining an extract rich in phenolic compounds, which was subsequently used in the preparation of an enriched bread. In particular, the effect of the enrichment percentage of phenolic extract has been evaluated in terms of antioxidant activity and phenolic content. A significant increase in the DPPH free-radical-inhibition potential and in the content of total flavonoids, in particular hesperidin, myricetin, and quercetin, has been observed to a greater extent in the bread enriched at 4% (w/v). In addition, a study of the digestive stability of the polyphenols in the 4% (w/v) enriched bread was carried out and compared with the control bread. The results obtained showed a higher content of total individual polyphenols in the functionalized bread at all digestive stages, although, due to changes in the pH of the medium and digestive enzymes, only hesperidin could be quantified in the duodenal stage, with a concentration as high as 150 $\mu g \cdot g^{-1}$. Thus, such utilization of mandarin peels opens the way to an ecological and low-cost alternative to synthetic additives, with the aim of producing enriched foodstuff with potential health benefits for consumers.

Supplementary Materials: The following supporting information can be downloaded at: https://www.mdpi.com/article/10.3390/antiox12091742/s1, Table S1: Analytical parameters, retention time, and mass spectral data for the identification and quantification of phenolic compounds using the cLC-ESI-MS method, Table S2: Analytical parameters, retention time, molecular formula, and mass spectral data for the identification and quantification of phenolic compounds using the HPLC-ESI-QTOF method.

Author Contributions: Conceptualization, E.G.-M., N.R.-C. and M.E.L.-G.; Data curation, E.G.-M., I.S., N.R.-C. and M.E.L.-G.; Formal analysis, E.G.-M. and I.S.; Funding acquisition, Y.M.; Investigation, E.G.-M. and I.S.; Methodology, E.G.-M., N.R.-C. and M.E.L.-G.; Project administration, Y.M.; Resources, N.R.-C. and M.E.L.-G.; Software, E.G.-M., N.R.-C. and M.E.L.-G.; Supervision, E.G.-M., N.R.-C., M.E.L.-G. and Y.M.; Validation, E.G.-M., N.R.-C. and M.E.L.-G.; Visualization, E.G.-M., N.R.-C. and M.E.L.-G.; Writing—original draft, E.G.-M.; Writing—review and editing, E.G.-M., N.R.-C. and M.E.L.-G. All authors have read and agreed to the published version of the manuscript.

Funding: This research was funded by the Community of Madrid/FEDER program [S2018/BAA-4393, AVAN-SECAL II-CM] and the Ministry of Science, Innovation and Universities [project PID 2020-114714RB-I00].

Institutional Review Board Statement: Not applicable.

Informed Consent Statement: Not applicable.

Data Availability Statement: All data are contained within the article and Supplementary Material.

Acknowledgments: We are grateful to the Analysis Service Unit facilities of ICTAN for the analysis of Liquid Chromatography and Mass Spectrometry.

Conflicts of Interest: The authors declare no conflict of interest.

References

1. Nawaz, R.; Safdar, N.; Ainee, A.; Jabbar, S. Development and Storage Stability Studies of Functional Fruit Drink Supplemented with Polyphenols Extracted from Lemon Peels. *J. Food Process. Preserv.* **2021**, *45*, e15268. [CrossRef]
2. Piechowiak, T.; Grzelak-Błaszczyk, K.; Bonikowski, R.; Balawejder, M. Optimization of Extraction Process of Antioxidant Compounds from Yellow Onion Skin and Their Use in Functional Bread Production. *LWT* **2020**, *117*, 108614. [CrossRef]
3. Dziki, D.; Różyło, R.; Gawlik-Dziki, U.; Świeca, M. Current Trends in the Enhancement of Antioxidant Activity of Wheat Bread by the Addition of Plant Materials Rich in Phenolic Compounds. *Trends Food Sci. Technol.* **2014**, *40*, 48–61. [CrossRef]
4. Silva, R.F.M.; Pogačnik, L. Polyphenols from Food and Natural Products: Neuroprotection and Safety. *Antioxidants* **2020**, *9*, 61. [CrossRef] [PubMed]
5. Leporini, M.; Loizzo, M.R.; Sicari, V.; Pellicanò, T.M.; Reitano, A.; Dugay, A.; Deguin, B.; Tundis, R. *Citrus* × *Clementina* Hort. Juice Enriched with Its by-Products (Peels and Leaves): Chemical Composition, in Vitro Bioactivity, and Impact of Processing. *Antioxidants* **2020**, *9*, 298. [CrossRef]
6. Wedamulla, N.E.; Fan, M.; Choi, Y.J.; Kim, E.K. Citrus Peel as a Renewable Bioresource: Transforming Waste to Food Additives. *J. Funct. Foods* **2022**, *95*, 105163. [CrossRef]
7. Li, W.; Li, Y.; Bi, J.; Ji, Q.; Zhao, X.; Zheng, Q.; Tan, S.; Gao, X. Effect of Hot Air Drying on the Polyphenol Profile of Hongjv (Citrus Reticulata Blanco, CV. Hongjv) Peel: A Multivariate Analysis. *J. Food Biochem.* **2020**, *44*, e13174. [CrossRef]
8. Taglieri, I.; Sanmartin, C.; Venturi, F.; Macaluso, M.; Bianchi, A.; Sgherri, C.; Quartacci, M.F.; De Leo, M.; Pistelli, L.; Palla, F.; et al. Bread Fortified with Cooked Purple Potato Flour and Citrus Albedo: An Evaluation of Its Compositional and Sensorial Properties. *Foods* **2021**, *10*, 942. [CrossRef]
9. Yaqoob, M.; Aggarwal, P.; Rasool, N.; Baba, W.N.; Ahluwalia, P.; Abdelrahman, R. Enhanced Functional Properties and Shelf Stability of Cookies by Fortification of Kinnow Derived Phytochemicals and Residues. *J. Food Meas. Charact.* **2021**, *15*, 2369–2376. [CrossRef]
10. Laganà, V.; Giuffrè, A.M.; De Bruno, A.; Poiana, M. Formulation of Biscuits Fortified with a Flour Obtained from Bergamot By-Products (*Citrus bergamia*, Risso). *Foods* **2022**, *11*, 1137. [CrossRef]
11. Castillo, A.; Celeiro, M.; Rubio, L.; Bañobre, A.; Otero-Otero, M.; Garcia-Jares, C.; Lores, M. Optimization of Bioactives Extraction from Grape Marc via a Medium Scale Ambient Temperature System and Stability Study. *Front. Nutr.* **2022**, *9*, 1008457. [CrossRef] [PubMed]
12. Gómez-Mejía, E.; Rosales-Conrado, N.; León-González, M.E.; Valverde, A.; Madrid, Y. A Combined Analytical-Chemometric Approach for the in Vitro Determination of Polyphenol Bioaccessibility by Simulated Gastrointestinal Digestion. *Anal. Bioanal. Chem.* **2022**, *414*, 2739–2755. [CrossRef] [PubMed]

13. Carbonell-Capella, J.M.; Buniowska, M.; Barba, F.J.; Esteve, M.J.; Frígola, A. Analytical Methods for Determining Bioavailability and Bioaccessibility of Bioactive Compounds from Fruits and Vegetables: A Review. *Compr. Rev. Food Sci. Food Saf.* **2014**, *13*, 155–171. [CrossRef] [PubMed]
14. AOAC International AOAC: Official Methods of Analysis. 1980. Available online: https://archive.org/details/gov.law.aoac.methods (accessed on 27 July 2023).
15. Gómez-Mejía, E.; Rosales-Conrado, N.; León-González, M.E.; Madrid, Y. Citrus Peels Waste as a Source of Value-Added Compounds: Extraction and Quantification of Bioactive Polyphenols. *Food Chem.* **2019**, *295*, 289–299. [CrossRef]
16. Gómez-Mejía, E.; Sacristán, I.; Rosales-Conrado, N.; León-González, M.E.; Madrid, Y. Effect of Storage and Drying Treatments on Antioxidant Activity and Phenolic Composition of Lemon and Clementine Peel Extracts. *Molecules* **2023**, *28*, 1624. [CrossRef]
17. Gómez-Mejía, E.; Vicente-Zurdo, D.; Rosales-Conrado, N.; León-González, M.E.; Madrid, Y. Screening the Extraction Process of Phenolic Compounds from Pressed Grape Seed Residue: Towards an Integrated and Sustainable Management of Viticultural Waste. *LWT* **2022**, *169*, 113988. [CrossRef]
18. International Council for Harmonisation ICH Topic Q 2 (R1) Validation of Analytical Procedures: Text and Methodology. 1995. Available online: https://www.ema.europa.eu/en/ich-q2r2-validation-analytical-procedures-scientific-guideline (accessed on 27 July 2023).
19. Rambla-Alegre, M.; Esteve-Romero, J.; Carda-Broch, S. Is It Really Necessary to Validate an Analytical Method or Not? That Is the Question. *J. Chromatogr. A* **2012**, *1232*, 101–109. [CrossRef]
20. Minekus, M.; Alminger, M.; Alvito, P.; Ballance, S.; Bohn, T.; Bourlieu, C.; Carrière, F.; Boutrou, R.; Corredig, M.; Dupont, D.; et al. A Standardised Static In Vitro Digestion Method Suitable for Food—An International Consensus. *Food Funct.* **2014**, *5*, 1113–1124. [CrossRef]
21. Gómez-Mejía, E.; Mikkelsen, L.H.; Rosales-Conrado, N.; León-González, M.E.; Madrid, Y. A Combined Approach Based on Matrix Solid-Phase Dispersion Extraction Assisted by Titanium Dioxide Nanoparticles and Liquid Chromatography to Determine Polyphenols from Grape Residues. *J. Chromatogr. A* **2021**, *1644*, 462128. [CrossRef]
22. Suo, G.; Sun, Z.; Sun, Y.; Xue, W.; Zhou, L.; Zhang, J.; Bao, X.; Zhu, Z.; Zhang, X. Rapid Determination of 30 Bioactive Constituents in XueBiJing Injection Using Ultra High Performance Liquid Chromatography-High Resolution Hybrid Quadrupole-Orbitrap Mass Spectrometry Coupled with Principal Component Analysis. *J. Pharm. Biomed. Anal.* **2017**, *137*, 220–228. [CrossRef]
23. Liu, N.; Li, X.; Zhao, P.; Zhang, X.; Qiao, O.; Huang, L.; Guo, L.; Gao, W. A Review of Chemical Constituents and Health-Promoting Effects of Citrus Peels. *Food Chem.* **2021**, *365*, 130585. [CrossRef] [PubMed]
24. Kruczek, M.; Gumul, D.; Korus, A.; Buksa, K.; Ziobro, R. Phenolic Compounds and Antioxidant Status of Cookies Supplemented with Apple Pomace. *Antioxidants* **2023**, *12*, 324. [CrossRef]
25. Blicharski, T.; Oniszczuk, A.; Olech, M.; Oniszczuk, T.; Wójtowicz, A.; Krawczyk, W.; Nowak, R. Puffed Cereals with Added Chamomile—Quantitative Analysis of Polyphenols and Optimization of Their Extraction Method. *Ann. Agric. Environ. Med.* **2017**, *24*, 222–228. [CrossRef]
26. Sagar, N.A.; Pareek, S.; Sharma, S.; Yahia, E.M.; Lobo, M.G. Fruit and Vegetable Waste: Bioactive Compounds, Their Extraction, and Possible Utilization. *Compr. Rev. Food Sci. Food Saf.* **2018**, *17*, 512–531. [CrossRef] [PubMed]
27. Tapia-Quirós, P.; Montenegro-Landívar, M.F.; Vecino, X.; Alvarino, T.; Luis Cortina, J.; Saurina, J.; Granados, M.; Reig, M. A Green Approach to Phenolic Compounds Recovery from Olive Mill and Winery Wastes. *Sci. Total Environ.* **2022**, *835*, 155552. [CrossRef] [PubMed]
28. Ameer, K.; Shahbaz, H.M.; Kwon, J.H. Green Extraction Methods for Polyphenols from Plant Matrices and Their Byproducts: A Review. *Compr. Rev. Food Sci. Food Saf.* **2017**, *16*, 295–315. [CrossRef] [PubMed]
29. Sharma, M.; Rahim, M.S.; Kumar, P.; Mishra, A.; Sharma, H.; Roy, J. Large-Scale Identification and Characterization of Phenolic Compounds and Their Marker–Trait Association in Wheat. *Euphytica* **2020**, *216*, 127. [CrossRef]
30. Garcia-Vallejo, M.C.; Solarte-Toro, J.C.; Ortiz-Sanchez, M.; Chamorro-Anaya, L.; Chamorro-Anaya, L.; Peroza-Piñeres, P.; Pérez-Cordero, A.; Cardona Alzate, C.A. Exploring the Production of Antioxidants and Biogas from Avocado (*Persea Americana* Var. Americana) Residues as an Alternative for Developing Rural Bioeconomies. *Sustain. Chem. Pharm.* **2023**, *33*, 101089. [CrossRef]
31. Teslić, N.; Bojanić, N.; Rakić, D.; Takači, A.; Zeković, Z.; Fišteš, A.; Bodroža-Solarov, M.; Pavlić, B. Defatted Wheat Germ as Source of Polyphenols—Optimization of Microwave-Assisted Extraction by RSM and ANN Approach. *Chem. Eng. Process.—Process Intensif.* **2019**, *143*, 107634. [CrossRef]
32. Banerjee, J.; Singh, R.; Vijayaraghavan, R.; MacFarlane, D.; Patti, A.F.; Arora, A. Bioactives from Fruit Processing Wastes: Green Approaches to Valuable Chemicals. *Food Chem.* **2017**, *225*, 10–22. [CrossRef]
33. Anticona, M.; Blesa, J.; Lopez-Malo, D.; Frigola, A.; Esteve, M.J. Effects of Ultrasound-Assisted Extraction on Physicochemical Properties, Bioactive Compounds, and Antioxidant Capacity for the Valorization of Hybrid Mandarin Peels. *Food Biosci.* **2021**, *42*, 101185. [CrossRef]
34. Cedola, A.; Palermo, C.; Centonze, D.; Nobile, M.A.D.; Conte, A. Characterization and Bio-Accessibility Evaluation of Olive Leaf Extract-Enriched "Taralli". *Foods* **2020**, *9*, 1268. [CrossRef] [PubMed]
35. Ferreira, S.S.; Silva, A.M.; Nunes, F.M. Citrus Reticulata Blanco Peels as a Source of Antioxidant and Anti-Proliferative Phenolic Compounds. *Ind. Crops Prod.* **2018**, *111*, 141–148. [CrossRef]

36. Safdar, M.N.; Kausar, T.; Jabbar, S.; Mumtaz, A.; Ahad, K.; Saddozai, A.A. Extraction and Quantification of Polyphenols from Kinnow (*Citrus reticulate* L.) Peel Using Ultrasound and Maceration Techniques. *J. Food Drug Anal.* **2017**, *25*, 488–500. [CrossRef] [PubMed]
37. Zulkifli, K.S.; Abdullah, N.; Abdullah, A.; Aziman, N.; Wan Saidatul, S.W.K. Bioactive Phenolic Compounds and Antioxidant Activity of Selected Fruit Peels. *Int. Proc. Chem. Biol. Environ. Eng. (IPCBEE)* **2012**, *49*, 66–70.
38. Hayat, K.; Zhang, X.; Chen, H.; Xia, S.; Jia, C.; Zhong, F. Liberation and Separation of Phenolic Compounds from Citrus Mandarin Peels by Microwave Heating and Its Effect on Antioxidant Activity. *Sep. Purif. Technol.* **2010**, *73*, 371–376. [CrossRef]
39. Geana, E.I.; Ciucure, C.T.; Apetrei, I.M.; Clodoveo, M.L.; Apetrei, C. Discrimination of Olive Oil and Extra-Virgin Olive Oil from Other Vegetable Oils by Targeted and Untargeted HRMS Profiling of Phenolic and Triterpenic Compounds Combined with Chemometrics. *Int. J. Mol. Sci.* **2023**, *24*, 5292. [CrossRef]
40. Lu, Y.; Luthria, D.; Fuerst, E.P.; Kiszonas, A.M.; Yu, L.; Morris, C.F. Effect of Processing on Phenolic Composition of Dough and Bread Fractions Made from Refined and Whole Wheat Flour of Three Wheat Varieties. *J. Agric. Food Chem.* **2014**, *62*, 10431–10436. [CrossRef]
41. Xiao, Y.; Yang, C.; Xu, H.; Zhang, J.; Zhang, L. Study on the Change of Flavonoid Glycosides to Aglycones during the Process of Steamed Bread Containing Tartary Buckwheat Flour and Antioxidant, α-Glucosidase Inhibitory Activities Evaluation in Vitro. *LWT* **2021**, *145*, 111527. [CrossRef]
42. Xu, X.; An, X. Study on Acrylamide Inhibitory Mechanism in Maillard Model Reaction: Effect of p-Coumaric Acid. *Food Res. Int.* **2016**, *84*, 9–17. [CrossRef]
43. Debelo, H.; Li, M.; Ferruzzi, M.G. Processing Influences on Food Polyphenol Profiles and Biological Activity. *Curr. Opin. Food Sci.* **2020**, *32*, 90–102. [CrossRef]
44. Arranz, S.; Saura Calixto, F. Analysis of Polyphenols in Cereals May Be Improved Performing Acidic Hydrolysis: A Study in Wheat Flour and Wheat Bran and Cereals of the Diet. *J. Cereal Sci.* **2010**, *51*, 313–318. [CrossRef]
45. Tenore, G.C.; Campiglia, P.; Giannetti, D.; Novellino, E. Simulated Gastrointestinal Digestion, Intestinal Permeation and Plasma Protein Interaction of White, Green, and Black Tea Polyphenols. *Food Chem.* **2015**, *169*, 320–326. [CrossRef] [PubMed]
46. Soares, M.J.; Sampaio, G.R.; Guizellini, G.M.; Figueira, M.S.; Pinaffi, A.C.D.C.; Soares Freitas, R.A.M.; Shahidi, F.; de Camargo, A.C.; Torres, E.A.F.D.S. Regular and Decaffeinated Espresso Coffee Capsules: Unravelling the Bioaccessibility of Phenolic Compounds and Their Antioxidant Properties in Milk Model System upon in Vitro Digestion. *LWT* **2021**, *135*, 110255. [CrossRef]
47. Celep, E.; Charehsaz, M.; Akyüz, S.; Acar, E.T.; Yesilada, E. Effect of in Vitro Gastrointestinal Digestion on the Bioavailability of Phenolic Components and the Antioxidant Potentials of Some Turkish Fruit Wines. *Food Res. Int.* **2015**, *78*, 209–215. [CrossRef] [PubMed]
48. Tagliazucchi, D.; Verzelloni, E.; Bertolini, D.; Conte, A. In Vitro Bio-Accessibility and Antioxidant Activity of Grape Polyphenols. *Food Chem.* **2010**, *120*, 599–606. [CrossRef]
49. Pyrzynska, K. Hesperidin: A Review on Extraction Methods, Stability and Biological Activities. *Nutrients* **2022**, *14*, 2387. [CrossRef]

antioxidants

MDPI

Article

Phenols Extraction from Sorghum Byproducts: Upcycling Strategies and Food Applications

Tiziana Amoriello [1,*], Francesco Mellara [1], Roberto Ciorba [2], Danilo Ceccarelli [2], Monica Amoriello [3], Federica Taddei [4] and Roberto Ciccoritti [2,*]

1 Consiglio per la Ricerca in Agricoltura e l'Analisi dell'Economia Agraria, Research Centre for Food and Nutrition, Via Ardeatina 546, 00178 Rome, Italy; francesco.mellara@crea.gov.it

2 Consiglio per la Ricerca in Agricoltura e l'Analisi dell'Economia Agraria, Research Centre for Olive, Citrus and Tree Fruit, Via di Fioranello 52, 00134 Rome, Italy; roberto.ciorba@crea.gov.it (R.C.); danilo.ceccarelli@crea.gov.it (D.C.)

3 Consiglio per la Ricerca in Agricoltura e l'Analisi dell'Economia Agraria, Central Administration, Via Archimede 59, 00197 Rome, Italy; monica.amoriello@crea.gov.it

4 Consiglio per la Ricerca in Agricoltura e l'Analisi dell'Economia Agrarian, Research Centre for Engineering and Agro-Food Processing, Via Manziana 30, 00189 Rome, Italy; federica.taddei@crea.gov.it

* Correspondence: tiziana.amoriello@crea.gov.it (T.A.); roberto.ciccoritti@crea.gov.it (R.C.)

Abstract: In this research, ultrasound-assisted extraction (UAE) coupled with response surface methodology was used to identify the optimal process parameters (temperature, time, and solvent composition (ethanol–water ratio)) for bioactive compounds extraction from stalks and debranning products. Extraction efficiency was assessed in terms of total phenolic compounds (TPCs) and antioxidant activity (AA), and phenolic profiles were identified using HPLC-DAD for the four samples of byproducts (two samples from stalks, C1 and C2, and two samples for debranning products, C3 and C4, from two different farms). The optimized extract containing the highest amount of TPC at different levels was used to enrich bread to evaluate the ability of extending their shelf life using a hyperspectral imaging device (935–1720 nm). Under the optimal conditions, the amounts of phenolics on average in stalk increased by about 79.5% and 47.0% in debranning products, whereas the relative AA increased by about 28.5% (C1 and C2 samples) and 63.0% (C3 and C4 samples) when UAE was applied with respect to the traditional technique. The characterization of stalk phenolic acids profile revealed that gallic, ferulic, and 4-coumaric acids were the prevalent ones. Otherwise, caffeic, syringic, and 3-coumaric acids were the most abundant in debranning products. As expected, enriched bread showed a significant increase in TPC and AA values without influence on organoleptic characteristics. Finally, enriched bread showed a shelf-life increase of about five days.

Keywords: ultrasound-assisted extraction; response surface methodology; phenolic profile; antioxidant activity; bread; shelf life; hyperspectral imaging; sensorial analysis; sorghum; solvents tested

1. Introduction

Sorghum, (*Sorghum bicolor* L.), is a cereal crop belonging to the Poaceae (Gramineae) family. It originated in Africa, and later spread widely through Asia, Australia, and America, due to its high adaptability to various climate and soil conditions, its high resistance to drought and salinity, low fertilizing rate, and high resistance to biotic and abiotic stress [1–3].

It is the fifth most important cereal crop worldwide, with a wide range of applications in the food, feed, fuel, and industrial sectors. Its adaptability and nutritional profile make it valuable for both human consumption and agricultural systems worldwide [2]. Correspondingly, sorghum can be diversified into four major categories, encompassing grain sorghum, sweet sorghum, forage sorghum, and biomass sorghum [2]. From a human food point of view, sorghum can be used for whole grain consumption, flatbreads and porridges, gluten-free products, malting and brewing, as well as syrup preparation [4]. Sorghum is a major component of livestock feed, especially in semi-arid regions where maize is less productive. The grain can be used in feed rations for poultry, swine, and cattle. Forage sorghums are cultivated for grazing, hay, or silage. Moreover, stover can be used as roughage for ruminants [5]. Sorghum has gained importance as a bioenergy crop, especially in the context of renewable energy and climate resilience [6]. Ethanol can be produced from high biomass and sugar-rich varieties (e.g., sweet sorghum) [7]. Sorghum is used in biogas plants and for combustion in biomass energy systems. Finally, sorghum can be used for various non-food industrial applications, such as for the development of bioplastics and packaging, adhesives and paper, and building materials [8]. The adaptability to dietary and industrial applications is due to its biochemical composition, which can vary a lot, and it can depend on genotype, environmental conditions (growth location, soil type, and climate), agronomic management, and processing [9]. It is a high-energy cereal primarily composed of complex carbohydrates, mainly starch, which accounts for most of its dry matter. Although starch in grain sorghum varies from 32.0 to 72.5 g 100 g^{-1}, it generally contains 20–30% amylose and 70–80% amylopectin [10]. Sorghum is also rich in protein (8−14 g 100 g^{-1}), fat (2−5 g 100 g^{-1}), insoluble fiber (6−15 g 100 g^{-1}), beneficial for digestive health and glycemic control, and bioactive components like vitamin B and fat-soluble vitamins (D, E, and K), minerals (iron, zinc, phosphorus, magnesium, and potassium), and phytochemicals and antioxidants, such as anthocyanins and polyphenols [2]. Therefore, sorghum can contribute to human health, due to its antioxidative, anti-inflammatory, and anticancer effects, as well as its free radical scavenging and high antioxidant activity [11].

The cultivation and the processing of sorghum generate several byproducts, which are not part of the primary harvested grain but have economic, agricultural, or industrial value when properly managed or processed. In particular, stalks are the residues of the aboveground biomass left after grain harvest, including stems and leaves. They are employed for livestock fodder (grazing, hay, or silage), for mulching and soil cover to reduce erosion, or as raw material for bioenergy (e.g., biogas, bioethanol, etc.) [12]. With regard to the processed waste, the outer layers of the sorghum grain that are removed during debranning are defined as debranning products. They can be used as animal feed, being rich in fiber and residual nutrients, as dietary fiber supplement in human nutrition, or as a source of antioxidants (especially phenolic compounds) [13]. Other types of waste can be the germ of grain, used as protein-rich feed ingredient or for oil extraction; the bagasse, i.e., the fibrous residue left after crushing the stalks of sweet sorghum to extract juice for syrup or ethanol production, used as biofuel, animal bedding or compost, or substrate for mushroom cultivation [14]. Finally, sorghum residues can also be used as soil amendments through composting or incorporation into the soil; biodegradable packaging using fiber composites; substrate for microbial fermentation or enzyme production; or as growth medium in biotech processes [15]. In the last few years, great attention has been paid to the byproducts phenolic compounds' recovery using green chemistry techniques and chemometric tools such as ultrasound-assisted extraction, coupled with response surface methodology (RSM). Indeed, UAE is considered a green, efficient, and non-thermal extraction technique that uses ultrasonic waves to enhance the recovery of bioactive compounds from plant materials, including agricultural byproducts like sorghum residues [16].

RSM is a statistical and mathematical tool useful to optimize complex processes, such as ultrasound-assisted extraction, by evaluating the relationships between multiple independent variables (process parameters) and one or more response variables (e.g., TPC, AA, etc.) [16].

In this study, stalks and debranning products from sorghum white hybrid were considered to extract polyphenols and to evaluate the antioxidant activity of the extracts. The extraction was carried out using green solvents, ethanol, and water at different ratios, by applying UAE, while RSM was used to optimize the process parameters (solvent composition, extraction time, and extraction temperature). Then, on the optimized extracts, phenolic acids compositions of two types of residues (stalks and debranning products) were analyzed using HPLC-DAD to evaluate the most abundant phenolic acids. The extract with the highest TPC was used to enrich bread in order to assess its effect on the shelf life of bread, considering the antibacterial properties of phenolic compounds (especially due to gallic and ferulic acids). The potential of the extract as a natural preservative and to extend bread shelf life by inhibiting bacterial growth was evaluated using a short-wave infrared (SWIR) hyperspectral imaging (HSI) device (935–1720 nm). Finally, consumers' sensory perception and acceptability of enriched bread were investigated.

2. Materials and Methods

2.1. Raw Materials

Sorghum byproducts were obtained by cultivation (stalks) and processing (debranning products) of white hybrid, named Artista, from an organic farm and an integrated farm in Latium, Italy (Table 1). All byproducts were collected at kernel maturation. Entire stalks (length about 1.60 m) were reduced in size, frozen with liquid nitrogen, and then ground with a laboratory mill (Retsch ZM 200, Retsch GmbH 42781 Haan, Retsch-Allee 1-5, Germany) to obtain fine flour with particle size of $\leq$500 μm. Sorghum grain was oven-dried at 35–36 °C until the moisture content was less than 12 g 100 g^{-1}, below which microbial growth is strongly inhibited [16]. Then, grain was debranned, and the resulting debranning products were ground with a laboratory mill (Retsch ZM 200, Retsch GmbH 42781 Haan, Retsch-Allee 1-5, Germany) to obtain fine flour with particle size of $\leq$500 μm. All samples were divided into two aliquots, the first for traditional analyses and the second one to optimize the ultrasound-assisted extraction.

Table 1. Samples of sorghum byproducts used in this study.

Sample	Type of Waste	Type of Farm
C1	Stalk	Organic
C2	Stalk	Integrated
C3	Debranning products	Integrated
C4	Debranning products	Organic

Commercial soft wheat flour (Petra Srl, Vighizzolo d'Este, PD, Italy), fresh compressed yeast, and salt for bread were purchased from a local market.

2.2. Proximate Composition

Proximate composition of raw materials was performed in triplicate and the data were expressed as g 100 g^{-1} on a dry weight basis (DW). Moisture, ashes, and proteins were determined by the ICC standard methods 110/1, 104/1, and 105/2, respectively [17]. Protein content was estimated using the nitrogen-to protein conversion factors of 6.25 for sorghum byproducts and 5.7 for wheat flour. Total dietary fiber (TDF) content was obtained using a reagent kit (supelco TDF100A, Merck, Darmstadt, Germany), according to the AOAC method (1990) [18].

2.3. Determination of Total Phenolic Content, Flavans, Pigment, and Antioxidant Activity

TPC of raw materials and extracts were measured using the Folin–Ciocalteu method, as reported by Ciccoritti et al. [19]. Results are expressed as mg of gallic acid equivalents (GAE) 100 g^{-1} of fresh weight (FW). The vanillin assay method was applied to total flavans content (TTFC) determination according to Sun et al. [20]. TFC was calculated from a calibration curve, using catechin as a standard and the results were expressed as milligram of catechin equivalents per 100 g of fresh weight (mg CAE 100 g^{-1} FW). Pigments, i.e., chlorophyll a (ChA), chlorophyll b (ChB), and yellow pigment (YPG) were determined according to Dere et al. [21]. ChA and ChB were expressed as micrograms per 100 g of fresh weight (μg 100 g^{-1} FW), whereas YPG as grams per 100 g of fresh weight (g 100 g^{-1} FW).

The antioxidant activity of the extracts was evaluated with 2,2-diphenyl-1-picrylhydrazyl (DPPH) and the data were expressed as milligram of Trolox equivalent per 100 g of fresh weight (mg TE 100 g^{-1} FW) [22]. All determinations were performed in triplicate.

2.4. Extraction of Soluble Phenolic Compounds by Sorghum Byproducts Using Ultrasound-Assisted Extraction and Optimization Procedure

Soluble phenolic compounds (hereinafter referred to as phenolic compounds) from the four sorghum byproducts samples were extracted using ultrasound-assisted extraction (UAE) by an ultrasonic bath (ElmasonicS30H, Elma Ultrasonic Technology, Singen, Germany). For each sample, 2.0 g of dried and fine-milled material was diluted with 40 mL of different solvents in a tube, mixed, and sonicated at 37 kHz. A mixture of ethanol and water (with different ratio) was used as green solvent for UAE, whereas acidified methanol: water (80:20, 0.1% HCl) was used for the traditional extraction technique, as previously reported by Iadecola et al. [16]. The heating power was set at 200 W.

A Box–Behnken design (BBD) with three process parameters as independent factors (green solvent composition, extraction time, and extraction temperature) was considered for UAE, with these being the factors that most influence extraction efficiency and allow high yield and phytochemical contents [23]. Each factor was coded at three levels, −1, 0, and +1 (Table 2).

Table 2. Box–Behnken design with coded and uncoded parameters of ultrasound-assisted extraction (UAE).

Run	X_1	X_2	X_3	X_1 (%)	X_2 (min)	X_3 (°C)
1	−1	−1	0	50	40	75
2	1	−1	0	80	40	75
3	−1	1	0	50	60	75
4	1	1	0	80	60	75
5	−1	0	−1	50	50	70
6	1	0	−1	80	50	70
7	−1	0	1	50	50	80
8	1	0	1	80	50	80
9	0	−1	−1	65	40	70
10	0	1	−1	65	60	70
11	0	−1	1	65	40	80
12	0	1	1	65	60	80
13	0	0	0	65	50	75
14	0	0	0	65	50	75
15	0	0	0	65	50	75

Legend: X_1 = green solvent composition (%); X_2 = extraction time (min); X_3 = extraction temperature (°C).

The green solvent composition (X_1) is an ethanol–water ratio (50–65–80%). Extraction time (X_2) varied between 40 min and 60 min. Extraction temperature (X_3) ranged from 70 to 80 °C. The values of factor levels were chosen by previous studies on cereals [14]. The maximum settable temperature of the ultrasound equipment was 80 °C; therefore, it was the maximum value for extraction temperature. Times up to 60 min were set because the pilot study demonstrated that longer extraction times did not increase yields and were not economically sustainable. The design included 15 runs (three at the central point); each run was replicated three times.

At the end of sonication, the tube was cooled in a box with water and ice for 10 min, then centrifuged at 1500× *g* for 20 min at 4 °C. Finally, each sample was filtered using a nylon syringe filter (0.45 μm) and the supernatants were immediately analyzed.

RSM was used to optimize the process parameters to carry out the maximum yield in phenols. The predicted TPC content was carried out using a second-order polynomial equation, as follows:

$$Y_i = \beta_0 + \sum_{i=1}^{3} \beta_i X_i + \sum_{i=1}^{3} \beta_{ii} X_i^2 + \sum_{ij,i<j} \beta_{ij} X_i X_j + e_i \quad (1)$$

where Y = TPC; X_1 = green solvent composition (%); X_2 = extraction time (min); X_3 = extraction temperature (°C); β_0 = intercept; β_i, β_{ii}, β_{ij} = linear, quadratic, and interactive coefficients, respectively; e_i = error term. Goodness of fit of the model was evaluated by the coefficient of determination R^2, the adjusted coefficient of determination ${R_{adj}}^2$, and the lack of fit value [16]. The optimization procedure was carried out using 3D plots and desirability functions, as described by Iadecola et al. [16].

2.5. Optimization of Antioxidant Activity by UAE Extracts

The extracts obtained with BBD (Table 2) were also used to identify the optimal extraction conditions to gain the highest antioxidant activity. For this purpose, the RSM and the optimization procedure were used as described in Section 2.4, considering the antioxidant activity as the response variable.

2.6. Profiling of Phenolic Acids by HPLC-DAD

Once extracted, phenolic acids (PAs) were analyzed by RP-HPLC, using a Kinetex C18 (150 × 2.1 mm i.d., 1.7 μm) from Phenomenex (Torrance, CA, USA), placed in a column oven set at 30 °C, and Agilent 1290 Infinity Binary LC with UV–Vis photodiode array detector (DAD G4212A) (Agilent, Milan, Italy), as reported by Amoriello et al. [24]. The detected phenolic acids included gallic, vanillic, 4-coumaric, ferulic, caffeic, syringic, 3-coumaric, and sinapic acids. All standards and sample solutions were analyzed in triplicate, and the content of PAs was expressed as micrograms per milliliter of extracted (μg mL^{-1}).

2.7. Bread-Making Process

The dough of bread used as control (P1) was made with 1000 g wheat flour (14% moisture basis), 750 g of water, 20 g of compressed baker's yeast, and 20 g of salt. Bread loaves were produced by replacing part of the water content with extract C1, as C1 had the highest phenols content. Hence, bread samples were produced by replacing part of the water content with 10% (P2) and 20% (P3) of extract. We chose to use the extract from the sample with the highest content of phenols, namely, C1. Therefore, an extract from C1 was produced under optimal extraction conditions. Then, the ethanol was evaporated under nitrogen gas flow, and the obtained dry sample was reconstituted with the same water quantity to recover all bioactive compounds extracted.

The ingredients were mixed for 10 min in a planetary bread mixer (Quick 20 by Sottoriva, Marano, Italy). Once the dough was formed, they were placed in closed plastic containers and left to rise in the fridge at 7 °C for 12 h. Then, the dough was scaled into four equal pieces, inserted into rectangular aluminum bread molds, and placed for 2 h in a fermentation cabinet at 30 °C with 85% relative humidity. At the end, they were baked for 10 min at 220 °C and for 30 min at 200 °C in a convection/steam oven. Baking tests were performed on each bread type by using four replicates.

2.8. Color Measurements

Color was measured on bread crumb and crust using a Chroma Meter CR-400 (Konica Minolta, Tokyo, Japan) and (CIELab) $L^*a^*b^*$ scale. The CIELab color space coordinates are the lightness L^*, from black 0 to white 100; the redness a^* from green (−100) to red (+100); and the yellowness b^* from blue (−100) to yellow (+100). The measurements took place on day 1, and the results are the average of measurements of four different points per sample.

2.9. Consumer Acceptance

The organoleptic perception was assessed by forty consumer volunteers aged between 20 and 62 years using a consumer test. Approximately 1 cm thick slices of bread for each type of bread were served on white plastic plates. After each tasting, a glass of water was provided for rinsing. Questions about taste, appearance, aroma, color, and overall acceptability of the breads were asked to the consumers. The intensity of each attribute was rated on a 7-point Hedonic scale (1 = dislike very much, 2 = dislike moderately, 3 = dislike slightly, 4 = neither like nor dislike, 5 = like slightly, 6 = like moderately, 7 = like very much), according to Moskowitz [25]. Mean values of all tests for each attribute gave the relative scores.

2.10. Evaluation of Raw Materials and Bread Shelf Life by Hyperspectral Images Analysis

The chemical profile of raw materials was analyzed using two different HIS devices: a portable Specim IQ hyperspectral camera (Specim, Spectral Imaging Ltd., Oulu, Finland), operating in the visible and near-infrared (VisNIR) regions between 400 nm and 1000 nm [26], and a SisuCHEMA Hyperspectral Chemical Imaging Analyser (SPECIM, Spectral Imaging Ltd., Oulu, Finland), ranging in the short-wave infrared regions (SWIR: 935–1720 nm) [27]. The shelf life of breads was evaluated using only the SWIR system, monitoring two slices of the three types of breads every day. The bread images acquisition was carried out on the second day (T1), third day (T2), fourth day (T3), and seventh day (T4) after cooking.

These instruments allow the acquisition of HSI images in reflectance mode, using IQ studio software (version 2021, Specim, Spectral Imaging Ltd., Oulu, Finland) for VisNIR camera, and Lumo-Scanner software (version 2022, Lumo-Scanner, Specim, Spectral Imaging Ltd., Oulu, Finland) for the SWIR system. The parameters of the VisNIR instrument were set as follows: spatial resolution: 512 × 512 pixels; spectral resolution: 7 nm; integration time: 3.0 ms. The parameters of the SWIR instrument were set as follows: spectral resolution: 8 nm; spatial resolution: 640 pixels; exposure time: 4.70 ms; frame rate: 15.20 Hz; positioning speed of the platform: 20.00 mm s^{-1}; scanning speed to 5.84 mm s^{-1}. The reflectance of each image was corrected using a calibrated white and dark reference, according to the following equation:

$$I = \frac{I_{raw} - I_B}{I_W - I_B}$$

where I = the corrected reflectance, I_{raw} = the original reflectance, I_B = the black reference, and I_W = the white reference.

The processing of HSI images was carried out using Evince software (version 2.7.12, Prediktera AB, Umea, Sweden). The processing of the HSI images consisted of three steps (Figure 1). The first step regards the image segmentation, for the removal of the background and the extraction of the pixels of each sample from the whole hyperspectral image, using principal component analysis (PCA). The second step consists of a baseline correction and a smoothing with the application of the first order Savitzky–Golay derivative (second-degree polynomial and seven-point window). In the third step, mean spectrum is obtained as average of the spectra related to all pixels for each sample, considering the overall hyperspectral image. Finally, first-derivative reflectance spectra were used to highlight chemical differences during the storage time.

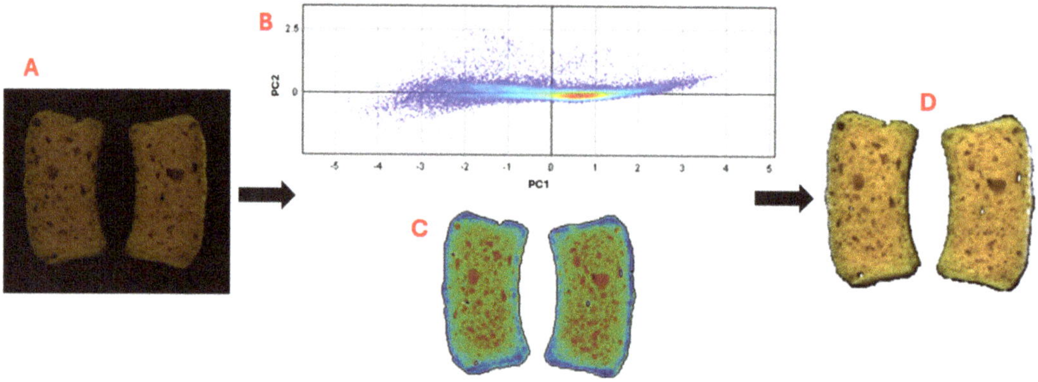

Figure 1. Example image of bread slices (**A**) before processing; PCA score plot of pixels (**B**); PCA score image (**C**); RGB image after processing (**D**).

2.11. Statistical Analysis

The results of all parameters were expressed as mean ± standard deviations (SD) for three replications. Analysis of variance (Kruskal–Wallis test) and the post hoc non-parametric Dunns' range test were performed, with the level of significance set at $p \leq 0.05$.

Principal component analysis (PCA) was carried out on spectral data for each type of bread and for each time to verify if the hyperspectral imaging device was able to recognize the presence of mold on bread. PCA was processed using the SPSS statistical software (Version 22.0; IBM Corp., Armonk, NY, USA).

3. Results and Discussion

3.1. Raw Material Characterization

3.1.1. Proximate Composition

Table 3 shows the biochemical composition of sorghum byproducts. Stalk samples showed high values of moisture, whereas values of debranning products (C3 and C4) were quite similar. The highest protein content was for C4 and the lowest for C1. The stalk samples were shown to be rich in minerals, in contrast to the bran fractions (Table 3). Stalk samples exhibited double the fiber content of debranning products. The results of the stalks were in accordance with Singh et al. [28], who analyzed the variation in carbohydrate and protein fractions in stover of sorghum cultivars. Regarding debranning products, Miafo et al. [29] reported that sorghum bran consists of 10 to 25% of the total whole grain and it is rich in dietary fiber (36 to 50% of total dietary fiber and 35 to 48% of insoluble dietary fiber). Our results are slightly lower. Moreover, sorghum bran can be a source of soluble dietary fiber with antioxidant properties, such as glucoarabinoxylans, as highlighted by Ayala-Soto et al. [30]. However, proximate composition of stalks and debranning products can be influenced by several factors like variety, agronomic management, growth stage, and environmental conditions during growth [31,32]. In fact, slight but significant differences in proximal composition were observed between samples from the two different management (organic C1–C4 and integrated C2–C3), except for TDF in stalk samples.

Table 3. Proximate composition (moisture, protein, ash, and total dietary fiber (TDF) of sorghum byproducts.

Sample	Moisture (g 100 g^{-1} FW)	Protein (g 100 g^{-1} DW)	Ash (g 100 g^{-1} DW)	TDF (g 100 g^{-1} DW)
C1	63.1 ± 0.5 ^{b}	8.1 ± 0.2 ^{b}	8.48 ± 0.03 ^{b}	60.4 ± 1.4 ^{a}
C2	69.6 ± 0.8 ^{a}	9.9 ± 0.2 ^{a}	9.03 ± 0.01 ^{a}	61.7 ± 0.3 ^{a}
C3	11.4 ± 0.3 ^{c}	10.5 ± 0.1 ^{d}	2.64 ± 0.01 ^{d}	32.1 ± 0.7 ^{b}
C4	11.7 ± 0.3 ^{c}	13.5 ± 0.1 ^{c}	4.00 ± 0.02 ^{c}	29.8 ± 0.4 ^{c}

Legend: FW = fresh weight; DW = dry weight; C1 = stalk from organic management; C2 = stalk from integrated management; C3 = debranning products from integrated management; C4 = debranning products from organic management; Results are expressed as mean ± standard deviation for three replications. Values with different letters in the same parameter are significantly different ($p \leq 0.05$).

The wheat flour proximal composition showed a moisture content of 8.8 g 100 g^{-1} DW, a protein content of 13.2 g 100 g^{-1} DW, an ash content of 3.92 g 100 g^{-1} DW, and a total dietary fiber content of 2.0 g 100 g^{-1} DW.

3.1.2. Characterization with HSI

Figure 2 depicts the average reflectance curves of the four samples of sorghum byproducts in the visible-light and near-infrared spectral regions. Curves of stalk samples and those of debranning product samples showed similar spectral profiles with slight differences. As reported by Huang et al. [33], the spectra reflected the chemical composition of the main components in the sorghum samples. In the visible range (400–780 nm), the average reflectance curves of C1 and C2 showed interesting peaks around 550 nm and 750 nm, whereas the spectra of C3–C4 displayed no obvious absorption peaks (Figure 2A). Spectra in the visible region mainly reflected the color information of the samples. The color characteristics of the stalks were strongly affected by several pigments, such as chlorophylls, whereas debranning products were characterized by different phenolic compounds, such as gallic acid and proanthocyanidins, and yellow pigment that could have contributed to the different absorption peak. The near-infrared region (800–1000 nm) revealed high absorption that could be assigned to third overtones of O–H and C–H, mainly related to carbohydrate and water content [34–36]. As illustrated in Figure 2B, six notable absorption peaks appeared at around 920, 980, 1020, 1130, 1480, and 1680 nm. The peaks at about 920 and 1480 nm correspond to the second and first vibrational overtones of the O–H bond, respectively, and their intensity variations primarily reflect differences in moisture content among the sorghum samples [34]. The absorption at around 980 nm can be attributed to the second overtone of O–H bond stretching and mainly associated with the presence of carbohydrates in sorghum [35]. The absorption feature at around 1020 nm can be primarily related to the second overtone of C–H bond stretching [36]. Similarly, the peak observed at around 1130 nm is originated from C–H stretching overtones and it is mainly linked to the carbohydrates and fats contents [37]. Absorption at around 1200–1300 nm is largely due to the second overtone stretching of C–H bonds, reflecting the presence of carbohydrates and lipids in sorghum [38]. The peak at 1480 nm is influenced by N–H bond absorption, which is typically associated with protein content [39]. The spectral profiles of various sorghum samples can exhibit significant differences across certain wavelength regions. By examining these spectral variations with the molecular bonds and functional groups corresponding to each absorption feature, it is possible to infer differences in the levels of water, carbohydrates, fats, and proteins among sorghum tissues, as previously reported by Hu et al. [40].

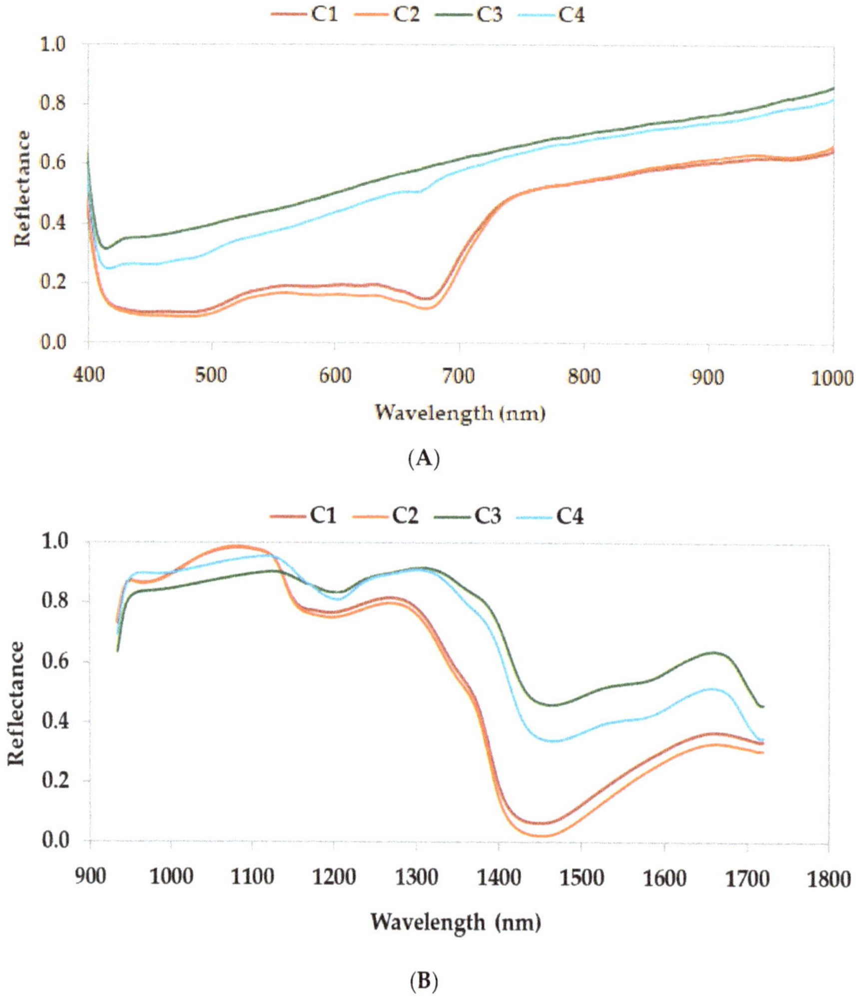

Figure 2. (**A**) VisNIR spectral profiles of different sorghums samples. (**B**) SWIR spectral profiles of different sorghum samples. Legend: C1 = stalk from organic management; C2 = stalk from integrated management; C3 = debranning products from integrated management; C4 = debranning products from organic management.

3.2. Optimization of UAE Process Parameters and Validation of the RSM Models

Based on the BBD, experimental tests (runs) were carried out to extract TPC by UAE. The results of the 15 tests for each of the 4 samples are reported in Table 4. The results of runs 13, 14, and 15 are equivalent, as expected from BBD.

With regard to the C1 sample (stalks from organic farming), the lowest mean value of TPC was recorded for run 9 (solvent composition = 65% ethanol/H_2O (*v/v*), extraction time = 40 min, extraction temperature = 70 °C), while the highest mean value was for run 11 (solvent composition = 65% ethanol/H_2O (*v/v*), extraction time = 40 min, extraction temperature = 80 °C). Regarding the C2 sample (stalks from integrated farming), the lowest mean TPC value was for run 2 (solvent composition = 80% ethanol/H_2O (*v/v*), extraction time = 40 min, extraction temperature = 75 °C), while the highest mean value was for run 12 (solvent composition = 65% ethanol/H_2O (*v/v*), extraction time = 60 min, extraction temperature = 80 °C). With regard to C3 sample (debranning products from organic farming), the lowest mean TPC value was recorded for runs 13–15 (solvent composition = 65% ethanol/H_2O (*v/v*), extraction time = 50 min, extraction temperature = 75 °C), while the highest mean value was recorded for run 2 (solvent composition = 80% ethanol/H_2O (*v/v*), extraction time = 40 min, extraction temperature = 75 °C). Regarding the C4 sample (debranning products from integrated farming), the lowest mean TPC value was for run 9 (solvent composition = 65% ethanol/H_2O (*v/v*), extraction time = 40 min, extraction temperature = 70 °C), while the highest mean value was for run 2 (solvent composition = 80% ethanol/H_2O (*v/v*), extraction time = 40 min, extraction temperature = 75 °C).

Table 4. Experimental and predicted response values (total phenolic compounds, TPC, in mg GAE 100 g^{-1} FW) in the extracts using response surface methodology (RSM).

	C1		C2		C3		C4	
Run	**TPC_{exp}**	**TPC_{RSM}**	**TPC_{exp}**	**TPC_{RSM}**	**TPC_{exp}**	**TPC_{RSM}**	**TPC_{exp}**	**TPC_{RSM}**
1	326 ± 2	324	234 ± 1	234	226 ± 3	227	257 ± 1	256
2	340 ± 4	343	228 ± 1	229	234 ± 4	233	288 ± 4	285
3	326 ± 1	323	248 ± 3	247	230 ± 4	231	278 ± 1	281
4	323 ± 6	324	256 ± 3	255	233 ± 1	232	259 ± 4	259
5	291 ± 6	292	235 ± 1	235	219 ± 5	218	265 ± 1	263
6	294 ± 3	292	256 ± 1	259	221 ± 4	222	260 ± 2	260
7	344 ± 2	346	264 ± 1	260	227 ± 2	226	253 ± 1	253
8	368 ± 5	366	241 ± 2	240	229 ± 1	230	262 ± 1	264
9	286 ± 8	286	250 ± 3	249	205 ± 1	205	265 ± 2	268
10	302 ± 1	302	267 ± 1	266	206 ± 3	206	277 ± 6	277
11	377 ± 2	376	249 ± 1	250	212 ± 1	212	275 ± 2	275
12	340 ± 3	340	270 ± 2	271	214 ± 2	214	267 ± 2	264
13	330 ± 1	330	252 ± 4	252	208 ± 1	208	221 ± 1	221
14	330 ± 1	330	252 ± 4	252	208 ± 1	208	221 ± 1	221
15	330 ± 1	330	252 ± 4	252	208 ± 1	208	221 ± 1	221

Legend: C1 = stalk from organic management; C2 = stalk from integrated management; C3 = debranning products from integrated management; C4 = debranning products from organic management; exp = experimental; RSM = response surface methodology. Results are expressed as mean ± standard deviation for three replications.

The regression models for the predicted response (TPC_{RSM}) for the four samples were the following:

$$TPC_{RSM\_C1} = -1870.99 - 2.38X_1 + 20.95X_2 + 40.40X_3 - 0.01X_1^2 - 0.17X_3^2 - 0.03X_1X_2 + 0.07X_1X_3 - 0.26X_2X_3$$

$$TPC_{RSM\_C2} = 1036.34 + 15.84X_1 - 2.11X_2 - 34.27X_3 - 0.05X_1^2 - 0.29X_3^2 + 0.02X_1X_2 - 0.15X_1X_3 - 0.02X_2X_3$$

$$TPC_{RSM\_C3} = -4.88 - 10.63X_1 - 3.76X_2 + 16.44X_3 + 0.08X_1^2 + 0.04X_2^2 - 0.11X_3^2 - 0.01X_1X_2 + 0.004X_1X_3 + 0.005X_2X_3$$

$$TPC_{RSM\_C4} = 5322.14 - 10.15X_1 - 17.04X_2 - 115.66X_3 + 0.09X_1^2 + 0.30X_2^2 + 0.78X_3^2 - 0.08X_1X_2 + 0.05X_1X_3 - 0.10X_2X_3$$

where X_1, X_2, and X_3 are the variables for green solvent composition, extraction time, and extraction temperature, respectively.

Table 5 exhibits the analysis of variance for the second-order polynomial equation for ultrasound-assisted extraction of total phenolic compounds, to evaluate the models' adequacy. The linear, quadratic, and two-factor interaction effect coefficients, the statistical significance (p-value), the coefficient of determination R^2, the adjusted coefficient of determination $R_{adj}{}^2$, and the lack of fit value were shown. All the models were highly significant ($p < 0.0001$), describing a high degree of correlation between the experimental and predicted values. In fact, all R^2 and $R_{adj}{}^2$ were higher than 0.95. Moreover, all p-values of lack of fit were not significant. Therefore, the models can be accepted.

Table 5. Analysis of variance for the second-order polynomial equation for ultrasound-assisted extraction of total phenolic compounds.

	C1		C2		C3		C4	
	Sum of Square	p-Value	Sum of Square	p-Value	Sum of Square	p-Value	Sum of Square	p-Value
X_1	370.01	<0.0001	0.20	0.8614	63.37	0.0015	57.20	0.0138
X_2	369.48	0.1711	1529.25	<0.0001	11.98	0.1261	2.88	0.5518
X_3	16,562.61	<0.0001	59.53	0.0064	242.57	<0.0001	34.26	0.0497
$X_1{}^2$	25.31	0.8805	770.88	<0.0001	2659.80	<0.0001	2692.59	<0.0001
$X_2{}^2$	0.29	<0.0001	0.01	0.9776	125.43	<0.0001	6711.89	<0.0001
$X_3{}^2$	136.81	0.0035	381.20	<0.0001	53.27	0.0031	2828.28	<0.0001
X_1 X_2	144.05	0.0028	88.13	0.0014	16.05	0.0794	1299.16	<0.0001
X_1 X_3	213.18	0.0005	976.22	<0.0001	0.58	0.7290	97.75	0.0021
X_2 X_3	1392.16	<0.0001	10.02	0.2262	0.40	0.7728	207.11	<0.0001
Residual	264.66		128.50		93.99		136.98	
Lack of fit	69.57	0.1308	39.35	0.0941	11.79	0.5044	55.02	0.0999
Pure error	195.09		89.15		82.21		81.96	
Total SS	19,475.60		3943.94		3281.72		12,582.01	
R^2	0.986		0.968		0971		0.9875	
$R_{adj}{}^2$	0.981		0.954		0.958		0.9819	
AAD								

Legend: X_1 = green solvent composition; X_2 = extraction time; X_3 = extraction temperature; Legend: C1 = stalk from organic management; C2 = stalk from integrated management; C3 = debranning products from integrated management; C4 = debranning products from organic management.

Experimental tests (runs) were carried out also for AA (Table 6). AA of sample C1 (stalks from organic farming) showed the lowest mean value at run 4 (solvent composition = 80% ethanol/H_2O (v/v), extraction time = 60 min, extraction temperature = 75 °C), while the highest mean value at run 5 (solvent composition = 50% ethanol/H_2O (v/v), extraction time = 50 min, extraction temperature = 70 °C) (Table 6). With regard to the C2 sample (stalks from integrated farming), the lowest mean value of antioxidant activity was obtained for run 6 (solvent composition = 80% ethanol/H_2O (v/v), extraction time = 50 min, extraction temperature = 70 °C), while the highest mean value was carried out for run 11 (solvent composition = 65% ethanol/H_2O (v/v), extraction time = 40 min, extraction temperature = 80 °C). Regarding C3 sample (debranning products from organic farming), the lowest mean value of AA was obtained for run 12 (solvent composition = 65% ethanol/H_2O (v/v), extraction time = 60 min, extraction temperature = 80 °C), while the highest mean value for runs 13–15 (solvent composition = 65% ethanol/H_2O (v/v), extraction time = 50 min, extraction temperature = 75 °C). With regard to the sample C4 (debranning products from integrated farming), the lowest mean value of AA was recorded for run 3 (solvent composition = 50% ethanol/H_2O (v/v), extraction time = 60 min, extraction temperature = 75 °C), while the highest mean value for run 9 (solvent composition = 65% ethanol/H_2O (v/v), extraction time = 40 min, extraction temperature = 70 °C).

The regression models for the predicted response (AA_{RSM}) for the four samples were as follows:

$$AA_{RSM\_C1} = 168.01 + 0.95X_1 + 2.09X_2 - 5.89X_3 + 0.002X_1^2 - 0.02X_2^2 + 0.04X_3^2 - 0.01X_1X_2 - 0.01X_1X_3 + 0.01X_2X_3$$

$$AA_{RSM\_C2} = 360.46 - 2.12X_1 + 0.56X_2 - 7.48X_3 - 0.002X_1^2 + 0.01X_2^2 + 0.05X_3^2 + 0.01X_1X_2 + 0.02X_1X_3 - 0.03X_2X_3$$

$$AA_{RSM\_C3} = 148.74 + 2.65X_1 + 0.01X_2 - 4.78X_3 - 0.02X_1^2 + 0.01X_2^2 + 0.03X_3^2 + 0.001X_1X_2 - 0.01X_1X_3 - 0.001X_2X_3$$

$$AA_{RSM\_C4} = -495.65 - 2.14X_1 + 3.86X_2 + 13.39X_3 - 0.003X_1^2 - 0.02X_2^2 - 0.10X_3^2 + 0.002X_1X_2 + 0.03X_1X_3 - 0.03X_2X_3$$

where X_1, X_2, and X_3 are the variables for green solvent composition, extraction time, and extraction temperature, respectively.

Table 6. Experimental and predicted response values (antioxidant activity, AA, in mg TE 100 g^{-1} FW) in the extracts using response surface methodology (RSM).

	C1		C2		C3		C4	
Run	AA_{exp}	AA_{RSM}	AA_{exp}	AA_{RSM}	AA_{exp}	AA_{RSM}	AA_{exp}	AA_{RSM}
1	20.2 ± 0.1	20.4	26.2 ± 0.4	26.4	20.9 ± 1.3	21.0	27.9 ± 0.1	28.0
2	20.7 ± 0.4	20.6	20.1 ± 0.1	20.1	22.3 ± 1.0	22.5	28.8 ± 0.7	28.7
3	23.9 ± 0.1	24.1	22.0 ± 0.8	22.1	18.6 ± 0.5	18.5	26.6 ± 0.5	26.7
4	19.1 ± 0.1	19.0	22.3 ± 0.3	22.2	20.7 ± 0.8	20.6	28.5 ± 0.9	28.4
5	25.6 ± 0.3	25.3	26.5 ± 0.4	26.2	19.2 ± 0.9	19.2	29.6 ± 0.4	29.7
6	24.5 ± 0.3	24.5	19.7 ± 0.7	19.7	21.9 ± 1.4	21.9	25.6 ± 0.2	25.9
7	25.2 ± 0.9	25.2	23.4 ± 0.3	23.4	19.7 ± 1.7	19.8	24.1 ± 0.9	23.9
8	20.8 ± 0.7	21.1	23.5 ± 0.1	23.7	20.8 ± 0.3	20.8	30.2 ± 0.7	30.1
9	22.1 ± 0.7	22.3	23.2 ± 0.2	23.3	26.7 ± 0.2	26.6	25.9 ± 0.9	25.7
10	22.4 ± 0.3	22.6	24.5 ± 0.4	24.7	24.3 ± 1.0	24.4	28.0 ± 0.4	27.8
11	20.0 ± 0.4	19.9	26.6 ± 0.3	26.4	26.5 ± 0.5	26.4	27.7 ± 0.2	27.9
12	21.8 ± 0.1	21.6	22.8 ± 0.1	22.7	24.0 ± 0.8	24.1	23.8 ± 0.4	24.1
13	22.6 ± 0.3	22.6	22.4 ± 0.6	22.4	23.4 ± 0.2	23.4	30.5 ± 0.2	30.5
14	22.6 ± 0.3	22.6	22.4 ± 0.6	22.4	23.4 ± 0.2	23.4	30.5 ± 0.2	30.5
15	22.6 ± 0.3	22.6	22.4 ± 0.6	22.4	23.4 ± 0.2	23.4	30.5 ± 0.2	30.5

Legend: C1 = stalk from organic management; C2 = stalk from integrated management; C3 = debranning products from integrated management; C4 = debranning products from organic management; exp = experimental; RSM = response surface methodology. Results are expressed as mean ± standard deviation for three replications.

ANOVA for AA (Table 7) showed high coefficient of determination R^2 (>0.93) and adjusted coefficient of determination $R_{adj}{}^2$ (>0.90) for all models, indicating a good agreement between the predicted and measured values.

Three-dimensional response surface plots were used to assess the effects of different combinations of levels of each pair of independent variables (X_1–X_3) on the overall response desirability (Figures 3 and 4) for TPC and AA. They can help visualize the interactions between variables. The desirability function ranges from 0.0 (undesirable) up to 1.0 (very desirable). Therefore, highly desirable values for TPC and AA are depicted in red for each pair of process variables. Simultaneous comparison of the desirability functions allowed estimation of the optimal extraction values for green solvent composition, extraction time, and extraction temperature, as reported in Table 8. The optimal conditions were determined by maximizing the response functions.

The comparison related to the two variables (TPC and AA) and the four samples can provide some general indications. The analysis of the models highlighted the possibility of obtaining an extract richer in phenols with a high ethanol content in solvent composition. This may be due to the fact that phenolic compounds are more soluble in an ethanol/water solution than in a pure solvent [16]. The extraction yield in TPC could increase due to the action of water that promotes the swelling of the cellular material, and therefore increases surface contact between plant matrix and solvent, with a consequent improvement of cell wall permeability [41,42]. At the same time, high temperatures can favor the extraction, increasing the release rate of the phytocompounds in the solvent, also taking into account the greater dissociation of the polyphenols bound to the membrane [43]. Moreover, time reduction is suggested for the preservation of thermolabile and/or unstable polyphenols, as well as for savings in the cost per unit volume of the extract [44,45]. Luo et al. [46] used UAE to extract TPC from red sorghum (*Sorghum bicolor* L.) bran. Although the authors considered different raw materials and different process factors and levels, some considerations may be common to the two studies. In fact, they observed that the yield of TPC increased as the ultrasonic time ascended, and an ethanol concentration of 30–70% was good for extracting TPC, with the best concentration at 50%. The importance of ethanol in the extraction of phenolic compounds was also highlighted by Barros et al. [47]. They used an accelerated solvent extractor (ASE) to extract polyphenols from black and tannin sorghum bran. The ASE at temperatures above 100 °C using water and ethanol/water (50% and 70%) solvent significantly improved the extraction of phenolic compounds from black sorghum bran compared to conventional extractions using the same solvents. Furthermore, the solvent at 70% ethanol: water ratio carried out the highest yield in TPC.

Table 7. Analysis of variance for the second-order polynomial equation for ultrasound-assisted extraction of antioxidant activity.

	C1		C2		C3		C4	
	Sum of Square	*p*-Value	Sum of Square	*p*-Value	Sum of Square	*p*-Value	Sum of Square	*p*-Value
X_1	24.54	<0.0001	36.27	<0.0001	13.20	0.0001	5.98	<0.0001
X_2	4.29	0.0001	5.21	<0.0001	19.12	<0.0001	2.90	0.0030
X_3	11.71	<0.0001	1.38	0.0133	0.26	0.5124	2.56	0.0049
X_1^2	1.32	0.0160	1.18	0.0201	110.66	<0.0001	4.67	0.0006
X_2^2	29.54	<0.0001	2.83	0.0009	8.45	0.0010	23.91	<0.0001
X_3^2	7.59	<0.0001	11.00	<0.0001	5.42	0.0060	41.28	<0.0001
$X_1 X_2$	14.06	<0.0001	19.97	<0.0001	0.28	0.4967	0.58	0.1462
$X_1 X_3$	5.58	<0.0001	23.81	<0.0001	1.39	0.1363	51.29	<0.0001
$X_2 X_3$	1.02	0.0315	13.12	<0.0001	0.01	0.9269	17.47	<0.0001
Residual	3.80		3.74		11.50		5.10	
Lack of fit	0.90	0.1925	0.54	0.4324	0.33	0.9153	0.78	0.4066
Pure error	2.90		3.20		11.16		4.32	
Total SS	106.48		120.64		178.62		148.20	
R^2	0.964		0.969		0.936		0.966	
R_{adj}^2	0.948		0.955		0.907		0.950	
AAD								

Legend: X_1 = green solvent composition, X_2 = extraction time, X_3 = extraction temperature; Legend: C1 = stalk from organic management; C2 = stalk from integrated management; C3 = debranning products from integrated management; C4 = debranning products from organic management.

Table 8. Optimal values of UAE process parameters for total phenolic compounds (TPC) and antioxidant activity (AA).

Sample	Response	X_1 (%)	X_2 (min)	X_3 (°C)
C1	TPC	80.0	40	80.0
	AA	50.0	55	80.0
C2	TPC	65.0	60	80.0
	AA	57.5	40	80.0
C3	TPC	80.0	40	77.5
	AA	65.0	40	70.0
C4	TPC	80.0	40	80.0
	AA	80.0	50	77.5

Legend: C1 = stalk from organic management; C2 = stalk from integrated management; C3 = debranning products from integrated management; C4 = debranning products from organic management.

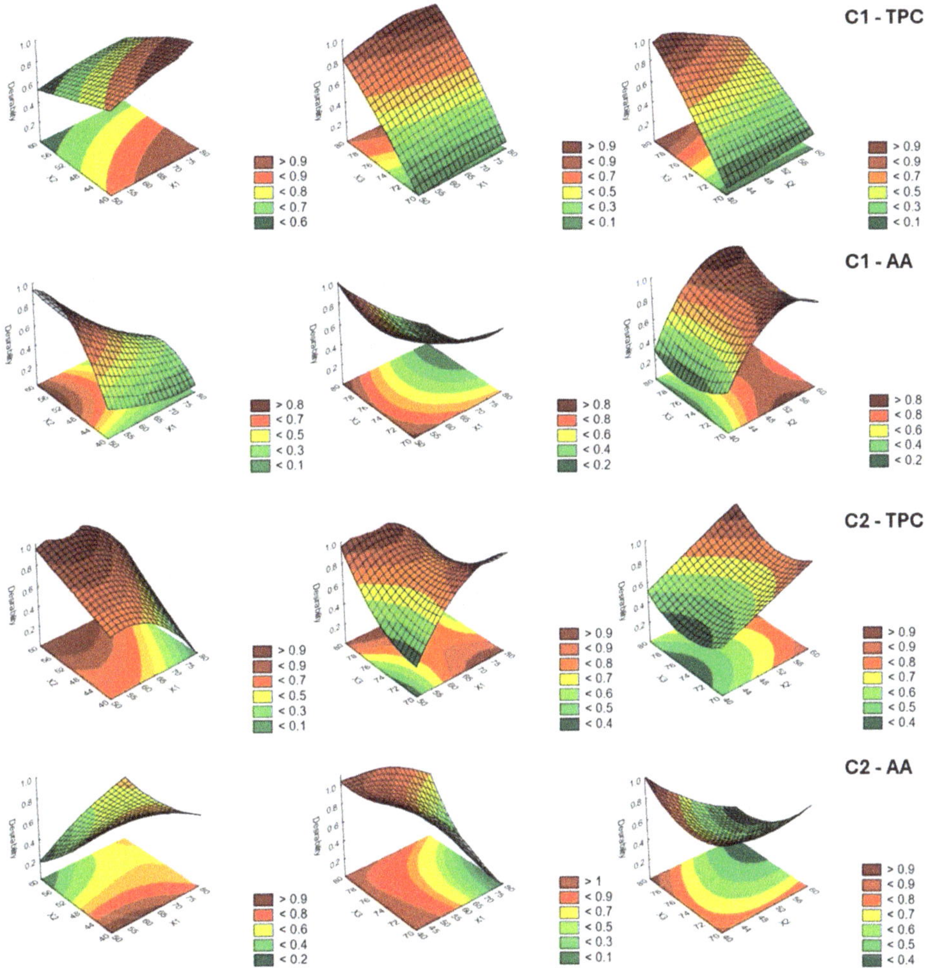

Figure 3. Response surface and contour plots of extracts of C1 and C2 samples for total phenolic compounds (TPC) and antioxidant activity (AA). Legend: C1 = stalk from organic management; C2 = stalk from integrated management.

AA showed its best performance at moderate times and low ethanol concentration, except for C4, and lower temperatures, especially for debranning products. Temperature can amplify solubility and diffusion through increased molecular motion while preventing degradation [42]. More concentrated ethanol can also extract non-antioxidant or pro-oxidant compounds, which dilute the antioxidant effect of the overall extracted pool [48]. Antioxidant compounds, especially polyphenols, are sensitive to oxidation. Longer extraction times expose them to oxygen, ultrasound, and heat for longer, increasing the risk of degradation. In addition, ultrasonic energy applied for long periods can generate free radicals (such as OH• radicals from water), which degrade antioxidant compounds.

Under the optimal conditions (Table 8), the extractions were repeated and compared to those obtained with the traditional method (Table 9).

All measurements showed higher TPC, TFC, and pigment contents and higher AA values with UAE in comparison with the traditional technique. Many studies confirmed the validity of the UAE extraction in obtaining a higher yield of phenols, pigment, and a corresponding antioxidant activity [16,44,49–51]. This is mainly due to the increase in the solute solubility, the favoring of cell disruption, the enhancing of mass transfer, and the improvement in solvent penetration [52–54].

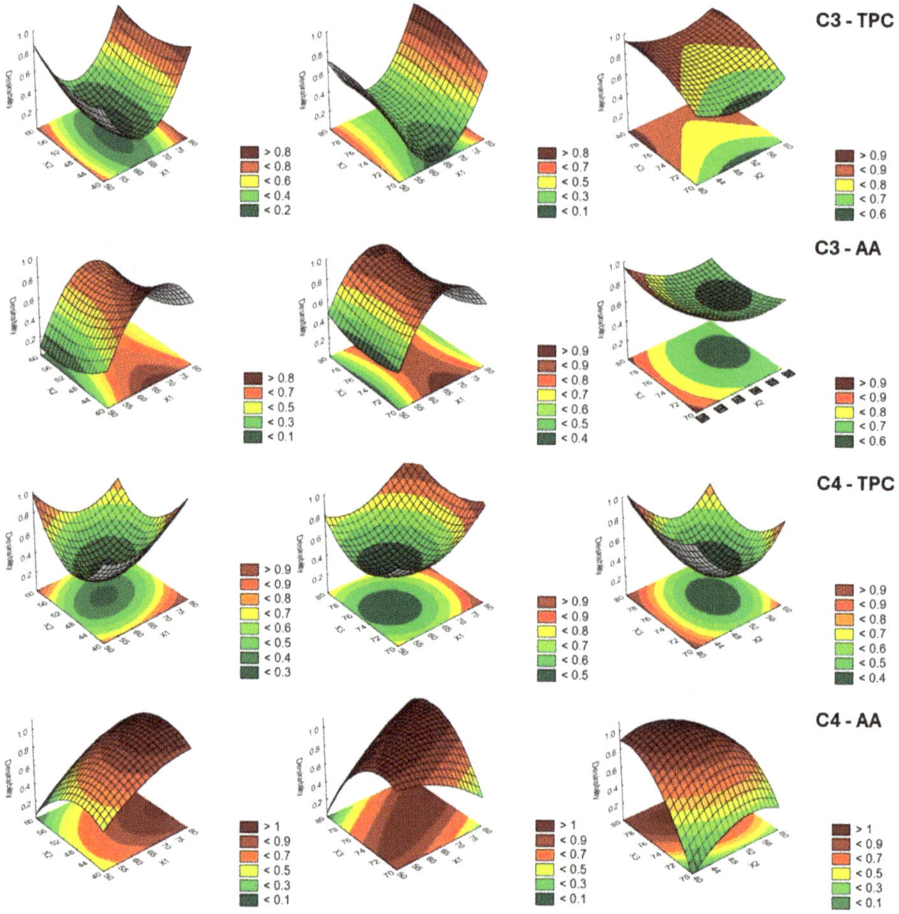

Figure 4. Response surface and contour plots of extracts of C3 and C4 samples for total phenolic compounds (TPC) and antioxidant activity (AA). Legend: C3 = debranning products from integrated management; C4 = debranning products from organic management.

3.3. *Characterization of Phenolic Acids Extract by HPLC-DAD*

HPLC chromatograms were used to investigate sorghum phenolic acids compositions among sorghum samples extracted with different ethanol: water ratios. In accordance with the retention time of commercially available phenolic standards, PAs were identified in sorghum extracts, most of which were more prominent under the detection wavelengths of 280 and 350 nm. The concentrations of phenolics in different extracting solvent procedures (ultrasound: UAE; traditional: TM) are shown in Table 10. The content of PAs significantly varied ($p \leq 0.05$) between different extraction systems and among sorghum samples. Many studies reported a different HPLC phenolic compounds profile when different extraction systems, sorghum genotypes, or histological tissues were studied [55–58].

All extracts with ethanol obtained from UAE procedures showed higher concentrations of PAs than those obtained from the classic extraction technique, except for vanillic acid in C4 and 4-coumaric acid in C3 and C4. A similar trend was reported by Hong et al. [55]. Generally, phenolics tend to be extracted in greater amounts using more polar solvents and applying physical treatment, such as microwave and ultrasounds. Differences in phenols profiles can strongly affect the potential biological activities of the extracts, including antimicrobial, antiproliferative, and proapoptotic effects against colon cancer cells [59]. In particular, Denardi-Souza et al. [59] reported a significant antimicrobial action of specific phenolic acids, such as gallic and ferulic acids, against different microorganisms, increasing bread shelf life.

Table 9. Comparison between results of ultrasound-assisted extraction (UAE) under optimal conditions and traditional method (TM) for total phenolic compounds (TPC), total flavans content (TFC), chlorophyll a (ChA), chlorophyll b (ChB), yellow pigment (YPG), and antioxidant activity (AA).

Sample	Extraction Method	TPC (mg GAE 100 g^{-1} FW)	TFC (mg CE 100 g^{-1} FW)	ChA (μg 100 g^{-1} FW)	ChB (μg 100 g^{-1} FW)	YPG (g 100 g^{-1} FW)	AA (mg TE 100 g^{-1} FW)
C1	TM	185 ± 1 ^{b}	12 ± 1 ^{b}	2882 ± 210 ^{b}	2493 ± 120 ^{b}	2.00 ± 0.02 ^{b}	20.5 ± 0.8 ^{b}
	UAE	382 ± 3 ^{a}	20 ± 2 ^{a}	3514 ± 62 ^{a}	2899 ± 42 ^{a}	6.8 ± 0.3 ^{a}	26.0 ± 0.4 ^{a}
C2	TM	163 ± 8 ^{b}	11 ± 1 ^{b}	2012 ± 154 ^{b}	1600 ± 85 ^{b}	1.60 ± 0.04 ^{b}	22.0 ± 1.0 ^{b}
	UAE	270 ± 2 ^{a}	18 ± 2 ^{a}	3510 ± 150 ^{a}	2642 ± 165 ^{a}	5.8 ± 0.4 ^{a}	26.6 ± 0.3 ^{a}
C3	TM	203 ± 2 ^{b}	1.0 ± 0.1 ^{b}	222 ± 12 ^{b}	339 ± 22 ^{b}	1.78 ± 0.04 ^{b}	16.5 ± 0.8 ^{b}
	UAE	295 ± 3 ^{a}	1.6 ± 0.2 ^{a}	459 ± 25 ^{a}	606 ± 46 ^{a}	1.92 ± 0.03 ^{a}	26.1 ± 0.2 ^{a}
C4	TM	162 ± 6 ^{b}	0.9 ± 0.1 ^{b}	323 ± 15 ^{b}	425 ± 31 ^{b}	2.00 ± 0.05 ^{b}	16.4 ± 0.3 ^{b}
	UAE	241 ± 2 ^{a}	1.5 ± 0.2 ^{a}	545 ± 19 ^{a}	778 ± 55 ^{a}	2.28 ± 0.09 ^{a}	27.1 ± 0.3 ^{a}

Legend: C1 = stalk from organic management; C2 = stalk from integrated management; C3 = debranning products from integrated management; C4 = debranning products from organic management; FW = fresh weight. Results are expressed as mean ± standard deviation for three replications. Values with different letters in the same parameter are significantly different ($p \leq 0.05$).

Table 10. Comparison of content of individuals phenolic acids (PAs) between conventional and UAE extraction from different byproducts. Data are expressed as mean values ± standard deviation.

Sample	Gallic Acid (μg/mL)	Vanillic Acid (μg/mL)	4-Coumaric Acid (μg/mL)	Ferulic Acid (μg/mL)	Caffeic Acid (μg/mL)	Syringic Acid (μg/mL)	3-Cumaric Acid (μg/mL)	Sinapic Acid (μg/mL)
C1								
UAE	14.6 ± 0.9 ^{a}	1.72 ± 0.08 ^{a}	3.9 ± 0.3 ^{a}	3.1 ± 0.1 ^{a}	-	-	-	-
TM	tr	tr	0.17 ± 0.02 ^{b}	0.52 ± 0.03 ^{b}	-	-	-	-
C2								
UAE	19.0±1.5 ^{a}	1.05 ± 0.01 ^{a}	4.1 ± 0.8 ^{a}	3.9 ± 0.2 ^{a}	-	-	-	-
TM	tr	Tr	0.14 ± 0.03 ^{b}	0.59 ± 0.05 ^{b}	-	-	-	-
C3								
UAE	-	0.10 ± 0.01 ^{b}	0.48 ± 0.02 ^{a}	0.41 ± 0.06 ^{a}	1.84 ± 0.07 ^{a}	0.72 ± 0.04 ^{a}	0.64 ± 0.03 ^{a}	0.10 ± 0.04 ^{a}
TM	-	0.20 ± 0.06 ^{a}	0.47 ± 0.06 ^{a}	0.24 ± 0.05 ^{b}	1.67 ± 0.04 ^{b}	Tr	0.12 ± 0.03 ^{b}	0.18 ± 0.05 ^{a}
C4								
UAE	-	0.20 ± 0.07 ^{a}	0.30 ± 0.05 ^{a}	0.6 ± 0.1 ^{a}	2.38 ± 0.01 ^{a}	0.70 ± 0.10 ^{a}	0.97 ± 0.01 ^{a}	0.10 ± 0.02 ^{a}
TM	-	0.21 ± 0.08 ^{a}	0.41 ± 0.02 ^{a}	0.3 ± 0.1 ^{b}	2.01 ± 0.09 ^{b}	0.10 ± 0.01 ^{b}	tr	tr

Legend: UAE = ultrasound-assisted extraction; TM = classic extraction technique; tr = trace values; C1 = stalk from organic management; C2 = stalk from integrated management; C3 = debranning products from integrated management; C4 = debranning products from organic management. Results are expressed as mean ± standard deviation for three replications. Values with different letters in the same parameter are significantly different ($p \leq 0.05$).

3.4. *Effect of Sorghum Stalk Optimal Extract on Bread*

Crumb and crust color characteristics for the three types of bread are shown in Table 11. Regarding the crust color, the enrichment with the extract significantly affected only the coordinate b^*: the yellowness was higher for P2. On the contrary, significant differences in all CIELab coordinates were observed among the bread crumbs. The luminosity, the redness, and the yellowness of the bread increased as the amount of extract increased. Color variation could be ascribed to the chemical composition of C1 extract (Table 10) used to enrich the dough, characterized by high amount of phenols, chlorophyll, and yellow pigment [60,61]. In particular, the red shift for enriched breads may be due to the presence of gallic acid in the extract, as emerged from chromatographic analysis. The increase in yellowness and luminosity may be ascribed to flavonoids, which are abundant in extracts from sorghum obtained with high amount of ethanol in solvent composition [55].

Table 11. Crumb and crust color characteristics for the three types of bread.

Bread	Crust			Crumb		
	L^*	a^*	b^*	L^*	a^*	b^*
P1	57.27 ± 0.85 [a]	7.33 ± 1.89 [a]	28.25 ± 1.55 [b]	58.33 ± 2.16 [b]	−6.08 ± 4.75 [b]	11.34 ± 0.30 [c]
P2	59.45 ± 1.20 [a]	5.49 ± 5.03 [a]	32.34 ± 1.70 [a]	61.36 ± 2.21 [ab]	2.15 ± 4.35 [a]	14.54 ± 0.89 [b]
P3	56.80 ± 2.41 [a]	8.72 ± 3.04 [a]	29.38 ± 1.19 [b]	62.46 ± 0.89 [a]	0.48 ± 0.22 [a]	17.46 ± 1.72 [a]

Legend: L^* = luminosity; a^* = redness; b^* = yellowness; P1 = control; P2 = bread with 10% of extract; P3 = bread with 20% of extract. Results are expressed as mean ± standard deviation for three replications. Values with different letters in the same parameter are significantly different ($p \leq 0.05$).

Processing and cooking can affect the concentrations of bioactive compounds in the final products, because these compounds can be thermolabile [24,62]. Therefore, TPC and AA were evaluated in breads to verify whether the different concentrations of the C1 extract brought about a significant increase in TPC and AA in P2 and P3 compared to the control bread (P1). Table 12 shows significant differences for both variables. The 10% enrichment produced an increase of 15.3% of TPC and 12.8% of AA. The effect of the extract on bread enriched at 20% was much more accentuated: increases of 12.8% of TPC and 79.5% of AA was observed. A similar trend was also observed by Chen et al. [63], who reported an increase in phenolic compounds and antioxidant activity in bread enriched with sorghum bran extract.

Table 12. Total phenolic compounds (TPC) and antioxidant activity (AA) for the three types of bread.

Bread	TPC (mg GAE 100 g^{-1} FW)	AA (mg TE 100 g^{-1} FW)
P1	23.6 ± 0.9 [c]	3.90 ± 0.09 [c]
P2	27.2 ± 0.6 [b]	4.40 ± 0.12 [b]
P3	30.0 ± 0.8 [a]	7.00 ± 0.10 [a]

Legend: P1 = control; P2 = bread with 10% of extract; P3 = bread with 20% of extract; FW = fresh weight. Results are expressed as mean ± standard deviation for three replications. Values with different letters for the same parameter are significantly different ($p \leq 0.05$).

One of the major problems that arise during the storage of bread is the appearance of mold, as it causes economic losses and dissatisfaction among consumers [64]. This is strictly related to the type of bread, the method, and the temperature of storage [65]. Various molds can appear in wheat bread, such as Penicillium, Aspergillus, Cladosporium, Mucorales and Neurospora [65–67].

Considering that sorghum byproducts showed a high amount of bioactive compounds, we verified if and to what extent the extract with the highest TPC content (C1) could influence the bread shelf life. Therefore, three types of bread were produced: a control (P1), a bread enriched with 10% extract (P2), and a bread enriched with 20% extract (P3). Bread samples were stored in sealed bags. Every day, hyperspectral image acquisitions were carried out with the SWIR camera, until the appearance of mold (Figure 5).

Significant differences were observed among the spectra of bread samples at different storage times. In particular, a high variation of spectra reflectance was observed at about 1150 and 1350 nm when mold appeared. A similar variation of SWIR signals was observed in wheat kernel and flour after fusarium infection by Alisaac et al. [68].

The mean spectra for each type of bread were calculated for four times, for which a principal component analysis was performed to verify the camera's ability to identify the appearance of mold, based on the change in the chemical composition of the spectra.

A score plot from principal component analysis performed on the mean spectra of each bread for four times (Figure 6) showed the similarities among all different types of bread during storage at room temperature (about 19 °C). The first two principal components accounted cumulatively for 98.9% of the explained variance: PC1 explained 90.7% and PC2 8.2% of the total variance. The score plot highlighted a discrimination between the spectra of the breads at times T1–T3 and those at T4, and especially those relating to the areas affected by mold in P1 and P2 breads. The separation was clearer for the control bread as the presence of mold at time T4 was extremely evident, compared to the P2 bread, which presented barely visible mold. In general, bread shelf life and spoilage depend on its moisture content [69]. However, in our study, all breads were made with the same addition of liquids part. Therefore, the behavior of P3 could be due to the addition of extract.

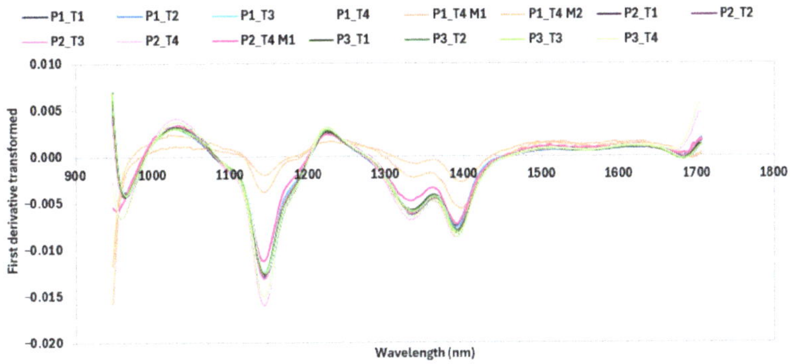

Figure 5. Mean spectra first derivative of each bread (P1 = control; P2 = bread with 10% of extract; P3 = bread with 20% of extract) at different storage days (T1 = second day after cooking; T2 = third day after cooking; T3 = fourth day after cooking; T4 = seventh day after cooking). The suffix M indicates the presence of mold.

These results confirmed that the natural extract with high amount of bioactive compounds could positively influence the maintenance of the bread product, and the ability of the HSI technique to conduct early inspection and monitor bread spoilage. Several studies attributed to the phenolic compounds an antimicrobial activity [70–72]. In particular, Borges et al. [73] and Chen et al. [74] ascribed to the phenolic acids, such as gallic and ferulic acids, the ability to destroy the integrity of microbial cell membranes, resulting in the leakage of intracellular substances. Furthermore, flavonoids can inhibit energy metabolism in cells and inhibit essential enzymes required for DNA and RNA replication, resulting in cell death [75].

Although there are many previous studies that have developed prediction models of food quality parameters using HSI data storage [76], few studies have investigated the potential of spectroscopic techniques to assess microbiological deterioration and shelf life of baked goods post-baking. Saleem et al. examined the microbial spoilage growth of sponge cake using a VisNIR hyperspectral camera (395–1000 nm); the method successfully allowed them to train the model to distinguish between healthy and spoiled samples with 98% accuracy [77]. Cevoli et al. used NIR spectroscopy coupled with principal component analysis to monitor the shelf life of a traditional Italian flat bread Piadina, improved with sourdough fermentation and enzymes, and to predict storage time [78]. Mehdizadeh et al. explored the ability of the VisNIR hyperspectral camera (400–950 nm) to evaluate bread texture over six days of storage, highlighting changes in crumb moisture, firmness, chewiness, cohesiveness, and springiness [79].

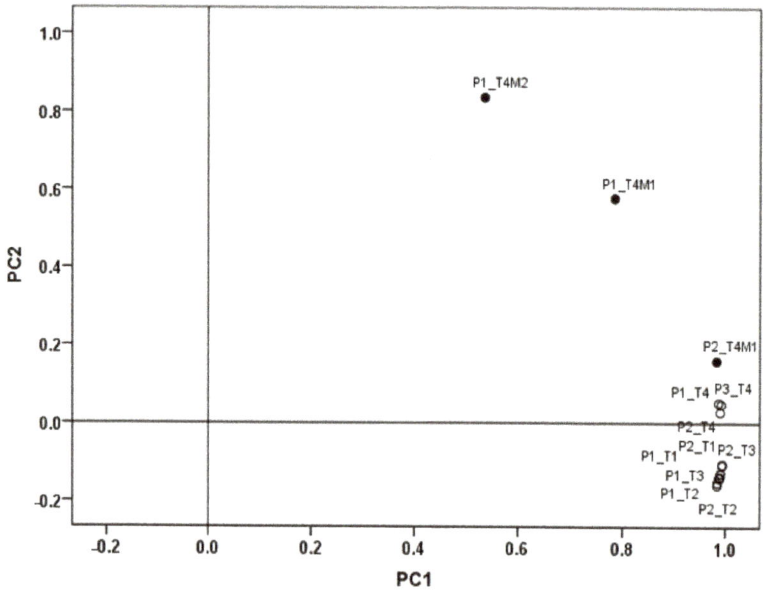

Figure 6. Score plot from principal component analysis performed on mean spectra of each bread (P1 = control; P2 = bread with 10% of extract; P3 = bread with 20% of extract) for 4 times (T1 = second day after cooking; T2 = third day after cooking; T3 = fourth day after cooking; T4 = seventh day after cooking). The suffix M and the solid circle indicate the presence of mold.

3.5. Sensorial Analysis

The mean intensity scores for organoleptic attributes for each type of bread are shown in Figure 7. The consumer test revealed the bread samples most preferred by consumers in terms of taste, color, aroma, appearance, and overall preference. No significant differences ($p < 0.05$) among breads were found for the overall acceptability and the sensorial attributes, except for aroma. The score of this attribute was significantly lower in P3 than those of the other two breads. This may be related to the grassy smell of the sorghum stalk extract.

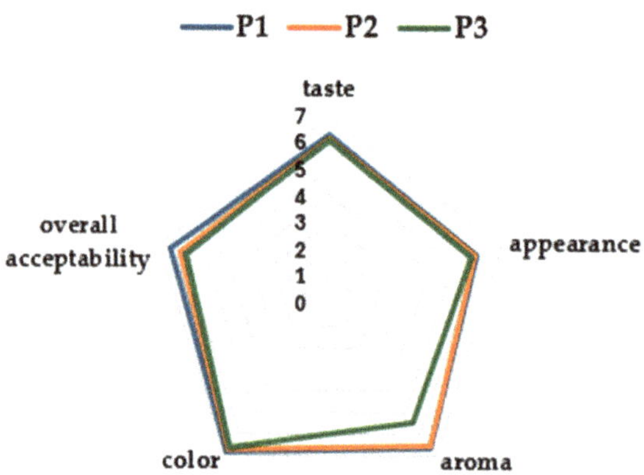

Figure 7. Sensory analysis of bread with different extracts enrichment (P1 = control; P2 = bread with 10% of extract; P3 = bread with 20% of extract).

Sensory analysis of bread, including its smell, is a crucial aspect of evaluating its quality and consumer appeal. The grass smell, which is perceived by consumers as a negative aspect, could be related to the presence of specific and not desired volatile compounds in the stalk extract. In the context of bread, the grass smell can be associated with a "green", "grass-like", or "vegetative" note, though less common than other bread aroma compounds (like those from yeast, sugars, and flour). Karl et al. analyzed samples of sorghum stems with leaves with online proton transfer reaction mass spectrometry and proton transfer ion trap mass spectrometry methods [80]. These samples released a large variety of oxygenated volatile organic compounds, including methanol, acetaldehyde, acetone, n-pentanal, methyl propanal, hexenol, hexanal, cis-3-hexenal, and trans-2-hexenal, which could be responsible for the lower score of aroma for P3 bread.

4. Conclusions

In the current agricultural and food industry, a pressing challenge is the reduction in waste production and the promotion of its reuse through the application of green technologies, such as UAE coupling with RSM and use of green solvents. Through RSM, we identified different optimal extraction conditions based on the type of residues (stalks or debranning products). Under optimal conditions, UAE resulted in over 80% higher phenolic yield and more than 25% greater antioxidant activity compared to conventional extraction methods. HPLC analysis revealed noteworthy phenolic acid profiles, with high levels of ferulic and gallic acids in stalks samples, and caffeic and 4-coumaric acids in debranning products. These compounds are known for their antioxidant and antimicrobial properties and could be used to obtain food with increased potential nutritional and prolonged shelf life.

Significant enhancements in total phenolic compounds and antioxidant activity were observed in bread enriched with the optimized extract from samples showing the maximum phenolic amount, along with an extension in shelf life.

Our findings highlighted that fine-tuning the physical parameters of the UAE process enhances the recovery of bioactive phenolic compounds, which are key to biological functionality. Consequently, these extracts show promise as additives or ingredients for natural, health-promoting products in food, pharmaceutical, and cosmetic industries. Nonetheless, further research is needed to explore the full range of eco-friendly extract applications. Moreover, transferring these applications at scale can involve further research to ensure the maximization of extraction efficiency and reproducibility.

Author Contributions: Conceptualization, T.A. and R.C. (Roberto Ciccoritti); methodology, T.A. and R.C. (Roberto Ciccoritti); software, T.A.; validation, T.A. and R.C. (Roberto Ciccoritti); formal analysis, T.A., F.M., R.C. (Roberto Ciorba), D.C., F.T., M.A. and R.C. (Roberto Ciccoritti); investigation, T.A., D.C., M.A. and R.C. (Roberto Ciccoritti); data curation, T.A., M.A., D.C., R.C. (Roberto Ciorba), F.T. and R.C. (Roberto Ciccoritti); writing—original draft preparation, T.A. and R.C. (Roberto Ciccoritti); writing—review and editing, T.A., D.C., M.A., F.T. and R.C. (Roberto Ciccoritti); funding acquisition, F.T. All authors have read and agreed to the published version of the manuscript.

Funding: This research was funded by Project SOUL Programma di Sviluppo Rurale 2014–2022, REGIONE LAZIO, Grant n. F87F23000190009.

Institutional Review Board Statement: Not applicable.

Informed Consent Statement: Not applicable.

Data Availability Statement: The original contributions presented in the study are included in the article; further inquiries can be directed to the corresponding author.

Conflicts of Interest: The authors declare no conflicts of interest.

References

1. Li, Z.K.; Li, X.L.; Yan, H.L.; Yan, J.C.; Lei, Z.P.; Ren, S.B.; Wang, Z.C.; Kang, S.G.; Shui, H.F. Two-step separation for enriching phenols and esters from base-catalyzed depolymerization of sorghum stalk. *Fuel* **2022**, *314*, 122739. [CrossRef]
2. Tanwar, R.; Panghal, A.; Chaudhary, G.; Kumari, A.; Chhikara, N. Nutritional, phytochemical and functional potential of sorghum: A review. *Food Chem. Adv.* **2023**, *3*, 100501. [CrossRef]
3. Sunoj, V.J.; Prasad, P.V.; Ciampitti, I.A.; Maswada, H.F. Narrowing diurnal temperature amplitude alters carbon tradeoff and reduces growth in C4 crop sorghum. *Front. Plant Sci.* **2020**, *11*, 1262. [CrossRef] [PubMed]
4. McGinnis, M.J.; Webster, M. Current and potential future uses of sorghum to increase nutrient density for human foods. *J. Food Sci.* **2024**, *89*, A42–A51. [CrossRef]
5. Xie, Q.; Xu, Z. Sustainable Agriculture: From Sweet Sorghum Planting and Ensiling to Ruminant Feeding. *Mol. Plant* **2019**, *12*, 603–606. [CrossRef]
6. Meena, K.; Visarada, K.; Meena, D.K. *Sorghum bicolor* (L.) Moench a multifarious crop -fodder to therapeutic potential and biotechnological applications: A future food for the millennium. *Future Foods* **2022**, *6*, 100188. [CrossRef]
7. Joy, S.P.; Krishnan, C. Modified organosolv pretreatment for improved cellulosic ethanol production from sorghum biomass. *Ind. Crops Prod.* **2022**, *177*, 114409. [CrossRef]
8. De Carvalho, A.P.A.; Silva, V.D.M.; Souza, P.T.F.; Garcia, C.F.; Queiroz, V.A.V.; Junqueira, R.G.; Garcia, M.A.V.T. Sorghum starch: Extraction, characterization and film development. *Mater. Today Commun.* **2024**, *39*, 109020. [CrossRef]
9. Taylor, J.; Duodu, K.G. *Sorghum and Millets: Chemistry, Technology, and Nutritional Attributes*; Elsevier Ink: Amsterdam, The Netherlands, 2018.
10. Lestari, E.G.; Herawati, H.; Suarni, S.; Ishaq, M.I.; Syahruddin, K.; Widiastuti, D.; Mulyati, A.H.; Yunita, R.; Haziman, M.L.; Suparjo. Nutritional profiling and selection of promising F3 sorghum genotypes from bioguma and Gando Keta crosses for food security and industrial applications. *Food Humanit.* **2025**, *4*, 100574. [CrossRef]
11. Chhikara, N.; Abdulahi, B.; Munezero, C.; Kaur, R.; Singh, G.; Panghal, A. Exploring the nutritional and phytochemical potential of sorghum in food processing for food security. *Nutr. Food Sci.* **2018**, *49*, 318–332. [CrossRef]
12. Dahunsi, S.O.; Adesulu-Dahunsi, A.T.; Osueke, C.O.; Lawal, A.I.; Olayanju, T.M.A.; Ojediran, J.O.; Izebere, J.O. Biogas generation from *Sorghum bicolor* stalk: Effect of pretreatment methods and economic feasibility. *Energy Rep.* **2019**, *5*, 584–593. [CrossRef]
13. Kumari, P.K.; Umakanth, A.V.; Narsaiah, T.B.; Uma, A. Exploring anthocyanins, antioxidant capacity and α-glucosidase inhibition in bran and flour extracts of selected sorghum genotypes. *Food Biosci.* **2021**, *41*, 100979. [CrossRef]
14. Pehlivan, U.; Ozdemir, S.; Ozer, H.; Dede, O.H. Fuel properties and incineration behavior of poultry litter blended with sweet sorghum bagasse and pyrolysis oil. *J. Environ. Manag.* **2024**, *357*, 120844. [CrossRef] [PubMed]
15. Barone, A.S.; Maragoni-Santos, C.; Marques de Farias, P.; Marcolongo Gomes Cortat, C.; Chieregato Maniglia, B.; Schmitz Ongaratto, R.; Ferreira, S.; Cavalcante Fai, A.E. Rethinking single-use plastics: Innovations, polices, consumer awareness and market shaping biodegradable solutions in the packaging industry. *Trends Food Sci. Technol.* **2025**, *158*, 104906. [CrossRef]
16. Iadecola, R.; Ciccoritti, R.; Ceccantoni, B.; Bellincontro, A.; Amoriello, T. Optimization of Phenolic Compound Extraction from Brewers' Spent Grain Using Ultrasound Technologies Coupled with Response Surface Methodology. *Sustainability* **2022**, *14*, 3309. [CrossRef]
17. International Association for Cereal Science and Technology. *ICC Standard Methods (Methods No. 105/2, 110/1, 104/1)*; ICC: Vienna, Austria, 2003.
18. AOAC. *Official Methods of Analysis*, 15th ed.; AOAC International: Arlington, VA, USA, 1990; Volume II, Section 985.29; p. 1105.
19. Ciccoritti, R.; Taddei, F.; Gazza, L.; Nocente, F. Influence of kernel thermal pre-treatments on 5-n-alkylresorcinols, polyphenols and antioxidant activity of durum and einkorn wheat. *Eur. Food Res. Technol.* **2021**, *247*, 353–362. [CrossRef]
20. Sun, B.; Ricardo-da-Silva, J.M.; Spranger, I. Critical factors of vanillin assay for catechins and proanthocyanidins. *J. Agric. Food Chem.* **1998**, *46*, 4267–4274. [CrossRef]
21. Dere, S.; Guneş, T.; Sivaci, R. Spectrophotometric determination of chlorophyll-A, B and total carotenoid contents of some algae species using different solvents. *Turk. J. Bot.* **1998**, *22*, 13–18.
22. Ciccoritti, R.; Ruggiero, G.; Ciorba, R.; Manetti, C.; Amoriello, M.; Amoriello, T. Shelf-life assessment of apricot fruit during cold storage by a portable visible and near-infrared hyperspectral imaging device. *Eur. Food Res. Technol.* **2025**, *251*, 545–558. [CrossRef]
23. Dai, J.; Mumper, R.J. Plant phenolics: Extraction, analysis and their antioxidant and anticancer properties. *Molecules* **2010**, *15*, 7313–7352. [CrossRef]
24. Amoriello, T.; Mellara, F.; Ruggeri, S.; Ciorba, R.; Ceccarelli, D.; Ciccoritti, R. Artichoke By-Products Valorization for Phenols-Enriched Fresh Egg Pasta: A Sustainable Food Design Project. *Sustainability* **2022**, *14*, 14778. [CrossRef]
25. Moskowitz, H.R. Utilitarian benefits of magnitude estimation scaling for testing product acceptability. In *Selected Sensory Methods: Problems and Approaches to Measuring Hedonics*; Kuznicki, J.T., Johnson, R.A., Rutkiewic, A.F., Eds.; American Society for Testing and Materials: Philadelphia, PA, USA, 1982.

26. Amoriello, T.; Ciorba, R.; Ruggiero, G.; Amoriello, M.; Ciccoritti, R. A Performance Evaluation of Two Hyperspectral Imaging Systems for the Prediction of Strawberries' Pomological Traits. *Sensors* **2024**, *24*, 174. [CrossRef] [PubMed]
27. Amoriello, T.; Mellara, F.; Amoriello, M.; Ciccoritti, R. Evaluation of Nutritional Values of Edible Algal Species Using a Shortwave Infrared Hyperspectral Imaging and Machine Learning Technique. *Foods* **2024**, *13*, 2277. [CrossRef] [PubMed]
28. Singh, S.; Venktesh Bhat, B.; Shukla, G.P.; Singh, K.K.; Gehrana, D. Variation in carbohydrate and protein fractions, energy, digestibility and mineral concentrations in stover of sorghum cultivars. *Trop. Grassl.-Forrajes Trop.* **2018**, *6*, 42–52. [CrossRef]
29. Miafo, A.P.T.; Koubala, B.B.; Kansci, G.; Muralikrishna, G. Free sugars and non-starchpolysaccharides phenolic acid complexes from bran, spent grain and sorghum seeds. *J. Cereal Sci.* **2019**, *87*, 124–131. [CrossRef]
30. Ayala-Soto, F.E.; Serna-Saldívar, S.O.; Welti-Chanes, J.; Gutierrez-Uribe, J.A. Phenolic compounds, antioxidant capacity and gelling properties of glucoarabinoxylans from three types of Sorghum brans. *J. Cereal Sci.* **2015**, *65*, 277–284. [CrossRef]
31. Stefaniak, T.R.; Dahlberg, J.A.; Bean, B.W.; Dighe, N.; Wolfrum, E.J.; Rooney, W.L. Variation in biomass composition components among forage, biomass, sorghum-sudangrass, and sweet sorghum types. *Crop Sci.* **2012**, *52*, 1949–1954. [CrossRef]
32. Galassi, E.; Taddei, F.; Ciccoritti, R.; Nocente, F.; Gazza, L. Biochemical and technological characterization of two C4 gluten-free cereals: *Sorghum bicolor* and *Eragrostis tef*. *Cereal Chem.* **2020**, *97*, 65–73. [CrossRef]
33. Huang, H.; Hu, X.; Tian, J.; Jiang, X.; Sun, T.; Luo, H.; Huang, D. Rapid and nondestructive prediction of amylose and amylopectin contents in sorghum based on hyperspectral imaging. *Food Chem.* **2021**, *359*, 129954. [CrossRef]
34. Yang, L.; Gao, H.; Meng, L.; Fu, X.; Du, X.; Wu, D.; Huang, L. Nondestructive measurement of pectin polysaccharides using hyperspectral imaging in mulberry fruit. *Food Chem.* **2021**, *334*, 127614. [CrossRef]
35. Zhang, H.; Ge, Y.; Xie, X.; Atefi, A.; Wijewardane, N.K.; Thapa, S. High throughput analysis of leaf chlorophyll content in sorghum using RGB, hyperspectral, and fluorescence imaging and sensor fusion. *Plant Methods* **2022**, *18*, 60. [CrossRef] [PubMed]
36. He, X.; Yan, C.; Jiang, X.; Shen, F.; You, J.; Fang, Y. Classification of aflatoxin B1 naturally contaminated peanut using visible and near-infrared hyperspectral imaging by integrating spectral and texture features. *Infrared Phys. Technol.* **2021**, *114*, 103652. [CrossRef]
37. Zhang, H.; Zhang, S.; Chen, Y.; Luo, W.; Huang, Y.; Tao, D.; Liu, X. Non- destructive determination of fat and moisture contents in Salmon (*Salmo salar*) fillets using near-infrared hyperspectral imaging coupled with spectral and textural features. *J. Food Compos. Anal.* **2020**, *92*, 103567. [CrossRef]
38. Peng, J.; Zhang, J.; Han, L.; Ma, X.; Hu, X.; Lin, T.; Chen, M. Determination of malathion content in sorghum grains using hyperspectral imaging technology combined with stacked machine learning models. *J. Food Compos. Anal.* **2024**, *135*, 106635. [CrossRef]
39. Huang, H.; Hu, X.; Tian, J.; Peng, X.; Luo, H.; Huang, D.; Wang, H. Rapid and nondestructive determination of sorghum purity combined with deep forest and near-infrared hyperspectral imaging. *Food Chem.* **2022**, *377*, 131981. [CrossRef]
40. Hu, X.; Dai, M.; Peng, J.; Zeng, J.; Tian, J.; Chen, M. Rapid sorghum variety identification by hyperspectral imaging combined with super-depth-of-field microscopy. *J. Food Compos. Anal.* **2025**, *137*, 106930. [CrossRef]
41. Dahmoune, F.; Nayak, B.; Moussi, K.; Remini, H.; Madani, K. Optimization of microwave-assisted extraction of polyphenols from *Myrtus communis* L. leaves. *Food Chem.* **2015**, *166*, 585–595. [CrossRef]
42. Zulkifli, M.Z.A.; Benjamin, M.A.Z.; Rosdan, M.D.E.M.; Saini, A.; Rusdi, N.A.; Awang, M.A. Optimisation of yield, flavonoids, and antioxidant activity via ultrasound-assisted extraction of bamboo leaves from *Dinochloa sublaevigata* S. Dransf. (Wadan) in Sabah, Malaysia. *Adv. Bamboo Sci.* **2025**, *10*, 100128. [CrossRef]
43. Yılmaz, M.; Karaaslan, M.; Vardin, H. Optimization of extraction parameters on the isolation of phenolic compounds from sour cherry (*Prunus cerasus* L.) pomace. *J. Food Sci. Technol.* **2015**, *52*, 2851–2859. [CrossRef]
44. Vilkhu, K.; Mawson, R.; Simons, L.; Bates, D. Applications and opportunities for ultrasound-assisted extraction in the food industry—A review. *Innov. Food Sci. Emerg. Technol.* **2008**, *9*, 161–169. [CrossRef]
45. Alara, O.R.; Abdurahman, N.H.; Ukaegbu, C.I. Extraction of phenolic compounds: A review. *Curr. Res. Food Sci.* **2021**, *4*, 200–214. [CrossRef] [PubMed]
46. Luo, X.; Cui, J.; Zhang, H.; Duan, Y.; Zhang, D.; Cai, M.; Chen, G. Ultrasound assisted extraction of polyphenolic compounds from red sorghum (*Sorghum bicolor* L.) bran and their biological activities and polyphenolic compositions. *Ind. Crops Prod.* **2018**, *112*, 296–304. [CrossRef]
47. Barros, F.; Dykes, L.; Awika, J.M.; Rooney, L.W. Accelerated solvent extraction of phenolic compounds from sorghum brans. *J. Cereal Sci.* **2013**, *58*, 305–312. [CrossRef]
48. García-Oms, S.; Sánchez-Bonet, D.; Belda-Antolí, M.; Padrón-Sanz, C.; Lloris-Carsi, J.M.; Cejalvo-Lapeña, D. Optimisation of a green ultrasound-assisted extraction (UAE) methodology for obtaining maximum antioxidant activity from red algae and determination of the co-extracted compounds. *J. Appl. Phycol.* **2024**, *36*, 1433–1444. [CrossRef]
49. Azmir, J.; Zaidul, I.S.M.; Rahman, M.M.; Sharif, K.M.; Mohamed, A.; Sahena, F.; Jahurul, M.H.A.; Ghafoor, K.; Norulaini, N.A.N.; Omar, A.K.M. Techniques for extraction of bioactive compounds from plant materials: A review. *J. Food Eng.* **2013**, *117*, 426–436. [CrossRef]

50. Virot, M.; Tomao, V.; Le Bourvellec, C.; Renard, C.M.C.G.; Chemat, F. Towards the industrial production of antioxidants from food processing by-products with ultrasound-assisted extraction. *Ultrason. Sonochem.* **2010**, *17*, 1066–1074. [CrossRef]
51. Manzoor, M.; Singh, J.; Gani, A.; Noor, N. Valorization of natural colors as health-promoting bioactive compounds: Phytochemical profile, extraction techniques, and pharmacological perspectives. *Food Chem.* **2021**, *362*, 130141. [CrossRef]
52. Das, A.K.; Adsare, S.R.; Das, M.; Kulthe, P.S. Advanced techniques in extraction of phenolics from cereals, pulses, fruits, and vegetables. In *Plant Secondary Metabolites, Volume Two*; Apple Academic Press: New York, NY, USA, 2017; pp. 53–102.
53. Kumar, K.; Srivastav, S.; Sharanagat, V.S. Ultrasound assisted extraction (UAE) of bioactive compounds from fruit and vegetable processing by-products: A review. *Ultrason. Sonochemistry* **2021**, *70*, 105325. [CrossRef]
54. Sethi, S.; Kaur, L.; Nath, P.; Yadav, D.N. Bioactive compounds and phytonutrients from cereals. In *Plant-Based Bioactive Compounds and Food Ingredients*; Apple Academic Press: New York, NY, USA, 2023; pp. 155–205.
55. Hong, S.; Pangloli, P.; Perumal, R.; Cox, S.; Noronha, L.E.; Dia, V.P.; Smolensky, D. A Comparative Study on Phenolic Content, Antioxidant Activity and Anti-Inflammatory Capacity of Aqueous and Ethanolic Extracts of Sorghum in Lipopolysaccharide-Induced RAW 264.7 Macrophages. *Antioxidants* **2020**, *9*, 1297. [CrossRef]
56. Dia, V.P.; Pangloli, P.; Jones, L.; McClure, A.; Patel, A. Phytochemical concentrations and biological activities of Sorghum bicolor alcoholic extracts. *Food Funct.* **2016**, *7*, 3410–3420. [CrossRef]
57. Moraes, É.A.; da Silva Marineli, R.; Lenquiste, S.A.; Steel, C.J.; de Menezes, C.B.; Queiroz, V.A.V.; Júnior, M.R.M. Sorghum flour fractions: Correlations among polysaccharides, phenolic compounds, antioxidant activity and glycemic index. *Food Chem.* **2015**, *180*, 116–123. [CrossRef] [PubMed]
58. Sohounhloue, D.C. Optimization of the Extraction of Sorghum's Polyphenols for Industrial Production by Membrane Processes. *Res. J. Recent Sci.* **2012**, *1*, 2502.
59. Denardi-Souza, T.; Luz, C.; Mañes, J.; Badiale-Furlong, E.; Meca, G. Antifungal effect of phenolic extract of fermented rice bran with *Rhizopus oryzae* and its potential use in loaf bread shelf life extension. *J. Sci. Food Agric.* **2018**, *98*, 5011–5018. [CrossRef] [PubMed]
60. Peng, X.; Ma, J.; Cheng, K.W.; Jiang, Y.; Chen, F.; Wang, M. The effects of grape seed extract fortification on the antioxidant activity and quality attributes of bread. *Food Chem.* **2010**, *119*, 49–53. [CrossRef]
61. Martins, Z.E.; Pinho, O.; Ferreira, I.M.; Jekle, M.; Becker, T. Development of fibre-enriched wheat breads: Impact of recovered agroindustrial by-products on physicochemical properties of dough and bread characteristics. *Eur. Food Res. Technol.* **2017**, *243*, 1973–1988. [CrossRef]
62. Oliviero, T.; Fogliano, V. Food design strategies to increase vegetable intake: The case of vegetable enriched pasta. *Trends Food Sci. Technol.* **2016**, *51*, 58–64. [CrossRef]
63. Chen, G.; Wang, J.; Li, Y. Extracts of sorghum bran, grape seed, and green tea: Chromatographic comparison of phenolic profiles and mitigation effect on acrylamide in antioxidant-fortified bread. *Food Chem. Adv.* **2022**, *1*, 100082. [CrossRef]
64. Bojnanská, T.; Kolesárová, A.; Cech, M.; Tancinová, D.; Urminská, D. Extracts with Nutritional Potential and Their Influence on the Rheological Properties of Dough and Quality Parameters of Bread. *Foods* **2024**, *13*, 382. [CrossRef]
65. Legan, J.D. Mould Spoilage of Bread: The Problem and Some Solutions. *Int. Biodeterior. Biodegrad.* **1993**, *32*, 33–53. [CrossRef]
66. Pateras, I. Bread Spoilage and Staling. In *Technology of Breadmaking*; Springer Ebooks: Boston, MA, USA, 1999; pp. 240–261.
67. Pitt, J.I.; Hocking, A.D. Ecology of Fungal Food Spoilage. In *Fungi Food Spoilage*; Springer: Cham, Switzerland, 2022; pp. 3–12.
68. Alisaac, E.; Behmann, J.; Rathgeb, A.; Karlovsky, P.; Dehne, H.W.; Mahlein, A.K. Assessment of *Fusarium* Infection and Mycotoxin Contamination of Wheat Kernels and Flour Using Hyperspectral Imaging. *Toxins* **2019**, *11*, 556. [CrossRef]
69. Alpers, T.; Kerpes, R.; Frioli, M.; Nobis, A.; Hoi, K.I.; Bach, A.; Becker, T. Impact of storing condition on staling and microbial spoilage behavior of bread and their contribution to prevent food waste. *Foods* **2021**, *10*, 76. [CrossRef] [PubMed]
70. Chen, H.; Tain, X.; Yu, Q.; Hu, W.; Chen, J.; Zhou, L. Sweet sorghum stalks extract has antimicrobial activity. *Ind. Crops Prod.* **2021**, *170*, 113746. [CrossRef]
71. Birhanu, S. Potential benefits of sorghum [*Sorghum bicolor* (L.) Moench] on human health: A review. *Int. J. Food Eng. Technol.* **2021**, *5*, 8–18. [CrossRef]
72. Magdoleen, G.; Daffalla Hussien, M. Phytochemical screening and antibacterial activities of *Sorghum bicolor* leaves derived from in vitro culture. *GSC Biol. Pharm. Sci.* **2020**, *10*, 65–72.
73. Borges, A.; Ferreira, C.; Saavedra, M.J.; Simões, M. Antibacterial Activity and Mode of Action of Ferulic and Gallic Acids against Pathogenic Bacteria. *Microb. Drug Resist.* **2013**, *19*, 256–265. [CrossRef]
74. Chen, H.; Xu, Y.; Chen, H.; Liu, H.; Yu, Q.; Han, L. Isolation and identification of polyphenols from fresh sweet sorghum stems and their antibacterial mechanism against foodborne pathogens. *Front. Bioeng. Biotechnol.* **2022**, *9*, 770726. [CrossRef]
75. Hiroyuki, H.; Tanimoto, K.; Tamura, Y.; Mizutani, K.; Kinoshita, T. Mode of Antibacterial Action of Retrochalcones from Glycyrrhiza Inflata. *Phytochemistry* **1998**, *48*, 125–129.
76. Ziani, I.; Bouakline, H.; El Guerraf, A.; El Bachiri, A.; Fauconnier, M.L.; Sher, F. Integrating AI and advanced spectroscopic techniques for precision food safety and quality control. *Trends Food Sci. Technol.* **2025**, *156*, 104850. [CrossRef]

77. Saleem, Z.; Hussain Khan, M.; Ahmad, M.; Sohaib, A.; Ayaz, H.; Mazzara, M. Prediction of Microbial Spoilage and Shelf-Life of Bakery Products through Hyperspectral Imaging. *IEEE Access* **2020**, *8*, 176986–176996. [CrossRef]
78. Cevoli, C.; Gianotti, A.; Troncoso, R.; Fabbri, A. Quality evaluation by physical tests of a traditional Italian flat bread Piadina during storage and shelf-life improvement with sourdough and enzymes. *Eur. Food Res. Technol.* **2015**, *240*, 1081–1089. [CrossRef]
79. Mehdizadeh, S.A.; Noshad, M.; Nouri, S.F. Non-destructive Detection of Bread Staleness Using Hyperspectral Images. *Innov. Food Technol.* **2023**, *10*, 299–317.
80. Karl, T.; Harre, F.; Warneke, C.; de Gouw, J.; Grayless, C.; Fall, R. Senescing grass crops as regional sources of reactive volatile organic compounds. *J. Geophys. Res.* **2005**, *110*, D15302. [CrossRef]

antioxidants

MDPI

Article

Bioactive Compounds of Shrimp Shell Waste from *Palaemon serratus* and *Palaemon varians* from Portuguese Coast

Maria Luz Maia [1,*], Clara Grosso [1], M. Fátima Barroso [1], Aurora Silva [1,2], Cristina Delerue-Matos [1] and Valentina Fernandes Domingues [1,*]

[1] REQUIMTE/LAQV, ISEP, Polytechnic of Porto, Dr. António Bernardino de Almeida, 4249-015 Porto, Portugal
[2] Nutrition and Bromatology Group, Department of Analytical and Food Chemistry, Faculty of Food Science and Technology, Ourense Campus, University of Vigo, E32004 Ourense, Spain
[*] Correspondence: maria.maia@graq.isep.ipp.pt (M.L.M.); vfd@isep.ipp.pt (V.F.D.); Tel.: +35-1228340500 (V.F.D.)

Abstract: The production and consumption of shrimp species create massive amounts of shrimp bio-waste. In this study, shrimp shell waste from *Palaemon serratus* and *Palaemon varians* from the Portuguese coast was characterized. Regarding the antioxidant capacity, the obtained values were between 4.7 and 10.4 mg gallic acid equivalents (GAE)/g dry weight (dw) for Total phenolic content (TPC); 3 and 7 mg ascorbic acid equivalents (AAE)/g dw for Ferric reducing antioxidant power assay (FRAP); 0.4 and 1.2 mg Trolox equivalent (TE)/g dw for 2,2-diphenyl-1-picryl-hydrazyl-hydrate free radical scavenging ($DPPH^{\bullet}$); 4 and 11 mg TE/g dw for 2,2′-azino-bis (3-ethylbenzothiazoline-6-sulfonic acid) radical scavenging activity ($ABTS^{\bullet +}$); and 72 and 130 mg TE/g dw for Oxygen radical absorbance capacity (ORAC). For the antimicrobial activity, shrimp shell waste from *P. varians* formed inhibition zones between 14 and 23 mm. Total carotenoid content values were in the range of 28 and 134 μg/g dw, and according to their HPLC-PAD profile, β-carotene and astaxanthin contents were between 0.3 and 7.6 μg/g dw and 1.1 and 26.1 μg/g dw, respectively. These studies are critical to recognizing the potential added value of shrimp shell waste as possible colorants and preservatives with antioxidant protection capacity to be used in the food industry.

Keywords: shrimp characterization; waste valorization; antioxidant activity; neuroprotective activity; antimicrobial activity

1. Introduction

Shrimps are crustaceans that are highly appreciated all over the world, suggested as high-quality food, and considered part of a balanced diet. The shrimp market has been growing over the years, which makes shrimps a valuable source of nutrients for the human population [1]. Shrimps are a good source of protein, vitamins, astaxanthin, and minerals such as phosphorus, calcium, selenium, copper, zinc, and iodine [2]. The Food and Agriculture Organization (FAO) establishes that shrimp consumption in several countries has been increasing globally. The FAO database reports that 12,611,809 tons of shrimp were consumed in 2020 in the world, and this value in Portugal was 28,835 tons. These data highlight the importance of shrimp in the global economy and also the amount of shell waste produced. Furthermore, Portugal's rate of consumption is higher than the worldwide average, with the quantity consumed per capita in 2020 being 2.83 kg in Portugal compared to the global average of 1.63 kg [3,4]. Regarding the capture of shrimp species in Portugal, in 2020 it reached 87 tons. This amount provided revenues of EUR 2,565,000 [5].

Depending on market demand, shrimps can be exported with or without the shell. All this consumption and production generates massive amounts of shrimp bio-waste. Usually, this waste comprises approximately 50% of the weight of raw shrimp [6]. The increase in the disposal of shrimp waste in the surrounding environment is a critical contribution to environmental pollution and health risks. Consequently, the processing and application of shrimp shell waste are crucial to reducing environmental pollution [6,7]. Pigments with high antioxidant capacities from shrimp shell wastes can be a good added value for new bioproducts, for instance, in the food industry, since shrimp shells are a good source of protein, minerals, carotenoids, such astaxanthin, a powerful antioxidant, and enzymes [7,8]. The shell composition of crustaceans, such as shrimp, can be slightly different depending on the species, season, and habitat; nevertheless, the main composition is calcium carbonate (20–50%), protein (20–40%), chitin (15–40%), and lipids (0–14%) with elevated contents of omega-3 fatty acids and pigments [9]. Several extractions have been performed to extract the pigments like carotenoids, and more specifically astaxanthin, from shrimp shell waste. Ethanol was considered suitable, effective, and safe to perform this extraction [10].

The current work aimed to explore the antioxidant, neuroprotective, and antimicrobial activities of shrimp shell waste. For that purpose, two shrimp species, *Palaemon serratus* and *Palaemon varians,* collected in different seasons and locations on the Portuguese coast, were studied. To the best of our knowledge, this is the first study assessing the influence of the seasons and sampling locations on the production of carotenoids in these two species from the Portuguese coast.

2. Materials and Methods

2.1. Reagents and Materials

Folin-Ciocalteu, 2,2-diphenyl-1-picryl-hydrazyl-hydrate free radical scavenging (DPPH), 6-hydroxy-2,5,7,8-tetramethylchroman-2-carboxylic acid (Trolox) dimethyl sulfoxide (DMSO), lactic acid, ascorbic acid, 2′,2′-azobis (2-amidinopropane) dihydrochloride (AAPH), α-glucosidase, α-amylase, butyrylcholinesterase (BuChE), acetylcholinesterase (AChE), 4-nitrophenyl-α-D-glucopyranoside, acarbose, Tris-HCl, potassium phosphate monobasic, potassium phosphate dibasic trihydrate, bovine serum albumin (BSA), galantamine, acarbose, starch, 3,5-dinitrosalicylic acid, and astaxanthin standard (≥97% (high performance liquid chromatography, HPLC), from *Blakeslea trispora*) were purchased from Sigma Aldrich (Steinheim, Germany). Gallic acid was obtained from Fluka (Steinheim, Germany). β-carotene standard (≥95% (HPLC) was from Extrasynthese, (Genay, France). Sodium hydroxide was from Labkem (Barcelona, Spain). Sodium carbonate was from Panreac (Barcelona, Spain). Potassium sodium tartrate tetrahydrate was from Scharlab (Barcelona, Spain). The culture media Mueller–Hinton broth (MHB) and Mueller–Hinton II agar were acquired from Sigma-Aldrich (Madrid, Spain). Ethanol absolute and butyl methyl ether were from Carlo Erba (Val de Reuil, France), and methanol was from Riedel-de Haën (Seelze, Germany). Ultrapure water resistivity of 18.2 MΩ cm, was from a Simplicity 185 water purification system (Millipore, Molsheim, France). All the solvents used were HPLC grade with the quality available (95–99%). All the spectrophotometric assays were performed in a Synergy HT W/TRF Multi Mode Microplate Reader with Gen5 2.0 software (BioTek Instruments, Winooski, VT, USA).

2.2. Samples

Shrimp shell waste from two different shrimp species from the Portuguese coast was analyzed. *P. serratus* was gathered at Figueira da Foz and Vila do Conde by local fishermen, and *P. varians* was from wild and aquaculture origins gathered in the Sado estuary. These two species are well described in the literature [11]. The sampling locations were chosen to represent different locations between the north and the center of Portugal. Northern waters are colder, and the Sado estuary represents a site with brackish water against the salted water from the other two locations (Figueira da Foz and Vila do Conde). Sampling was carried out in autumn and spring between 2017 and 2019, according to the period allowed for the capture [12]. The shell was separated from the edible portion of the shrimp and analyzed.

2.3. Extraction Procedure

Shrimp shells were dehydrated at 41 °C (Excalibur, model 4926T, Dublin, Ireland) for 48 h and grounded to obtain reduced particles. Preliminary extractions were carried out where different solvents (Ethanol, 50% Ethanol and 70% Acetone), different solid: solvent ratios (5 g:50 mL and 5 g:100 mL), and different temperatures (room temperature and 40 °C) were tested. The best condition was 5 g of shrimp shell and 50 mL of absolute ethanol solution under agitation for 2 h at room temperature. In terms of Total Phenolic Content (TPC), this extraction was not statistically different from the other three conditions: with absolute ethanol using 100 mL (instead of 50 mL) at room temperature or applying 40 °C, and the extraction performed with acetone, 5 g/50 mL of solid-solvent ratio and 40 °C. Moreover, considering Ferric Reducing Antioxidant Power (FRAP) assays, extractions performed with absolute ethanol were statistically and significantly different from all the others performed. Altogether, considering three fundamental aspects related to the extraction processes, such as the environmental impact of using higher volumes of solvent, the costs associated with the use of temperature, and that ethanol is considered a GRAS solvent (Generally recognized as safe), the extraction condition using absolute ethanol, at room temperature, and with a solid–solvent ratio of 5 g/50 mL was selected. After that, the content was filtered with filter paper and then evaporated at 40 °C under a vacuum and protected from light in a rotary evaporator.

Calibration standards for all the analyses were prepared daily, and all extracts were analyzed in triplicate. An $r^2 \geq 0.99$ was found for all calibration curves.

2.4. Chemical Characterization of the Extracts

2.4.1. Total Phenolic Content

TPC determination was performed based on the Folin–Ciocalteu procedure [13]. Gallic acid (GA) was used as standard, and the absorbance was measured at 760 nm. TPC was expressed as mg of GA equivalents per g of dry weight (dw) of extract (mg GAE/g extract dw).

2.4.2. Total Carotenoids Content

Total Carotenoids Content (TC) determination in the methanolic extracts was assessed by a colorimetric method and expressed in µg/g dw [14]. Contents were calculated using Equation (1), where A_{480} and A_{750} were the absorbances recorded at 480 and 750 nm, respectively:

$$\text{Carotenoid } (\mu g/mL) = 4 \times (A_{480} - A_{750}) \tag{1}$$

2.4.3. High Performance Liquid Chromatography (HPLC) with A Photodiode Array Detector (PDA)

The eluents used in the HPLC unit (Shimadzu, Kyoto, Japan) equipped with a photodiode array detector (PDA) model SPD-M20A were filtered through a 0.22 µm nylon membrane filter (Fioroni Filters, Ingré, France) using a vacuum pump (Dinko D-95, Barcelona, Spain) and degassed for 15 min in an ultrasonic bath (Sonorex Digital 10P, Bandelin DK 255P, Germany). Twenty µL of each shrimp shell extract were injected on an analytical HPLC with a low-pressure quaternary pump (model LC-20AT), a degasser (model DGU-20A5R), an auto-sampler (model SIL-20AT), and a column oven (model CTU-20AC). The gradient and column were previously described [15] and were used with some modifications. Briefly, compound separation was achieved using a C30 YMC Carotenoid S-5µm (25.0 × 0.46 cm; 5 µm particle size) column (Kyoto, Japan). The solvent system consisted of methanol (A) and MTBE (B) starting with 95% A, using a gradient to obtain 70% A at 30 min, 50% A at 60 min, and again 95% A at 65 min. The solvent flow rate was 0.9 mL/min. Chromatograms were recorded at 450 nm, and data were processed on LabSolutions software. Compounds were identified by comparing their UV–vis spectra and retention times with standards injected in the same conditions.

2.5. Biological Activity of the Extracts

2.5.1. Antioxidant Capacity

Ferric Reducing Antioxidant Power

FRAP determination was performed according to the previously developed method by Paz et al. [13]. Ascorbic acid (AA) was used as the standard, and the absorbance was measured at 593 nm. FRAP results were expressed as mg of AA equivalents per g dw of extract (mg AAE/g dw).

2,2-Diphenyl-1-Picryl-Hydrazyl-Hydrate Free Radical Scavenging

$DPPH^{\bullet}$ scavenging activity was performed as previously described [16]. Trolox solution was used as the standard, and the absorbance was measured at 517 nm. The results were expressed as mg of Trolox equivalents per g of dw of extract (mg TE/g dw). Inhibition (%) of DPPH activity was calculated after subtracting the respective blanks. The results were also expressed as the concentration needed to inhibit a biological process by 50% values (IC_{50}).

2,2′-Azino-Bis (3-Ethylbenzothiazoline-6-Sulfonic Acid) Radical Scavenging Activity

2,2′-azino-bis (3-ethylbenzothiazoline-6-sulfonic acid) radical scavenging activity ($ABTS^{\bullet+}$) was determined according to Correia et al. [17]. A trolox solution was used as the standard and the absorbance was measured at 734 nm [17]. The results were expressed as mg of Trolox equivalents per g of dw of extract (mg TE/g dw). Inhibition (%) of $ABTS^{\bullet+}$ scavenging activity was calculated. The results were also expressed as IC_{50} values.

Oxygen Radical Absorbance Capacity

Oxygen radical absorbance capacity (ORAC) was performed as previously described [18]. Trolox solution was used as the standard. Briefly, disodium fluorescein (FL) was added to sample dilutions, and the resulting mixture was equilibrated for 30 min at 37 °C. Then, the reaction was initiated by the addition of AAPH, and the fluorescence was recorded. The results were expressed as mg of Trolox equivalents per g of extract (mg TE/g dw).

2.5.2. Enzyme Inhibition

AChE and BuChE Inhibition Activities

AChE and BuChE inhibition activities of shrimp shell extracts were determined according to Ellman's method [19] with slight modifications. Briefly, samples were dissolved in 50 mM Tris–HCl buffer (pH 8) with 10% MeOH. Then, 25 µL of the samples previously dissolved were added to the wells with 125 µL of 3 mM DTNB reagent, 50 µL of 50 mM Tris–HCl buffer (pH 8) with 0.1% of BSA, 25 µL of ATCI/BTCI, and 25 µL of 0.44 U/mL of AChE or 0.40 U/mL of BuChE. The initial slopes of the reaction were calculated at 405 nm and the Tris–HCl buffer with 10% of MeOH was used as a negative control. The values for inhibitory activity were calculated. Galantamine was used as the positive control (IC_{50} = 0.92 µg/mL against AChE and IC_{50} = 4.92 µg/mL against BuChE).

α-Glucosidase Inhibition Activity

α-Glucosidase inhibition activity of shrimp shell extracts was determined as previously described [20]. Samples were dissolved in potassium phosphate buffer 10 mM (pH 7), then 50 µL were added to the wells. Next, 130 µL of buffer was added, plus 100 µL of enzyme substrate (4-nitrophenyl-α-D-glucopyranoside 2.5 mM) and 20 µL of α-glucosidase. The microplate was incubated at 37 °C, and the reaction slopes were calculated recording the absorbance at 405 nm for 10 min. Potassium phosphate buffer 10 mM was used as the negative control and acarbose as a positive control (IC_{50} = 302 µg/mL), and the values for inhibitory activity were calculated.

α-Amylase Inhibition Activity

α-Amylase inhibition activity of shrimp shell extracts was determined as previously described [21]. Samples were dissolved in 20 mM sodium phosphate buffer (pH 6.9 with 6 mM sodium chloride). Briefly, 100 µL of the sample plus 100 µL of 1% starch solution in buffer were incubated at 25 °C for 10 min. Next, 100 µL of α-amylase (8 mg/mL) was added and incubated again at 25 °C for 10 min. After adding 200 µL of dinitro alicyclic acid (DNS) color reagent, the reaction was stopped by incubating at 100 °C for 5 min.

After the samples cooled down, 50 µL was removed from each tube and transferred to a microplate and 200 µL of water was added to each well. Absorbance was measured at 540 nm. Acarbose was used as the positive control. Sodium phosphate buffer 20 mM (pH 6.9 with 6 mM sodium chloride) was used as a negative control, and the values for inhibitory activity were calculated.

2.5.3. Antimicrobial Activity

The shrimp shell extracts were dissolved in DMSO (45 mg/mL), and the evaluation of antimicrobial activity was performed as described previously [22]. The antimicrobial properties of the shrimp shell extracts were tested against the following bacterial strains: Gram-positive *Escherichia coli* (NCTC 9001) that were supplied by Microbiologics, Minnesota USA, and *Pseudomonas aeruginosa* (ATCC 10145), *Salmonella enteritidis* (ATCC 13676), Gram-negative *Staphylococcus aureus* (ATCC 25923), and *Bacillus cereus* (ATCC 14579) were provided by Selectrol (Buckingham, UK). The determination of antimicrobial activity was achieved via Petri dish culture and measurement of the inhibition by the production of halos after the addition of the extracts [23]. Primarily, the bacteria were inoculated with MHB and were left to grow between 12 h and 24 h at 37 °C. Employing UV spectrometry at 600 nm, the number was set between 1 and 2 $\times$ 10^8 colony forming units (CFUs). For that purpose, an absorbance between 0.09 and 0.110 of the McFarland scale was used. Briefly, 50 µL of the cultivated inoculum of the different bacteria was deposited and streaked. The Petri dish was divided into 4 quadrants, and 15 µL of 40% lactic acid was added as a positive control. In the remaining quadrants, 15 µL of the extract was added, and 15 µL of DMSO was added as a negative control in the center of the Petri dish and incubated for 24 h at 37 °C. The halos resulting from the inhibition were measured using a pachymeter in millimeters [24].

2.6. Statistical Analysis

All the experiments were repeated at least three times and presented as mean$\pm$standard deviation (SD). The statistical significance of the difference between the two groups was assessed by the nonparametric Mann–Whitney test, whereas the differences between more than two groups were assessed by Kruskal–Wallis one-way analysis of variance using Graph Pad Prism Software, version 6. The IC_{50} values were calculated also using Graph Pad Prism Software, version 6. The Pearson correlation coefficient was used to evaluate the correlation between different elements analysed. For that, SPSS Inc., version 22.0 was used (SPSS Inc., Chicago, IL, USA). Differences were considered statistically significant for $p < 0.05$.

3. Results

3.1. Chemical Characterization of the Extracts

Table 1 displays the TPC and TC values for the various locations and seasons; all data are reported in g dw of extract.

Figures 1–4, and Figures S2–S5 display the comparison between seasons, species, and locations of sampling. Regarding seasons, all samples collected in spring were compared with those collected in autumn. For species comparison, all *P. serratus* samples were compared with those of *P. varians*, regardless of their location or season. Finally, all samples of *P. serratus* (spring + autumn) collected in Figueira da Foz, Vila do Conde and of *P. varians* (Spring + Autumn) collected in the Sado estuary were treated as independent groups.

Table 1. Total phenolic content (TPC) and total carotenoids (TC); (A)-aquaculture; (W)-wild; GAE-gallic acid equivalents.

Location of Sampling and Season	Species	TPC			TC		
		mg GAE/g			μg/g		
Figueira da Foz, Spring	*Palaemon serratus*	8.1	±	0.7	80	±	9
Figueira da Foz, Autumn		9	±	1	134	±	11
Vila do Conde, Spring		6.4	±	0.4	52	±	3
Vila do Conde, Autumn		10.4	±	0.7	127	±	8
Sado estuary (A), Spring	*Palaemon varians*	5.0	±	0.4	50	±	3
Sado estuary (A), Autumn		9.0	±	0.5	28	±	5
Sado estuary (W), Spring		4.7	±	0.3	42	±	2
Sado estuary (W), Autumn		9.9	±	0.6	32	±	3

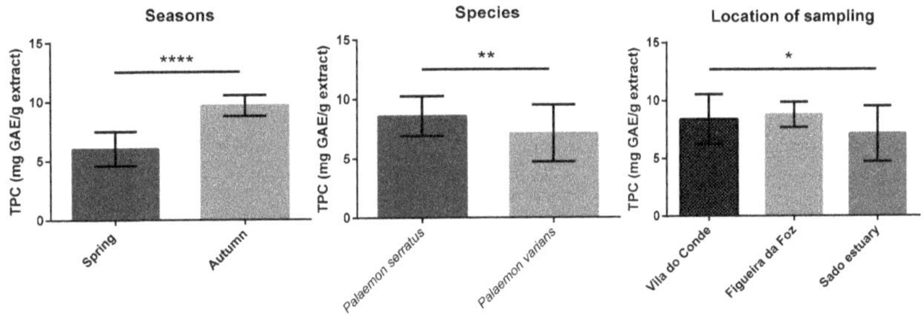

Figure 1. Differences in TPC content between seasons, species, and locations. Columns correspond to mean of the concentration ± SD. Significantly different, **** $p < 0.0001$; ** $p < 0.01$, * $p < 0.05$.

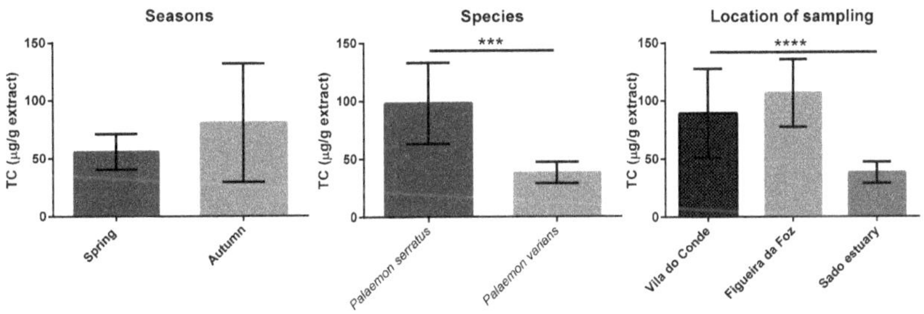

Figure 2. Differences in TC content between seasons, species, and locations. Columns correspond to mean of the concentration ± SD. Significantly different, **** $p < 0.0001$, *** $p < 0.001$.

For TPC content, the mean values ranged between 4.7 and 10.4 mg GAE/g dw. Regarding the influence of season, species, and location of sampling, as shown in Figure 1, the values were significantly higher in autumn (9.7 mg GAE/g dw, $p < 0.0001$), in *P. serratus* (8.6 mg GAE/g dw, $p < 0.01$), and collected from Figueira da Foz (8.8 mg GAE/g dw, $p < 0.05$), respectively.

TC average values ranged between 28 and 134 μg/g dw (Table 1). Statistically significant differences were observed concerning the species and locations of sampling (Figure 2). The values were higher in *P. serratus* at 98 μg/g dw ($p < 0.0001$) and Figueira da Foz at 107 μg/g dw ($p < 0.0001$).

Regarding the HPLC profile of the analyzed shrimp shell extract, β-carotene, and astaxanthin were identified and quantified, and an example of a chromatogram is presented in Figure S1. β-carotene and astaxanthin concentrations obtained in the shrimp extracts are presented in Figures S2 and S3. β-carotene mean values ranged between 0.3 and 7.6 μg/g dw. Regarding the different seasons, the values were significantly higher in spring at 4.1 μg/g dw ($p < 0.001$), and for different species and locations of sampling, no statistically significant differences were observed (Figure S2). Concerning astaxanthin, the mean values ranged between 1.1 and 26.1 μg/g dw. This time, no significative differences were observed for the different seasons (spring and autumn), whereas significative differences were observed when compared between different species and different locations of the sampling (Figure S3). Regarding shrimp species, the values were higher in *P. serratus* 17.3 μg/g dw ($p < 0.0001$), and, in the case of location of sampling, the values were higher in Vila do Conde 18.8 μg/g dw ($p < 0.001$).

3.2. Biological Activity of the Extracts

The results regarding FRAP, DPPH$^{\bullet}$, ABTS$^{\bullet+}$, and ORAC measurements are presented in Table 2 for the different locations and seasons. All the results are presented by g dw of extract.

Table 2. FRAP, RSA, and ORAC.; (A)-aquaculture; (W)-wild; AAE-ascorbic acid equivalents; TE-Trolox equivalents.

Location of Sampling and Season	Species	FRAP	DPPH		ABTS		ORAC
		mg AAE/g	mg TE/g	IC_{50} (mg/mL)	mg TE/g	IC_{50} (mg/mL)	mg TE/g
Figueira da Foz, Spring	*Palaemon serratus*	6 ± 1	0.5 ± 0.1	5.9	6 ± 2	0.5	76 ± 14
Figueira da Foz, Autumn		6 ± 2	0.5 ± 0.2	2.0	7 ± 2	0.5	75 ± 23
Vila do Conde, Spring		3 ± 2	0.7 ± 0.3	4.9	6 ± 2	0.3	72 ± 8
Vila do Conde, Autumn		7 ± 1	0.5 ± 0.1	4.3	4 ± 2	0.6	94 ± 35
Sado estuary (A), Spring	*Palaemon varians*	5 ± 1	0.4 ± 0.1	8.2	11 ± 4	0.3	96 ± 17
Sado estuary (A), Autumn		6 ± 2	1.2 ± 0.2	1.7	7 ± 2	0.5	79 ± 13
Sado estuary (W), Spring		5.1 ± 0.7	0.7 ± 0.2	3.6	6 ± 4	0.3	130 ± 21
Sado estuary (W), Autumn		6 ± 2	0.9 ± 0.3	2.0	7 ± 2	0.5	87 ± 20

Regarding FRAP, the mean values were between 3 and 7 mg AAE/g dw (Table 2). As presented in Figure S4, the values were significantly higher in autumn as well, with a value of 6.3 mg AAE/g dw ($p < 0.0001$). For species and location, no statistically significant differences were observed.

Concerning DPPH$^{\bullet}$ scavenging activity, the mean values ranged between 0.4 and 1.2 mg TE/g dw, and for IC_{50} values ranged between 1.7 and 8.2 mg/mL (Table 2). Figure 3 shows that the values were significantly higher in autumn as well at 0.79 mg TE/g dw ($p < 0.05$), in *P. varians*, 0.79 mg TE/g dw ($p < 0.01$), and in Sado estuary, 0.79 mg TE/g dw ($p < 0.05$).

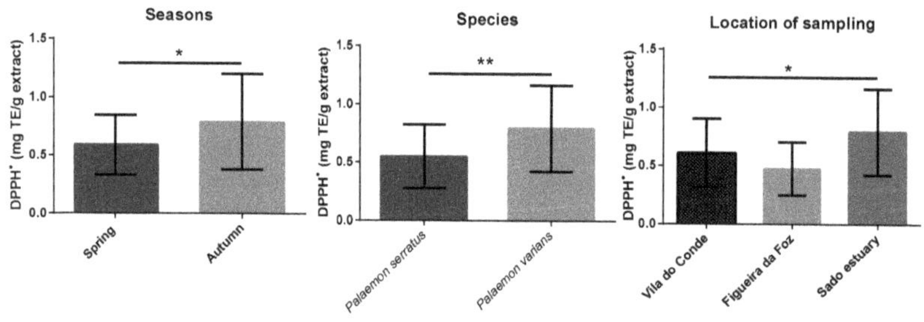

Figure 3. Differences of DPPH$^{\bullet}$ scavenging activity between seasons, species, and locations. Columns correspond to mean of the concentration ± SD. Significantly different, ** $p < 0.01$, * $p < 0.05$.

ABTS$^{\bullet+}$ scavenging activity mean values were between 4 and 11 mg TE/g dw, with IC_{50} values ranging from 0.3 to 0.6 mg/mL. In the case of ORAC mean values, these ranged between 72 and 130 mg TE/g dw (Table 2). As well as for DPPH$^{\bullet}$, Figures 4 and S5 show that the values for ABTS$^{\bullet+}$ and ORAC were significantly higher in *P. varians*,

7.3 mg TE/g dw ($p < 0.05$) and 98.8 mg TE/g dw ($p < 0.001$), respectively, and in Sado estuary, 7.3 mg TE/g dw ($p < 0.01$), and 98.8 mg TE/g dw ($p < 0.01$), respectively.

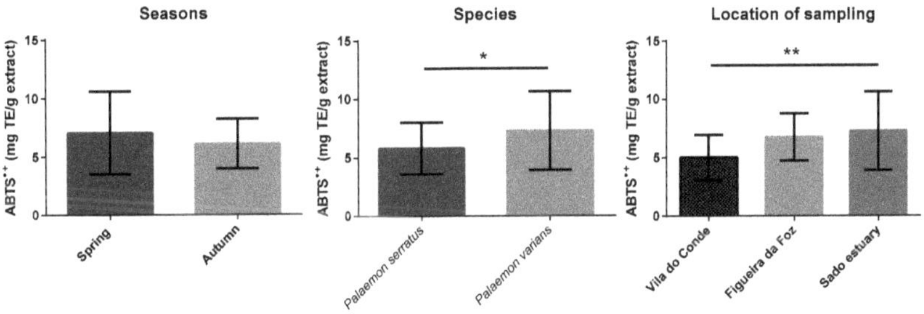

Figure 4. Differences of $ABTS^{\bullet +}$ scavenging activity between seasons, species, and locations. Columns correspond to mean of the concentration ± SD. Significantly different, ** $p < 0.01$, * $p < 0.05$.

3.3. Enzyme Inhibition

Concerning the determination of the enzyme inhibition by the shrimp shell extracts, the IC_{50} values were not possible to calculate due to the weak inhibition power of the extracts. Concentrations of the shrimp shell extracts tested were between 600 and 150 µg/mL for AChE and BuChE, between 250 and 20 µg/mL for α-glucosidase, and between 380 and 20 µg/mL for α-amylase. AChE and BuChE inhibitions were lower than 15% for 600 µg/mL of the extract. Concerning α-glucosidase, the inhibition was lower than 20% for 250 µg/mL of the extract, and for α-amylase the inhibition was lower than 10% concerning the concentration of 380 µg/mL of the extract.

3.4. Antimicrobial Activity

The results regarding the inhibition zones obtained for the shrimp shell extracts against several bacteria are presented in Table S1. The classification proposed by the Clinical and Laboratory Standards Institute was used for this assay, where the diameter of the inhibition growth measured allows the classification of bacteria as resistant (R, ≤ 14 mm), intermediate (I, 15–19 mm), or susceptible (S, ≥ 20 mm) [23].

Only the shrimp shell extracts from the Sado estuary (*P. varians*) formed inhibition zones. In the case of *P. aeruginosa*, both wild and aquaculture origin extracts were able to develop inhibition zones ranging from 14 to 20 mm (Table S1). *B. cereus* and *S. enteritidis* were also significative inhibited by *P. varians* shells extract (aquaculture origin). The inhibition zones in the case of *B. cereus* varied between 21 and 23.3 mm and for *S. enteritidis* ranged between 18 and 20 mm (Table S1). The results also demonstrate that the tested extracts do not show any activity against *E. coli* and *S. aureus*.

3.5. Correlations between Elements Analyzed

The data described in Table S2 show a strong Pearson correlation ($0.5 < |r| < 1$) and $p < 0.05$ between the levels of the elements analyzed. Positive correlations were found between the values of TPC and FRAP and also between the values of TC and astaxanthin. However, negative correlations were found between the values of $DPPH^{\bullet}$ scavenging and astaxanthin and also between values of FRAP and β-carotene.

4. Discussion

Regarding chemical characterization (TPC and TC), higher values were obtained for *P. serratus*, in autumn, and in Figueira da Foz, and astaxanthin values were also higher in *P. serratus*. Some of these results could be explained by the size of the shrimp because *P. serratus* was between 4 and 9 cm, *P. varians* was between 2 and 4 cm, and their metabolic rate could be different. *P. serratus*, in this case, seems to be producing more phenolic and carotenoid compounds (total and astaxanthin). Carotenoid retention was previously described to be dependent on the species analyzed and their reproduction cycle [25,26].

Seasonal variation of the TC could also be explained by changes in the quantity and quality of the algae available to the shrimp diet [25]. The results found in this work were slightly lower than the previously reported TPC value of 38 mg GAE/g dw [27]. The differences in the TPC values found between this study and previously reported ones might be attributed to variances in shrimp species or changes in the sampling site. The study of Shiekh et al. [27] used shrimp shells from a fish market in Jeddah, Saudi Arabia, and the solvent used in the extraction was methanol, whereas the current study used shrimps from the Portuguese coast and ethanol as the extraction solvent. So, as shown in the current study, different locations and species can have different impacts on TPC values. Regarding TC, a previous study reported TC mean values lower than the values determined in the present study [28], in this previous study, three shrimp species, *Farfantepenaeus brasiliensis*, *F. subtilis*, and *Litopenaeus schmitti* from the Brazilian coast were analyzed, and the obtained TC values in ethanol:acetone (1:1) shrimp extracts were between 2 and 9 μg/g [28]. Furthermore, a TC of 43 μg/g was obtained when using the shrimp species *Litopenaeus vannamei* from Brazil and the extraction performed in n-hexane:isopropanol (60:40) [29]. Another study presented similar TC values to the ones described in the present study: TC of 80 μg/g for *Trachysalambria curvirostris* [30]. This species was sampled on the coast of China, and the extraction solvent used was acetone.

β-carotene values were higher in spring, and concerning the shrimp species, β-carotene and astaxanthin were higher in *P. serratus*. Astaxanthin mean values ranged between 1.1 and 26.1 μg/g dw in this study, and a value of 5.8 μg/g of astaxanthin in the shells of *Pandalus borealis* shrimp species, using ethanol and ultrasound equipment for the extraction, was reported [31]. The value reported is in the range of the values reported in the present study, and in the case of *P. serratus*, the values have higher printing value in their potential waste. High values of carotenoids, such as β-carotene and astaxanthin, have been linked to lower risks of cardiovascular and degenerative diseases [26], so the consumption or use of products with high values of these carotenoids could be beneficial to health.

The biological activity of the extracts varied between the analysis performed, $ABTS^{\bullet+}$ and ORAC values were higher in spring, whereas FRAP and $DPPH^{\bullet}$ values were higher in autumn. Concerning the shrimp species, $DPPH^{\bullet}$, $ABTS^{\bullet+}$, and ORAC values were higher in *P. varians*. That was the species from the estuary, so from brackish waters. Values of FRAP reported previously for shrimp shells were around 7.3 and 16.3 mg TE/g [32]. In that study [32], shrimps were from a Canadian company, and the solvent used was an ethylenediaminetetraacetic acid buffer. Regarding the shrimp muscle, the values were around 1.5 mg TE/g [33], and this result was obtained from the shrimp specie *Pandalus borealis* caught in the Norwegian sea. These results valorize the shrimp shell waste, and the values reported in the present study are similar to the values described for shrimp shells. Previous results for $DPPH^{\bullet}$ scavenging activity in shrimp shell waste were around 3 and 4.5 mg/g [32], slightly above the values shown in the present study. Regarding $ABTS^{\bullet+}$, values around 6 and 13 mg TE/g were reported [32], which are in accordance with the values described in the present work. Concerning ORAC for shrimp muscle samples, the value reported is around 38.8 mg TE/g [33]. This value is lower than the values reported in this study for shrimp shells, which valorizes shrimp shell waste.

Positive or negative correlations were found between some of the parameters analyzed. Positive correlations were found between TPC and FRAP values, and this was described previously in herbs, spices, and pulses [34,35]. This indicates that phenolic compounds could be major contributors to antioxidant power. In the same way, when TC values raise, astaxanthin values also increase in the shrimp shell samples, this could indicate that the total value of carotenoids is particularly influenced by the amount of the carotenoid astaxanthin. Negative correlations were found between $DPPH^{\bullet}$ values and astaxanthin. This was an unexpected result because astaxanthin is known for its antioxidant capacity. Nevertheless, a negative correlation between DPPH and other carotenoids was described previously for fruit samples [36]. Similarly, a negative correlation was found between FRAP and β-carotene. A previous study reported a negative correlation between FRAP and carotenoids [37]. In the case of the present work, the negative correlation was particularly with carotenoid β-carotene.

Regarding the study of shrimp shell waste as a potential enzyme inhibitor, a previous work studied a shrimp shell deproteinized bioactive hydrolysate from *Metapenaeus monoceros*. Using this hydrolysate, the authors reached 100% of AChE inhibition at 620 μg/mL and 100% of α-amylase inhibition at 400 μg/mL [38]. Conversely, in the present study, similar concentrations only inhibited 15% and 10% of AChE and α-amylase activity, respectively. Moreover, the acetone and dichloromethane extracts from by-products (heads, shells, and tails) of *Pandalus borealis*, *Pandalus hypsinotus*, and *Pandalopsis japonica*, characterized by carotenoid contents between 6.79 and 11.12 mg/g, displayed moderate AChE and BuChE inhibitions [39]. The authors reported IC_{50} in the range of 200–940 μg/mL against AChE and 670–2050 μg/mL against BuChE. These differences could be explained by the different extraction procedures used or can be justified by the differences between the shrimp species itself.

P. varians demonstrated good antimicrobial activity against *B. cereus*, *P. aeruginosa*, and *S. enteritidis*. Instead, *P. serratus* did not demonstrate any antimicrobial activity. These phenomena could be explained by the fact that *P. varians* is the specie from the Sado estuary. Brackish water, probably with high levels of bacteria, may increase the antimicrobial activity by adaptive responses, and although the shrimps have the same genera, they are classified into two different species and so can exhibit different antimicrobial activity [40]. Shrimp shell from a fish market in Dammam city, Saudi Arabia was extracted using methanol and previously evaluated [41] against some of the bacteria tested in the present study (*E. coli*, *S. aureus*, and *P. aeruginosa*), and the results for *P. aeruginosa* (18 mm) were similar to the presented results for *P. varians* from aquaculture origin. Concerning *S. aureus*, the results are similar to the previous results reporting no formed inhibition zone. However, the shrimp shell extract was not able to form an inhibition zone for *E. coli*, whereas the study from Gumgumjee et al. [41] presented a value of 30 mm, which can probably be explained by differences between the strains or extraction procedures [41].

5. Conclusions

The analysis of bioactive compounds from natural sources is nowadays of high importance. Shrimp shell waste analyzed in this study presented a significant antioxidant capacity with values in the range of previous works reported. The results demonstrate that, for the parameters evaluated, significant differences between the variables analyzed (species, seasons, and locations of sampling) were observed. All the findings of this work reveal the potential application of shrimp shell waste in new bioproducts. This incorporation could remarkably raise the antioxidant capacity of the products and improve their color making them more appealing to the food industry.

Supplementary Materials: The following supporting information can be downloaded at: https://www.mdpi.com/article/10.3390/antiox12020435/s1. Figure S1: Chromatogram of the sample Vila do Conde spring containing astaxanthin (1) and β-carotene (2) obtained in the PDA detector; Figure S2: Differences of β-carotene content between seasons, species, and locations; Figure S3: Differences of astaxanthin content between seasons, species, and locations; Figure S4: Differences of FRAP content between seasons, species, and locations; Figure S5: Differences of ORAC content between seasons, species, and locations; Table S1: Average diameter of inhibition zone (mm) of shrimp shell; Table S2: Positive and negative strong correlations between the elements analyzed.

Author Contributions: Conceptualization, M.L.M., C.G. and M.F.B.; Methodology, M.L.M. and A.S.; Validation, M.L.M., C.G. and M.F.B.; Investigation, M.L.M.; Statistical analysis, M.L.M.; Writing—original draft, M.L.M.; Writing—review & editing, C.G., M.F.B., A.S., C.D-M. and V.F.D.; Resources, C.D.-M.; Supervision, V.F.D. All authors have read and agreed to the published version of the manuscript.

Funding: This work was financially supported by Portuguese national funds through projects UIDB/50006/2020, UIDP/50006/2020, and LA/P/0008/2020, from the Fundação para a Ciência e a Tecnologia (FCT)/Ministério da Ciência, Tecnologia e Ensino Superior (MCTES). The authors also thank FCT and the European Union's H2020 Research and Innovation Programme for funding through the project SYSTEMIC—An integrated approach to the challenge of sustainable food systems: adaptive and mitigatory strategies to address climate change and malnutrition.

Institutional Review Board Statement: Not applicable.

Informed Consent Statement: Not applicable.

Data Availability Statement: Not applicable.

Conflicts of Interest: The authors declare no conflict of interest.

References

1. Maia, L.; Almeida, A.; Soares, C.; Silva, L.M.S.; Delerue-Matos, C.; Calhau, C.; Fernandes, V. Minerals and fatty acids profile of Northwest Portuguese coast shrimps. *J. Food Compos. Anal.* **2022**, *112*, 104652. [CrossRef]
2. Dayal, J.S.; Ponniah, A.G.; Khan, H.I.; Babu, E.P.M.M.; Ambasankar, K.; Vasagam, K.P.K.K. Shrimps—A nutritional perspective. *Curr. Sci.* **2013**, *104*, 1487–1491.
3. FAO Food Supply—Livestock and Fish Primary Equivalent. FAOSTAT 2021. Available online: https://www.fao.org/faostat/en/#data/FBS (accessed on 27 December 2022).
4. FAO The State of World Fisheries and Aquaculture—Contributing to Food Security and Nutrition for All. Food and Agriculture Organization of the United Nations. 2016. Available online: https://www.fao.org/3/i5555e/i5555e.pdf (accessed on 27 December 2022).
5. INE Fishery Statistics. Stat. Port. 2020. Available online: https://www.ine.pt/xportal/xmain?xpid=INE&xpgid=ine_publicacoes&PUBLICACOESpub_boui=280980980&PUBLICACOESmodo=2 (accessed on 27 December 2022).
6. Fawwaz, M.; Pratama, M.; Hasrawati, A.; Sukmawati; Widiastuti, H.; Rahmawati; Abidin, Z. Total carotenoids, antioxidant and anticancer effect of penaeus monodon shells extract. *Biointerface Res. Appl. Chem.* **2021**, *11*, 11293–11302. [CrossRef]
7. Muniyappan, J.; Varadharajan, V.; Namadevan, P. Biochemical Screening and Determination of Bioactive Components of Commercially Cultured Pacific White Shrimp Penaeus vannamei. *Pharmacogn. Res.* **2019**, *11*, 140–146. [CrossRef]
8. Pattanaik, S.S.; Sawant, P.B.; Xavier, K.A.M.; Dube, K.; Srivastava, P.P.; Dhanabalan, V.; Chadha, N.K. Characterization of carotenoprotein from different shrimp shell waste for possible use as supplementary nutritive feed ingredient in animal diets. *Aquaculture* **2020**, *515*, 734594. [CrossRef]
9. Šimat, V.; Rathod, N.B.; Čagalj, M.; Hamed, I.; Mekinić, I.G. Astaxanthin from Crustaceans and Their Byproducts: A Bioactive Metabolite Candidate for Therapeutic Application. *Mar. Drugs* **2022**, *20*, 206. [CrossRef]
10. Chintong, S.; Phatvej, W.; Rerk-Am, U.; Waiprib, Y.; Klaypradit, W. In vitro antioxidant, antityrosinase, and cytotoxic activities of astaxanthin from shrimpwaste. *Antioxidants* **2019**, *8*, 128. [CrossRef]
11. González-Ortegón, E.; Cuesta, J.A. An illustrated key to species of *Palaemon* and *Palaemonetes* (Crustacea: Decapoda: Caridea) from European waters, including the alien species *Palaemon macrodactylus*. *J. Mar. Biol. Assoc. United Kingdom* **2006**, *86*, 93–102. [CrossRef]
12. DRE Portaria n.o 1102-E/2000. Diário da República n.o 270/2000, 2o Supl. Série I-B 2000-11-22 2000, 12–16. Portaria n.° 1102-E/2000, de 22 de Novembro 2000. Available online: https://dre.pt/dre/detalhe/portaria/1102-e-2000-284922 (accessed on 23 November 2021).
13. Paz, M.; Gúllon, P.; Barroso, M.F.; Carvalho, A.P.; Domingues, V.F.; Gomes, A.M.; Becker, H.; Longhinotti, E.; Delerue-Matos, C. Brazilian fruit pulps as functional foods and additives: Evaluation of bioactive compounds. *Food Chem.* **2015**, *172*, 462–468. [CrossRef]
14. Stengel, D.B.; Walker, J.M.; Connan, S. Natural Products From Marine Algae. *Methods Mol. Biol.* **2015**, *1308*, 1–37.
15. Fernandes, F.; Barbosa, M.; Oliveira, A.P.; Azevedo, I.C.; Sousa-Pinto, I.; Valentão, P.; Andrade, P.B. The pigments of kelps (Ochrophyta) as part of the flexible response to highly variable marine environments. *J. Appl. Phycol.* **2016**, *28*, 3689–3696. [CrossRef]
16. Barroso, M.F.; Ramalhosa, M.J.; Alves, R.C.; Dias, A.; Soares, C.M.D.; Oliva-Teles, M.T.; Delerue-Matos, C. Total antioxidant capacity of plant infusions: Assessment using electrochemical DNA-based biosensor and spectrophotometric methods. *Food Control* **2016**, *68*, 153–161. [CrossRef]
17. Castro-correia, C.; Maia, M.L.; Norberto, S.; Costa-santos, C. Can Antioxidative Status Be Involved in Type 1 Diabetes? *J. Clin. Med. Res.* **2017**, *9*, 998–1001. [CrossRef]
18. Soares, C.; Paíga, P.; Marques, M.; Neto, T.; Carvalho, A.P.; Paiva, A.; Simões, P.; Costa, L.; Bernardo, A.; Fernández, N.; et al. Multi-step subcritical water extracts of *Fucus vesiculosus* L. And *Codium tomentosum* stackhouse: Composition, health-benefits and safety. *Processes* **2021**, *9*, 893. [CrossRef]
19. Ellman, G.L.; Courtney, K.D.; Andres, V.; Featherstone, R.M. A new and rapid colorimetric determination of acetylcholinesterase activity. *Biochem. Pharmacol.* **1961**, *7*, 88–95. [CrossRef]
20. Vinholes, J.; Grosso, C.; Andrade, P.B.; Gil-Izquierdo, A.; Valentão, P.; De Pinho, P.G.; Ferreres, F. In vitro studies to assess the antidiabetic, anti-cholinesterase and antioxidant potential of *Spergularia rubra*. *Food Chem.* **2011**, *129*, 454–462. [CrossRef]

21. Lordan, S.; Smyth, T.J.; Soler-Vila, A.; Stanton, C.; Paul Ross, R. The α-amylase and α-glucosidase inhibitory effects of Irish seaweed extracts. *Food Chem.* **2013**, *141*, 2170–2176. [CrossRef]
22. Sokovicx', M.; Glamočlija, J.; Marin, P.D.; Brkić, D.; Van Griensven, L.J.L.D. Antibacterial effects of the essential oils of commonly consumed medicinal herbs using an in vitro model. *Molecules* **2010**, *15*, 7532–7546. [CrossRef]
23. Clinical and Laboratory Standards Institute. *Performance Standards for Antimicrobial Disk Susceptibility Tests: Approved Standard*, 11th ed.; Clinical and Laboratory Standards Institute: Wayne, PA, USA, 2012; Volume 32.
24. Lourenço-Lopes, C.; Fraga-Corral, M.; Soria-Lopez, A.; Nuñes-Estevez, B.; Barral-Martinez, M.; Silva, A.; Li, N.; Liu, C.; Simal-Gandara, J.; Prieto, M.A. Fucoxanthin's Optimization from Undaria pinnatifida Using Conventional Heat Extraction, Bioactivity Assays and In Silico Studies. *Antioxidants* **2022**, *11*, 1296. [CrossRef]
25. Yanar, Y.; Çelik, M.; Yanar, M. Seasonal changes in total carotenoid contents of wild marine shrimps (*Penaeus semisulcatus* and *Metapenaeus monoceros*) inhabiting the eastern Mediterranean. *Food Chem.* **2004**, *88*, 267–269. [CrossRef]
26. Carvalho, C.C.C.R.; Caramujo, M.J. Carotenoids in aquatic ecosystems and aquaculture: A colorful business with implications for human health. *Front. Mar. Sci.* **2017**, *4*, 93. [CrossRef]
27. Shiekh, H.M.; Gumgumjee, N.M.; Danial, E.N. Antifungal and antioxidant activities of methanol extract of chitin, chitosan and shrimp shell waste. *Int. J. Pharm. Phytopharm. Res.* **2018**, *8*, 25–30.
28. López, A.M.Q.; Dos Santos, F.A.R.; Martins, E.S.; Silva, A.L.D.S.; Dos Santos, E.C.L. Pink and white shrimps from the Brazilian coast: Pigment identification, antioxidant activity and microbial quality under different freezing-times. *Food Sci. Technol.* **2021**, *41*, 447–457. [CrossRef]
29. Seabra, L.M.A.J.; da Silva Chaves Damasceno, K.S.F.; da Silva, C.R.; de Carvalho Gomes, C.; Pedrosa, L.F.C. Total carotenoids in white shrimp (*Litopenaeus vannamei*) waste. *Rev. Ceres* **2014**, *61*, 130–133. [CrossRef]
30. Su, F.; Liu, J. The carotenoid characteristics of the important wild shrimp *Trachysalambria curvirostris* (Stimpson, 1860) in China. *J. Oceanol. Limnol.* **2019**, *37*, 706–712. [CrossRef]
31. Hu, J.; Lu, W.; Lv, M.; Wang, Y.; Ding, R.; Wang, L. Extraction and purification of astaxanthin from shrimp shells and the effects of different treatments on its content. *Rev. Bras. Farmacogn.* **2019**, *29*, 24–29. [CrossRef]
32. Ambigaipalan, P.; Shahidi, F. Bioactive peptides from shrimp shell processing discards: Antioxidant and biological activities. *J. Funct. Foods* **2017**, *34*, 7–17. [CrossRef]
33. Jensen, I.J.; Hogne, A.; Maehre, H.K.; Elvevoll, E.O. Changes in antioxidative capacity of saithe (Pollachius virens) and shrimp (*Pandalus borealis*) during in vitro digestion. *J. Agric. Food Chem.* **2009**, *57*, 10928–10932. [CrossRef]
34. Maizura, M.; Aminah, A.; Wan Aida, W.M. Total phenolic content and antioxidant activity of kesum (*Polygonum minus*), ginger (*Zingiber officinale*) and turmeric (*Curcuma longa*) extract. *Int. Food Res. J.* **2011**, *534*, 529–534.
35. Parikh, B.; Patel, V.H. Total phenolic content and total antioxidant capacity of common Indian pulses and split pulses. *J. Food Sci. Technol.* **2018**, *55*, 1499–1507. [CrossRef]
36. Rey, F.; Zacarías, L.; Rodrigo, M.J. Carotenoids, vitamin c, and antioxidant capacity in the peel of mandarin fruit in relation to the susceptibility to chilling injury during postharvest cold storage. *Antioxidants* **2020**, *9*, 1296. [CrossRef]
37. Singh, B.K.; Koley, T.K.; Maurya, A.; Singh, P.M.; Singh, B. Phytochemical and antioxidative potential of orange, red, yellow, rainbow and black coloured tropical carrots (*Daucus carota* subsp. sativus Schubl. & Martens). *Physiol. Mol. Biol. Plants* **2018**, *24*, 899–907. [CrossRef]
38. Mechri, S.; Sellem, I.; Bouacem, K.; Jabeur, F.; Laribi-Habchi, H.; Mellouli, L.; Hacène, H.; Bouanane-Darenfed, A.; Jaouadi, B. A biological clean processing approach for the valorization of speckled shrimp *Metapenaeus monoceros* by-product as a source of bioactive compounds. *Environ. Sci. Pollut. Res.* **2020**, *27*, 15842–15855. [CrossRef]
39. Kim, S.B.; Yoon, N.Y.; Shim, K.B.; Lim, C.W. Antioxidant and cholinesterase inhibitory activities of the By-Products of three pandalid shrimps. Fish. *Aquat. Sci.* **2014**, *17*, 421–425. [CrossRef]
40. Pellizzoni, M.; Ruzickova, G.; Kalhotka, L.; Lucini, L. Antimicrobial activity of different *Aloe barbadensis* Mill. and *Aloe arborescens* Mill. leaf fractions. *J. Med. Plants Res.* **2012**, *6*, 1975–1981. [CrossRef]
41. Gumgumjee, N.M.; Shiekh, H.M.; Danial, E.N. Antioxidant and Antibacterial Activity of Chitin, Chitosan and Shrimp Shells from Red Sea for Pharmaceutical Uses. *Int. J. Pharm. Res. Allied Sci.* **2018**, *7*, 1–8.

antioxidants

Article

Valorization of Olive Leaf Polyphenols by Green Extraction and Selective Adsorption on Biochar Derived from Grapevine Pruning Residues

Melissa Prelac [1], Nikola Major [1,*], Danko Cvitan [1], Dominik Anđelini [1], Maja Repajić [2], Josip Ćurko [2], Tvrtko Karlo Kovačević [1], Smiljana Goreta Ban [1], Zoran Užila [1], Dean Ban [1] and Igor Palčić [1]

[1] Institute of Agriculture and Tourism, Karla Huguesa 8, 52440 Poreč, Croatia; melissa@iptpo.hr (M.P.); danko@iptpo.hr (D.C.); dominik@iptpo.hr (D.A.); tvrtko@iptpo.hr (T.K.K.); smilja@iptpo.hr (S.G.B.); zoran@iptpo.hr (Z.U.); dean@iptpo.hr (D.B.); palcic@iptpo.hr (I.P.)

[2] Department of Food Engineering, University of Zagreb, Faculty of Food Technology and Biotechnology, Pierottijeva 6, 10000 Zagreb, Croatia; maja.repajic@pbf.unizg.hr (M.R.); josip.curko@pbf.unizg.hr (J.Ć.)

* Correspondence: nikola@iptpo.hr

Abstract: Given today's increasingly intensive agriculture, one key problem area considers the valorization and reuse of wastes from food and agricultural production with minimal impact on the environment. Due to its physicochemical characteristics, biochar (BC) derived from grapevine pruning residue has shown considerable potential for use as an adsorbent. High-value phytochemicals found in abundance in the olive leaf (OL) can be employed in many different industrial sectors. The potential application of BC in the removal of specific polyphenolic components from OL extracts has been investigated in the present study. Water, as the most available and greenest of solvents, was investigated as to its use in the extraction of polyphenols, which was carried out by comparing maceration, ultrasound-assisted extraction, and microwave-assisted extraction, considering different temperatures and solid-to-liquid (s/l) ratios. The BC adsorption capacity of selected polyphenols was fitted with both the Langmuir and Freundlich isotherm models. The Freundlich model fitted better relative to OL polyphenols adsorption. Oleuropein was the most abundant compound identified in the extracts, obtaining the highest K_f value (20.4 (mg/g) × (L/g)^n) and R^2 coefficient (0.9715) in the adsorption on the biochar's surface. The optimum conditions in the dosage experiment suggest the use of 0.5 g of BC using 3 g/L extracts, with an exception for oleuropein and hydroxytyrosol, for which the highest biochar dose (2.5 g) performed better. Considering the compounds' concentrations and the BC dose, BC from grapevine pruning residues demonstrated a potential use in the uptake of specific polyphenols from olive leaves, making it a promising adsorbent for such applications.

Keywords: adsorption; bioactive compounds; green extraction; sustainable agriculture; waste management

1. Introduction

The main role of agricultural production is to supply food to the ever-growing population, but at the same time, it has a negative impact on the environment, considering the use of pesticides and fertilizers, the emissions of various gases, and the production of biomass residues [1–3]. Biomass residues are usually rich in compounds that can be used for different purposes, such as in the food, chemical, and pharmaceutical industries [4,5].

The olive tree (*Olea europea* L.) is commonly grown for its fruit, which is used in olive oil production. According to Eurostat [6], the European Union counted 4.49 million ha under olive trees in 2017, mainly in the Mediterranean area, with Spain and Italy leading the production of the fruit. Olive pomace, olive mill wastewater, and branches and leaves are the main biomass residues from olive oil production and olive-tree growing. To achieve higher and healthier yields, pruning is performed, as an agro-technical measure, to remove the excess branches and leaves [7–9]. The production of olive leaves and branches from pruning has been estimated to be 25 kg per olive tree [10]. In most cases, the obtained biomass is improperly disposed of, incinerated or spread across the field [9], with a resulting series of negative environmental effects, such as emissions of greenhouse gases; air, water, and soil contamination; and waste of resources [11]. Olive biomass is considered a byproduct with no value [12], but different authors [13–15] have reported high polyphenolic concentrations in olive residues. Secoiridoids, in particular oleuropein and its derivatives, followed by hydroxytyrosol, are the main olive leaf components, a list which also includes other polyphenols and simple phenolics (caffeic acid, tyrosol), triterpenes, oleanolic acid, and flavonoids (i.e., rutin, apigenin, kaempferol, and luteolin) [16,17].

The concentrations of the extracted bioactive compounds depend on the olive variety and, mostly, on the extraction technique [18]. Different solvents are used in the extraction of bioactive compounds to achieve better performance, extraction, and yields [19]. Classic extraction procedures often involve the use of unsustainable solvents such as methanol, acetonitrile, or hexane [14]. To reduce the impact on the environment and to contribute to the fight against climate change, the European Commission adopted the European Green Deal strategy, including the Chemicals Strategy for Sustainability Towards a Toxic-Free Environment [20], with reducing human and environmental risks posed by certain hazardous chemicals as one of the strategy's goals.

The use of eco-friendly chemicals, as well as the development of green extraction technologies, are challenges for researchers. Many studies have reported the high extraction of bioactive compounds using green solvents such as ethanol [21], acetone [19], or natural deep eutectic solvents (NADES) [22]. However, water is the most naturally available solvent, covering more than 70% of the Earth's surface. Because of its polarity, low supply costs, easy availability, and low environmental impact, water could be a potential solution in bioactive compounds extraction. To improve aqueous extraction and achieve better yields, different technologies are used nowadays, such as microwave-assisted extraction (MAE) or ultrasound-assisted extraction (UAE) [12]. When choosing the extraction technology, it is necessary to take into account various factors such as temperature, extraction time, and solid-to-liquid ratio [23].

Viticulture in the Mediterranean region represents 40% of the total area under grapevine production worldwide [24], generating huge amounts of residues due to agro-technical measures [25]. Pyrolysis is a common decomposition method for biomass under anaerobic conditions and in a temperature range of 300–900 °C [26], representing a potential solution for viticulture biomass valorization by its encouragement of the circular economy. The product of pyrolysis is biochar, described as a carbon rich, heterogeneous solid material characterized by a porous structure and low polarity [27,28]. It has a wide application in environmental remediation due to its strong adsorption capacity [26,27]. Biochar (BC) from lignin or cellulose-rich plants could form more porous structures [26], making it more suitable for the removal of compounds. Furthermore, due to its properties such as large surface area, the presence of negatively charged organic functional groups, and its cation exchange capacity, it is considered to be an efficient adsorbent [28–30]. Several authors have reported biochar's capacity in the removal of pollutants and phenols [26,29,31].

The aim of this research was to evaluate water as a green solvent in the extraction of polyphenols from olive leaves and the potential of BC from grapevine pruning residues in the adsorption of bioactive compounds from olive leaf extracts. Using three different extraction techniques, maceration (MAC), MAE, and UAE, in addition to solid-to-liquid ratio (s/l) and temperature modulation, the polyphenolic profiles and antioxidant capacities of the obtained extracts were investigated. The BC produced from grapevine pruning residues was tested as an adsorbent for polyphenolic compounds from the obtained olive leaf extract using Langmuir and Freundlich isotherm models.

2. Materials and Methods

2.1. Plant Material

Olive leaves (*O. europea* L.) were collected in June 2022 (approximately 1 kg of leaves was collected in total) from an experimental olive plantation at the Institute of Agriculture and Tourism, Poreč, Croatia. The leaves were air-dried at 30 °C until they reached a constant weight (Memmert UF160, Schwabach, Germany), and ground in an ultra-centrifugal mill (Retsch ZM 200, Haan, Germany) to a 0.2 mm fine powder.

2.2. BC Production

Residues from grapevine pruning destined for biochar (BC) production were gathered at the Institute of Agriculture and Tourism in Poreč, Croatia. These residues originated from an experimental vineyard featuring the 'Istrian Malvasia' cultivar (*Vitis vinifera* L.). The canes underwent pyrolysis using a Kon-Tiki system, with the peak temperature reaching 400 °C. The resulting biochar was subjected to air drying at a constant temperature of 30 °C (Memmert UF160, Schwabach, Germany), followed by grinding in a mortar mill (Retsch, RM 200, Haan, Germany). The powder was subsequently sifted through a test sieve to achieve particle sizes ranging from 125 to 250 μm. The details of the production process and the characterization of the produced biochar is reported in Prelac et al. [29].

2.3. The Extraction of Polyphenolic Compounds

To investigate the potential of water as a sole solvent for the extraction of polyphenolic compounds from olive leaves, an experiment with a balanced design was set up with s/l ratio and temperature as the main factors, with five levels each, and with three replications. The samples were fused with 25 mL of distilled water at 20 °C to obtain s/l ratios of 1:25, 1:50, 1:100, 1:250, and 1:500, using 1, 0.5, 0.25, 0.1, and 0.05 g of olive leaves, respectively. The investigated extraction temperatures were 30, 45, 60, 75, and 90 °C, achieved by either an ultrasonic bath (40 kHz, 300 W ultrasound power, 400 W heater power, MRC 250 H, Holon, Israel), a microwave unit with the power set at 800 W (Milestone Ethos Up, Sorisole, Italy), or a water bath (GFL 1013, Burgwede, Germany). Each extraction lasted for a period of 30 min, including a 5 min pre-heating phase, and the samples were then left to cool for 24 h. Following this, the extract underwent centrifugation at 16,000× *g* for 5 min using a Domel Centric 350 centrifuge (Železniki, Slovenia). The resulting supernatant was filtered through a 0.22 μm syringe filter, and the extracts were subsequently stored at −18 °C until analysis.

2.4. Analysis of Polyphenolic Compounds in Olive Leaf Extracts

The polyphenolics analysis was performed on a Shimadzu Nexera UPLC-PDA instrument consisting of two pumps (LC -40DX3, Shimadzu, Kyoto, Japan), a degasser (DGU-405, Shimadzu, Kyoto, Japan), a controller (SCL-40, Shimadzu, Kyoto, Japan), an autosampler (SIL-40CX3, Shimadzu, Kyoto, Japan), a diode array detector (SPD-M40, Shimadzu, Kyoto, Japan), and a heated column compartment (CTO-40C, Shimadzu, Kyoto, Japan). The column for separation of the analytes was a Poroshell 120 EC-C18 2.7 μm (2.1 mm × 150 mm) (Agilent, Palo Alto, CA, USA). The column temperature was set at 40 °C. A flow rate of 0.4 mL/min was established. The binary gradient elution of mobile phases A and B followed this sequence: 0–18 min, transitioning from 98% A to 40% A; 18–20 min, 40% A to 20% A; 20–21 min, 20% A to 2% A; 21–24 min, maintaining 2% A; 24–25 min, 2% A to 98% A; and 25–30 min, 98% A. Solvent A was water, while solvent B was methanol, both containing 0.2% acetic acid (*v/v*). The entire run's duration was 30 min. The polyphenolics detected in olive leaf extracts included 11 compounds, but due to low concentrations, only hydroxytyrosol, luteolin-7-*O*-glucoside, apigenin-7-glucoside, and oleuropein were further investigated. Polyphenolic compounds were quantified using calibration curves obtained with serial standard dilutions of hydroxytyrosol (y = 28,440.06x − 4 455.44, R^2 = 0.9999), apigenin-7-glucoside (y = 29,478.83x + 29 675.27, R^2 = 0.9999), and oleuropein (y = 16,109.34x − 369.53, R^2 = 0.9999). Luteolin-7-*O*-glucoside was quantified using luteolin-4-*O*-glucoside (y = 53,613.20x + 20,071.95, R^2 = 0.9998). Quantification of hydroxytyrosol and oleuropein was performed at 280 nm, while apigenin-7-*O*-glucoside and luteolin-7-*O*-glucoside were quantified at 360 nm. The results were expressed in μg/g dry weight (DW) of olive leaves.

2.5. Antioxidant Capacity of Olive Leaf Extracts

The assay for DPPH radical scavenging activity was conducted following the method outlined by Brand-Williams et al., with certain modifications [32]. The reaction mixture comprised 200 μL of freshly prepared 0.02M DPPH radical and 100 μL of the extract. The well-plate was placed in the dark at 25 °C for 30 min, and the antioxidant capacity values were measured at an absorbance of 517 nm (Tecan Infinite 200 Pro M Nano+, Männedorf, Switzerland) after the specified reaction time. The results were calculated against a Trolox calibration curve (ranging from 20 to 100 μM, y = −13.47x + 13.407; R^2 = 0.9998) and expressed as μmol of Trolox equivalents per gram of dry weight (μmol TE/g DW).

For the ferric reducing antioxidant power assay (FRAP), the procedure followed that of Benzie and Strain, with some adjustments [33]. The reaction mixture consisted of 100 μL of extract and 200 μL of freshly prepared FRAP reagent. The well-plate was stored in the dark at 25 °C for 10 min, and absorbance was measured at 593 nm (Tecan Infinite 200 Pro M Nano+, Männedorf, Switzerland). FRAP values were calculated using a Trolox calibration curve (ranging from 20 to 100 μM; y = 6.82156x + 0.02291; R^2 = 0.9999) and expressed as μmol TE/g DW.

The oxygen radical absorbance capacity (ORAC) was investigated according to the description of Ou et al., with slight modifications [34]. In summary, 37.5 μL of extracts were mixed with 225 μL of freshly prepared 4 μM fluorescein solution, and the reaction mixture was incubated at 37 °C for 30 min. Subsequently, 37.5 μL of freshly mixed AAPH was added to the incubated mixture. Excitation (485 nm) and emission (528 nm) wavelengths were measured for 120 min (Tecan Infinite 200 Pro M Nano+, Männedorf, Switzerland). ORAC values were calculated from a Trolox calibration curve (ranging from 4 to 20 μM; y = 0.0404x − 0.0005, R^2 = 0.9999) and expressed as μmol TE/g DW.

2.6. Adsorption Capacity of BC Derived from Grapevine Pruning Residues

Based on the experimental data, olive leaf extract obtained by UAE at 90 °C and an s/l ratio of 1:100 was used for further experiments with BC adsorption. The first adsorption experiment was carried out by fusing batches of 10 mg BC with olive leaf extract at concentrations ranging from 5 to 50 mg/L to determine the capacity of BC to adsorb polyphenols. In the second adsorption experiment, the effect of BC dosage on the adsorption of polyphenolic compounds was investigated by using BC at dosages of 0.5, 1.0, 1.5, 2.0, and 2.5 g/L, and fusing it with olive leaf extract at a concentration of 3 g/L.

The mixtures underwent rotation for a duration of 24 h at 25 °C using the Biosan Multi RS60 apparatus (Riga, Latvia). Afterward, the samples were filtered through a 0.22 μm nylon filter into an HPLC vial, and analyses were carried out on an LC-ESI-QqQ system from Shimadzu, in Kyoto, Japan. This instrumentation included a column oven compartment (Nexera CTO-40C), an autosampler (Nexera SIL-40CX3), two solvent delivery units (Nexera LC-40DX3), and a QqQ mass spectrometer (LCMS8045). To identify targeted compounds, specific ions and retention times were compared with analytical standards. The separation of these compounds was accomplished by injecting 1 μL of the extract onto a C18, 2.1 mm × 150 mm, 2.7 μm core-shell column from Advanced Materials Technology in Wilmington, DE, USA. The oven temperature was maintained at 40 °C. The binary gradient elution of mobile phases occurred as follows: 0 min to 1 min, 98% A; 1 min to 16 min, 98% A to 40% A; 16 min to 21 min, 40% A to 0% A; 21 min to 24 min, 0% A; 24 min to 25 min, 0% A to 98% A; and 25 min to 30 min, 98% A. In this gradient, mobile phase A consisted of water, and mobile phase B comprised methanol, both containing 0.1% acetic acid (*v*/*v*). The flow rate was set at 0.30 mL/min. The LC-ESI-QqQ analysis revealed 31 polyphenolic compounds in the olive leaf extract. After the adsorption on the

BC, only the compounds with the highest concentrations were fitted with the isotherm models. The studied compounds were vanillic acid-4-glucoside, hydroxytyrosol, luteolin-7-*O*-glucoside, luteolin-7-*O*-rutinoside, apigenin-7-*O*-glucoside, and oleuropein. The results were expressed in μg/g DW.

The results of the first experiment were fitted with the Langmuir and Freundlich isotherms to better understand the adsorption dynamics of the polyphenolics on the surface of the grapevine-pruning-residue BC. The Langmuir isotherm is explained as follows [35]:

$$1/q_{eL} = 1/q_{max} + 1/(K_L \times q_{max}) \times 1/\gamma_e \tag{1}$$

where q_{eL} represents the amount of adsorbate concentration in the solid phase at equilibrium (mg/g), $1/q_{max}$ is the slope of linear equation, $1/(K_L \times q_{max})$ is the y-intercept, K_L signifies the affinity constant (L/mg), q_{max} is the maximum monolayer adsorption capacity (mg/g), and γ_e is the amount of adsorbate concentration in the liquid phase at equilibrium (mg/L). The equation was plotted as $1/q_{eL}$ vs. $1/\gamma_e$, and the coefficient of determination (R^2) was calculated. Additionally, the R_L factor was calculated to determine the favorability of Langmuir isotherms, as described below:

$$R_L = 1/(1 + K_L \times \gamma_0) \tag{2}$$

where K_L is the affinity constant (L/mg), and γ_0 is the initial concentration of the adsorbate (mg/L).

The Freundlich isotherms were calculated using the equation below and plotted as $\log q_{eF}$ vs. $\log \gamma_e$. The Freundlich isotherm constant ($K_F/(mg/g) \times (L/g)^n$), adsorption intensity (n), and R^2 were calculated using the plot.

$$\log q_{eF} = \log K_F + 1/n \times \log \gamma_e \tag{3}$$

2.7. Statistical Analysis

Statistical analysis of the data was conducted through Statistica 13.4 (Tibco, Inc., Palo Alto, CA, USA) using analysis of variance (ANOVA) and Tukey's post hoc test, considering significant differences at a *p*-value of $\leq$0.05 for the comparison of group mean values. Furthermore, the graphs depicting the relationship between temperature and s/l ratio in the extracted data were generated using the Distance Weighted Least Square algorithm in Statistica 13.4 (Tibco, Inc., Palo Alto, CA, USA).

3. Results

3.1. The Influences of Extraction Method, Temperature, and Solid-to-Liquid Ratio on Olive Leaves' Polyphenolic Compound Content and Antioxidant Capacity

The polyphenols detected in olive leaf extracts included 11 compounds, but due to low concentrations, only hydroxytyrosol, luteolin-7-*O*-glucoside, apigenin-7-glucoside, oleuropein, and their sum were further analyzed.

The effects of temperature against s/l ratio on polyphenolic profile while using MAC, UAE, and MAE are shown in Figures 1–3. In general, all investigated compounds yielded better at 75 °C or above. Higher yields of hydroxytyrosol were obtained at extraction temperatures of 75 and 90 °C, with no influence of s/l ratio when MAC (Figure 1a) and UAE (Figure 1b) were applied. On the contrary, MAE (Figure 1c) yielded better at all temperatures used, with visible s/l ratio influence; s/l ratios of 1:25 and 1:50 were more favorable when temperatures from 45 to 90 °C were used. The s/l ratios from 1:50 to 1:100 yielded better at 30 °C, while 1:25 achieved the lowest yield at the same temperature.

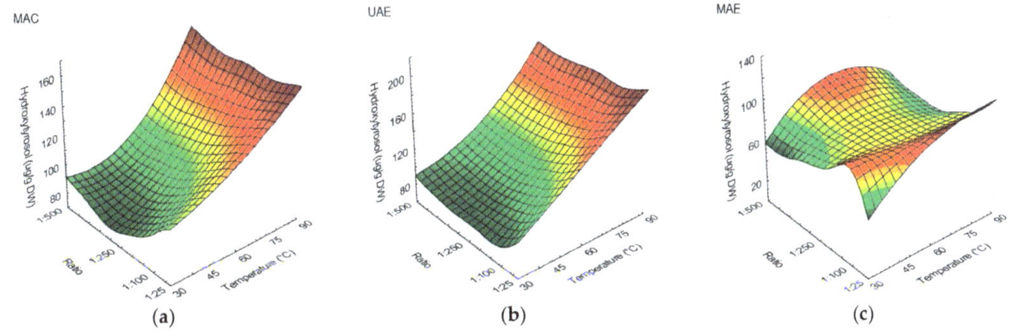

Figure 1. Response surface plots showing the influence of temperature against s/l ratio in olive leaf extracts on the content of hydroxytyrosol (µg/g DW): (**a**) extraction performed using MAC; (**b**) extraction performed using UAE; (**c**) extraction performed using MAE.

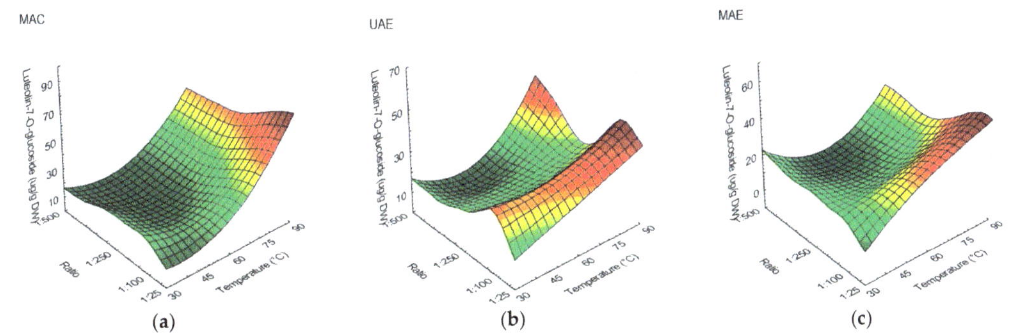

Figure 2. Response surface plots showing the influence of temperature against s/l ratio in olive leaf extracts on the content of luteolin-7-*O*-glucoside (µg/g DW): (**a**) extraction performed using MAC; (**b**) extraction performed using UAE; (**c**) extraction performed using MAE.

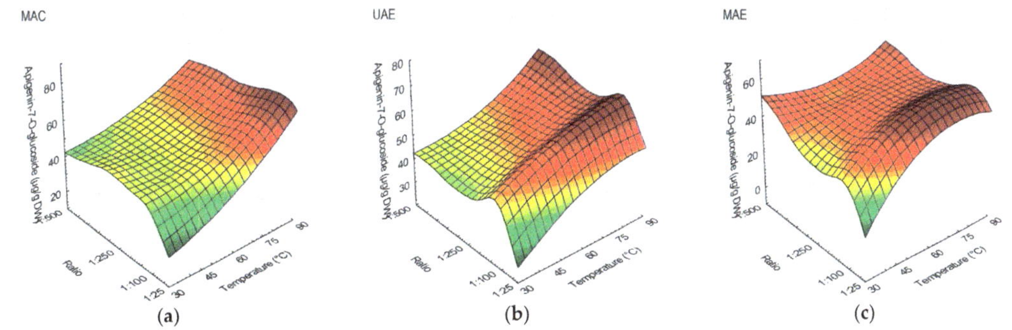

Figure 3. Response surface plots showing the influence of temperature against s/l ratio in olive leaf extracts on the content of apigenin-7-*O*-glucoside (µg/g DW): (**a**) extraction performed using MAC; (**b**) extraction performed using UAE; (**c**) extraction performed using MAE.

As for luteolin-7-*O*-glucoside, there was an evident effect of s/l ratio and temperature on the extraction yield. The highest yield of luteolin-7-*O*-glucoside was detected at 90 °C when applying MAC with s/l ratio from 1:25 to 1:250, while the lowest yield was obtained using s/l ratio 1:500 at 45, 75, and 90 °C (Figure 2a). In UAE application, s/l ratio 1:100 performed better in all temperatures used, while s/l ratio 1:500 obtained the lowest amount of luteolin-7-O-glucoside (Figure 2b), except when the temperature was set at 75 or 90 °C. When applying MAE at a temperature of 30 °C, the influence of ratio on the yield of the investigated compound was visible (Figure 2c). Specifically, as the s/l ratio decreased, the concentration of the investigated compound increased. The opposite trend was observed at 60 °C; the concentration of the compound increased as the ratio increased. Furthermore, at temperatures of 45, 75, and 90 °C, an increase in yield was recorded at ratios of 1:50 and 1:100; when reducing the ratio, the yield would also decrease.

The yield of apigenin-7-O-glucoside was affected by temperature in MAC application, performing better at 90 °C with no visible s/l ratio influence (Figure 3a). As for UAE, comparable results were obtained from 60 to 90 °C, and with ratios starting from 1:50 or less (Figure 3b). MAE obtained the lowest amount of apigenin-7-O-glucoside when utilizing 30 °C and an s/l ratio of 1:25, in comparison with other methods, while the highest yields were observed at 45 °C and with s/l ratios of 1:100 and 1:250, 60 °C and s/l ratio 1:25, and 75 and 90 °C with s/l ratios of 1:50 and 1:100 (Figure 3c).

Oleuropein was the compound found most abundantly in olive leaves, and accordingly, the sum of polyphenolics resulted in a similar trend. MAC and UAE obtained higher yields in similar conditions, with visible temperature and s/l ratio influences on the yield. MAC performed better at 75 and 90 °C when s/l ratios of 1:250 or 1:500 were used (Figure 4a,d), while in the application of UAE, similar results were obtained at temperatures of 60, 75, and 90 °C (Figure 4b,e). MAE has obtained higher yields of oleuropein and polyphenolics at 30 °C, with results comparable to those at 75 and 90 °C (Figure 4c,f). Overall, MAC has extracted the highest yield of total polyphenolics (3037 ± 22 μg/g DW) at 90 °C and an s/l ratio of 1:500, followed by UAE using an s/l ratio of 1:500 at 60 °C (2476 ± 22 μg/g DW), 75 °C (2383 ± 29 μg/g DW), and 90 °C (2405 ± 22 μg/g DW). As for MAE, the highest yield was observed at 30 °C and with a 1:500 s/l ratio (1582 ± 122 μg/g DW).

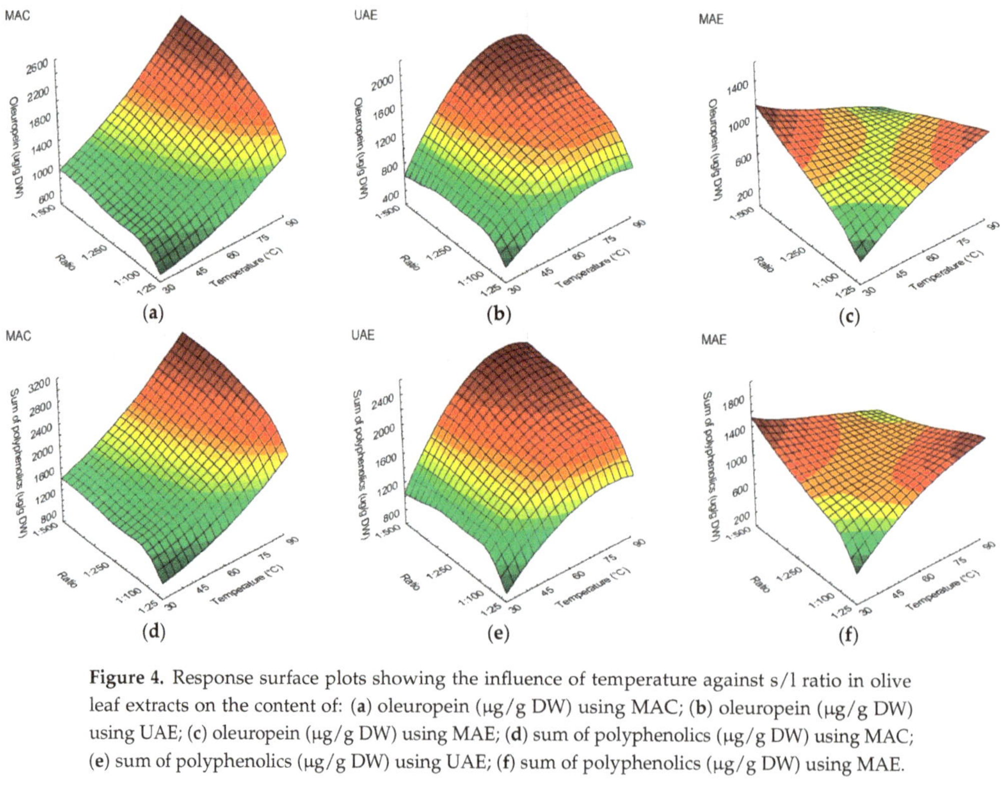

Figure 4. Response surface plots showing the influence of temperature against s/l ratio in olive leaf extracts on the content of: (**a**) oleuropein (μg/g DW) using MAC; (**b**) oleuropein (μg/g DW) using UAE; (**c**) oleuropein (μg/g DW) using MAE; (**d**) sum of polyphenolics (μg/g DW) using MAC; (**e**) sum of polyphenolics (μg/g DW) using UAE; (**f**) sum of polyphenolics (μg/g DW) using MAE.

The results for the antioxidant capacity followed the polyphenolics profiles results. The results are available in Supplementary Table S1. The results have shown the influences of s/l ratio and temperature in ORAC assays when MAC and UAE were applied. MAC results have shown an effect of temperature and s/l ratio at temperatures from 30 to 60 °C. The highest yield was obtained at 90 °C and with an s/l ratio of 1:100. In the case of UAE, there was an evident influence of those two parameters; the yield was increasing as the temperature increased and ratio decreased. MAE resulted in comparable values within the group, obtaining a higher yield at 75 °C and an s/l ratio of 1:100, and a lower yield at 30 °C and with an s/l ratio of 1:25. DPPH assay results have shown the influence of temperature when MAC was applied, yielding better at 75 and 90 °C. On the contrary, UAE yielded better at temperature range from 45 to 60 °C, while MAE obtained higher values at 45 and 75 °C, regardless of the s/l ratio. FRAP assay results suggested the use of MAC at 90 °C using an s/l ratio of 1:25, and UAE at 75 °C with the same ratio. As for MAE, the results were comparable within the group, but indicated obtaining higher yields at 75–90 °C and an s/l ratio of 1:25.

3.2. *Adsorption Capacity*

3.2.1. Langmuir and Freundlich Isotherms

The adsorption results of polyphenolic compounds from the first experiment were fitted with the Langmuir and Freundlich isotherm models in order to understand and determine the process of the adsorption of the targeted compounds onto BC. Figure 5 shows the Langmuir isotherm models for vanillic acid-4-glucoside, hydroxytyrosol, luteolin-7-*O*-glucoside, luteolin-7 *O*-rutinoside, apigenin-7-*O*-glucoside, and oleuropein, as well as the sum of polyphenols, with the R^2 coefficients ranging from 0.549 to 0.999. Freundlich isotherm models are shown in Figure 6, where the R^2 ranges from 0.854 to 0.999.

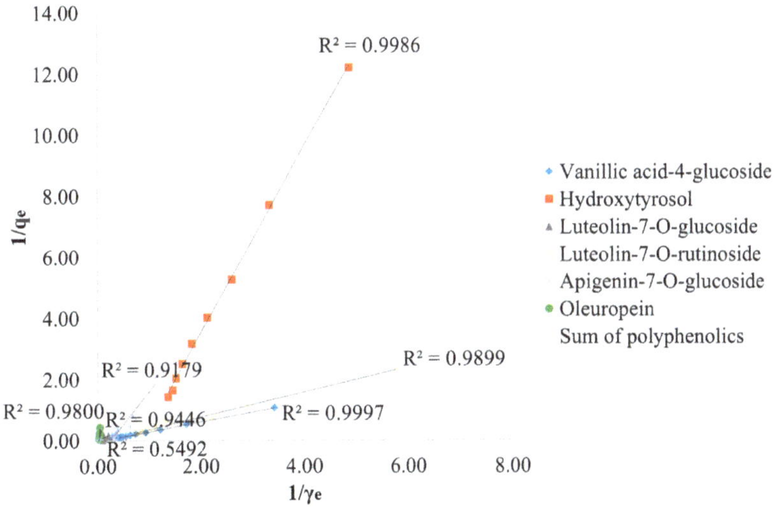

Figure 5. Langmuir adsorption isotherms for the adsorption of specific compounds by biochar are expressed in terms of key parameters, among which R^2 represents the coefficient of determination, q_e signifies the amount of adsorbate concentration in the solid phase at equilibrium (mg/g), and γ_e denotes the amount of adsorbate concentration in the liquid phase at equilibrium (mg/L).

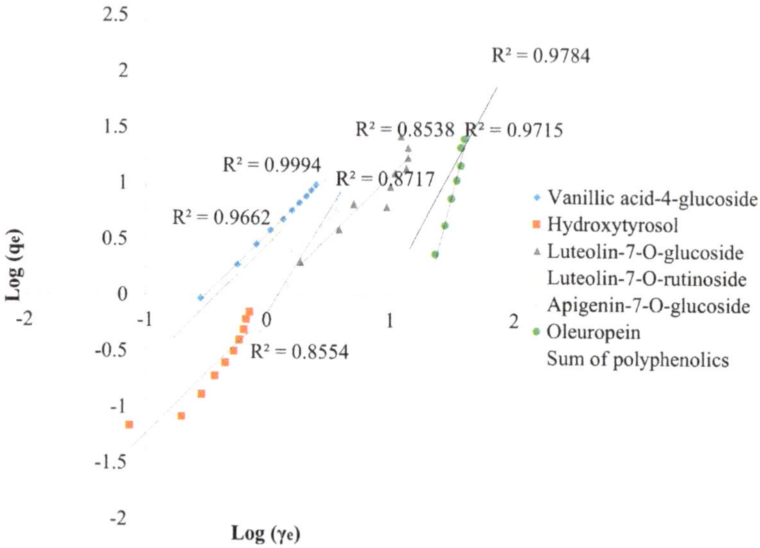

Figure 6. The Freundlich adsorption isotherms for the adsorption of specific compounds by biochar are characterized by key parameters, among which R^2 represents the coefficient of determination, q_e indicates the amount of adsorbate concentration in the solid phase at equilibrium (mg/g), and γ_e signifies the amount of adsorbate concentration in the liquid phase at equilibrium (mg/L).

As shown in Table 1, all investigated compounds obtained R^2 coefficients higher than 0.90, suggesting the suitability of the Langmuir model for the above-mentioned compounds' adsorption, with the exception of luteolin-7-*O*-glucoside, for which the R^2 was 0.5492. However, the other obtained parameters should also be considered in the adsorption model suitability determination. The Langmuir model was not suitable for vanillic acid-4-glucoside, luteolin-7-*O*-rutinoside, apigenin-7-*O*-glucoside, and oleuropein due to negative K_L and R_L values. Furthermore, the Langmuir model fitted better only in hydroxytyrosol and total polyphenolics adsorption. Total adsorption of polyphenols obtained a twofold-higher maximum monolayer adsorption capacity (q_{max}), followed by hydroxytyrosol and the highest affinity constant (K_L), respectively. The Freundlich model was more favorable for all investigated compounds, resulting in $R^2 \geq 0.854$. The highest R^2 coefficient was obtained in vanillic acid-4-glucoside adsorption (0.999), followed by total polyphenols (0.978) and oleuropein (0.972). The highest adsorption capacity (K_f) was reached with oleuropein (20.4 (mg/g) × (L/g)^n). The 1/n values were in a range between 0 and 1 for all investigated compounds.

Table 1. Parameters of Langmuir and Freundlich models for targeted olive-leaf polyphenolic compounds adsorbed by grapevine-pruning-residues biochar.

	Parameters	VA-4-g	Hyty	L-7-g	L-7-r	A-7-g	Olp	Sum
Langmuir isotherm	q_{max} (mg/g)	1.54	3.08	1.21	2.44	0.47	0.05	6.83
	K_L (L/mg)	−0.28	0.38	102	−10.1	−4.17	−41.20	9.64
	R_L	(−2.62)–(−0.01)	0.05–0.35	0.00–0.91	(−105)–(−0.02)	(−0.66)–(−0.05)	0.00–1.32	0.02–0.50
	R^2	0.999	0.999	0.549	0.990	0.918	0.980	0.945
Freundlich isotherm	K_f (mg/g) × (L/g)^n	0.32	1.20	1.44	0.40	1.35	20.4	9.49
	1/n	0.93	0.80	0.78	0.89	0.48	0.21	0.47
	R^2	0.999	0.855	0.854	0.966	0.872	0.972	0.978

VA-4-g—Vanillic acid-4-glucoside; Hyty—Hydroxytyrosol; L-7-g—Luteolin-7-*O*-glucoside; L-7-r—Luteolin-7-*O*-rutinoside; A-7-g—Apigenin-7-*O*-glucoside; Olp—Oleuropein; Sum—Sum of polyphenols.

3.2.2. Effects of BC Dosages in Polyphenolic Adsorption

Figure 7 illustrates the outcomes of the experiment conducted with various biochar (BC) dosages while maintaining a consistent concentration of olive leaf extract (3 g/L). The results are presented in terms of milligrams of the targeted compound adsorbed per gram of BC and the overall amount of adsorbed compound under different BC dosages. Notably, the 0.5 g BC dosage exhibited the highest adsorption for all compounds, demonstrating a diminishing trend as the BC quantity increased. In the total adsorption capacity experiment, the influence of BC dosages on adsorption was evident after reaching equilibrium for all investigated compounds, excluding vanillic acid-4-glucoside and luteolin-7-*O*-rutinoside.

Specifically, the maximum amount adsorbed per gram of BC for vanillic acid-4-glucoside was observed at the 0.5 g BC dosage (11.6 mg vanillic acid-4-glucoside/g BC), gradually decreasing to 2.28 mg vanillic acid-4-glucoside/g BC with an increase in BC dosage (Figure 7a). However, the total amount of vanillic acid-4-glucoside adsorbed remained consistent, ranging from 5.71 to 5.78 mg, indicating no significant impact of BC dosages on overall adsorption (Figure 7a).

As shown in Figure 7b, the highest amount of hydroxytyrosol adsorbed per g of BC was observed when 0.5 g of BC was used (0.62 mg hydroxytyrosol/g BC), decreasing to 0.19 mg hydroxytyrosol/g BC as the BC dosage increased, while the total amount of hydroxytyrosol adsorbed increased as the BC dosage did, ranging from 0.31 mg at 0.5 g of BC to 0.48 mg of hydroxytyrosol when 2.5 g of BC was applied.

Luteolin-7-*O*-glucoside adsorption results per g of BC were the highest among other individual compounds, ranging from 26.2 to 4.94 mg (Figure 7c). The total adsorption values obtained a a s/l zag pattern, suggesting the influence of BC dosage on adsorption; the highest amounts of luteolin-7-*O*-glucoside were adsorbed using 0.5 (13.1 mg), 1.5 (13.8 mg), and 2.5 g (12.4 mg) of BC, as shown in Figure 7c.

As for luteolin-7-*O*-rutinoside, the highest amount adsorbed per g of BC was obtained with the application of 0.5 g of BC (5.29 mg luteolin-7-*O*-rutinoside/g of BC), with adsorption per g of BC decreasing as the dosage increased (Figure 7d). The total adsorption capacity demonstrated no influence on luteolin-7-*O*-rutinoside adsorption when different BC dosages were applied, with values ranging from 2.65 to 2.72 mg (Figure 7d).

Apigenin-7-*O*-glucoside results followed the trends of luetolin-7-*O*-glucoside, obtaining the highest adsorption when 0.5 g of BC was applied (10.9 mg apigenin-7-*O*-glucoside/g BC) and showing a decreasing trend as the BC dosage increased, as well as a similar zig-zag pattern in the total-adsorption-capacity experiment. The dosage of 2.5 g of BC adsorbed the highest amount of apigenin-7-*O*-glucoside (8.18 mg), as shown in Figure 7e.

Oleuropein values for the adsorption experiment per g of BC resulted in highest adsorption when 0.5 g of BC was applied (11.9 mg oleuropein/g BC), with decreases in the adsorbed amount of the compound as the dosage of BC increased. The total adsorption values obtained a linear increasing trend, adsorbing 5.95 mg of oleuropein with 0.5 g BC dosage, with an increase to 15.5 mg when 2.5 g of BC was applied, suggesting an evident effect of BC dosage on the adsorption of polyphenols. Both results are shown in Figure 7f.

In Figure 7g, the results for the sum of polyphenols are shown. The BC dosage of 0.5 g followed the previous adsorption compounds trend by adsorbing the highest amount of total polyphenols (89.4 mg/g BC), with a decrease in the amount of adsorbed compound to 23.6 mg/g BC when 2.5 g of BC was applied. The total adsorption experiment obtained a linear relationship between the adsorbed amount of polyphenols and BC dosage, ranging from 44.7 mg of polyphenols when 0.5 g of BC was used, to, after a slight increase at 2.5 g of BC, 58.9 mg of polyphenols.

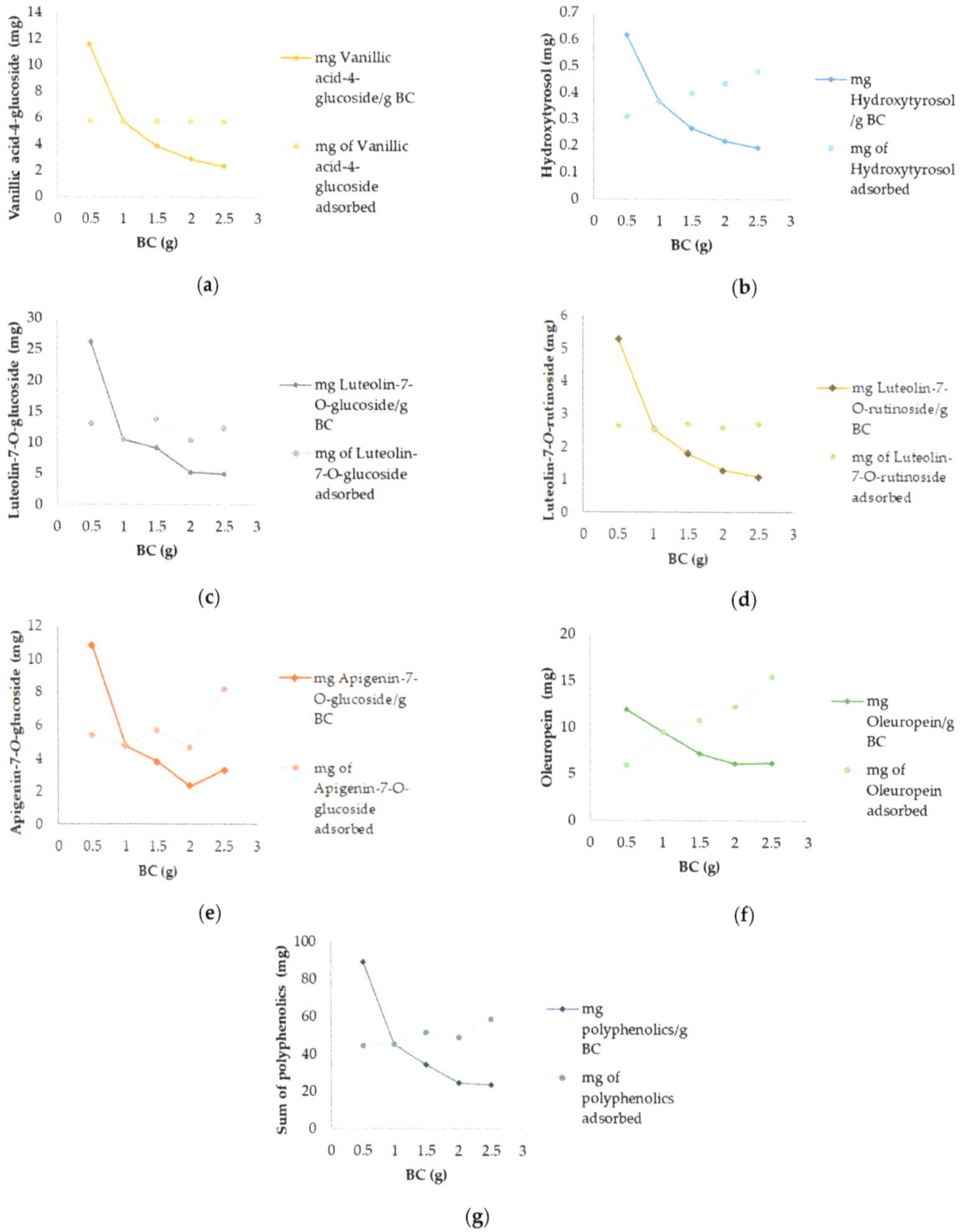

Figure 7. Influences of different biochar (BC) dosages in adsorption of polyphenolic compounds from olive leaf extracts with 24 h contact: (**a**) vanillic acid-4-glucoside; (**b**) hydroxytyrosol; (**c**) luteolin-7-*O*-glucoside; (**d**) luteolin-7-*O*-rutinoside; (**e**) apigenin-7-*O*-glucoside; (**f**) oleuropein; (**g**) sum of polyphenolics.

4. Discussion

In this study, olive leaves were used as a source material rich in bioactive compounds, water as a solvent for extractions, and BC from grapevine pruning residues as an adsorbent, in order to utilize agricultural-production and food biomass and wastes, leading to a sustainable production, and obtain an eco-friendly approach in extraction and adsorption processes.

The extraction of natural compounds is a demanding process in which a non-toxic solvent should be used, especially if it is carried out for food purposes [36,37]. Water is considered to be one of the greenest solvents used in extraction processes. The number of experiments in which water was used as an environmentally friendly solvent has increased [38]. Benincasa et al. investigated the effects of different water types in the extraction of high-valued compounds from olive leaves, stating that ultrapure water stimulates the migration process of oleuropein from the leaves to the solution more than micro-filtered or osmosis-treated water [14]. In our previous work, detailed observation of water as a green solvent was given, and the study reported the efficiency of its use as a solvent in the extraction of polyphenols from onion peels [39]. In order to extract a higher amount of polyphenols from olive leaves, different techniques are usually applied, with regard given to the extraction temperature and solvent as important parameters for the recovery of phenols [37].

In this work, three different methods were used (MAC, UAE, and MAE), with different temperature and ratio levels investigated. Five temperatures (30, 45, 60, 75, and 90 °C) and five s/l ratios (1:25, 1:50, 1:100, 1:250, and 1:500) were examined, with the aim being to reduce the energy consumption and obtain a high yield of bioactive compounds by reducing the use of solvents and increasing the use of biomass. As the results suggested, the highest yields of polyphenols and highest antioxidant activity were obtained at temperatures of 75 or 90 °C, regardless of the extraction method, probably due to cell-wall disruption caused by high temperatures [40]. Khemakhem et al. have reported an improvement in total phenolic content, antioxidant activity, and oleuropein amounts by increasing the temperature from 10 to 70 °C in olive leaf extractions, using the conventional extraction method and UAE [41]. Furthermore, in another research effort [42], different temperature ranges, times and s/l ratios in conventional aqueous olive leaf extractions were investigated. The optimal conditions for the highest yield of phenolic compounds were found to be 90 °C for 70 min, and at an s/l ratio of 1:100. To minimize the use of solvent, the authors suggested the use of an s/l ratio of 1:60 for obtaining 80% of the total phenolic compounds and maximized antioxidant capacity. A similar trend was observed in this study in the antioxidant activity assays: the highest yield in ORAC was obtained at 90 °C and an s/l ratio of 1:100 for MAC and UAE, while MAE obtained better results at 75 °C. UAE and MAE performed similarly in the DPPH assay, with better yields at temperatures from 45 to 60 °C, and 45 to 75 °C, respectively. In MAC, higher temperatures were needed, ranging from 75 to 90 °C. Finally, FRAP results suggested the use of a temperature range from 75 to 90 °C and an s/l ratio of 1:25 to achieve higher values. According to the results, high temperature is not a limiting factor in the extraction of polyphenols from olive leaves, considering the obtained high yield and preserved antioxidant capacity.

However, when observing the individual compounds and their yields, the influences of the extraction method itself, temperature, and ratio were noticeable. In hydroxytyrosol extraction, an evident influence of temperature was noticeable in MAC and UAE applications. The highest yield was obtained when 75 or 90 °C were used. As for MAE, an s/l ratio effect was observed, yielding better at 45 to 90 °C and using ratios of 1:25 or 1:50. Luteolin-7-*O*-glucoside and apigenin-7-glucoside were extracted in higher amounts at temperatures from 45 to 90 °C when MAE was used, as well as when MAC was used at 90 °C with ratios from 1:25 to 1:250. As for UAE in luteolin-7-*O*-glucoside extraction, the highest yield was achieved using an s/l ratio of 1:100 at all investigated temperatures, suggesting the possibility of reducing energy consumption if lower temperatures are applied, while temperatures from 60 to 90 °C were more favorable in apigenin-7-*O*-glucoside extraction.

The main compound found in olive leaves was oleuropein, which is in accordance with previous results [43–46]. Accordingly, the sum of polyphenols performed similarly to oleuropein. The highest yield was obtained when using MAC or UAE at temperatures between 60 and 90 °C and with an s/l ratio of 1:250 to 1:500, while MAE performed better at 30 °C, providing an eco-friendly extraction due to lower energy consumption. According to Goldsmith et al., this phenomenon agrees with mass transfer principles: the gradient concentration is higher when there is more solvent present, leading to higher diffusion rates [42]. The amounts of the extracted compounds in this study were lower in comparison with other papers where 80%-methanol [43], ethanol: water (1:1) [47] or distilled water [48] were used. This phenomenon could be explained by the olive leaves' collecting period having caused a decrease in the amount of polyphenols in a certain growing period [47–50]. Furthermore, the phenolic profiles and concentrations, as well as the antioxidant activity, are influenced by many factors, like seasoning age, climatic conditions, geographical position, cultivar, genetic factors [43,51], and exposure to low air temperatures [52]. Likewise, extraction conditions such as temperature, contact time, solvent, s/l ratio, and sample preparation also influence the polyphenolic content of the extract [17,53]. However, in the study conducted by Benincasa et al. with different water types, the amount of extracted oleuropein was almost threefold lower when compared with results in this study, while the concentration of hydroxytyrosol was fourfold higher in 24 h contact time [14]. The amount of hydroxytyrosol could increase during maturation or treatment due to oleuropein degradation [37]. This data indicates the appropriateness of the methods studied in this work for the aqueous extraction and preservation of higher concentrations of oleuropein.

Although in several works [37,54,55], innovative extraction methods such as MAE and UAE performed better than conventional methods, in this research, among all studied extraction techniques, MAE obtained the lowest yield of the investigated compounds. For instance, in this work, MAC has extracted a twofold higher amount of polyphenols at conditions of 90 °C and an s/l ratio of 1:500 if compared to the highest yield obtained by MAE (30 °C, s/l ratio of 1:500). In the research of da Rosa et al., MAC, UAE, and MAE were compared as to the recovery of bioactive compounds from Brazilian olive leaves [12]. The authors concluded that MAE was more efficient than the other two investigated methods. Valinger et al. also compared the efficiency of three methods of bioactive compounds' extraction from olive leaves using conventional extraction, MAE, and microwave–ultrasound-assisted extraction, using water as a solvent and with an s/l ratio of 1:50 [56]. The combination of microwaves and ultrasounds obtained the best results when a temperature of 60 °C was used, while MAE performed better at 80 °C. Furthermore, Vizzarri et al. obtained important results in polyphenolic extraction from olive leaves in applying UAE by mixing 1.5 kg of dried leaves in 3 L of distilled water [57]. The results were almost 10-fold higher than in this work, suggesting a higher s/l ratio for a better extraction. However, in Lama-Muñoz et al. the conventional Soxhlet extraction method showed better performance in most of the variables analyzed from olive leaves when compared to the innovative pressurized liquid extraction [18]. Sánchez-Gutiérrez et al. obtained higher phenolic yield and antioxidant activity in conventional extraction as compared to MAE [58]. Finally, conventional extraction such as MAC is considered more suitable for extracting polar compounds such as oleuropein derivatives, apigenin-rutinoside, and luteolin-glucosides [52], a determination which was confirmed in this study.

Adsorption is a process in which soluble substances in the liquid phase transfer onto the surface or onto the bulk of the solid adsorbent [59], and it occurs by the formation of the physical or chemical bonds between a porous solid medium and a mixture of liquid or gas multi-component fluid [60]. The adsorption isotherm models describe the interaction mechanisms between the adsorbent and the adsorbate at constant temperature [60]. The Langmuir and Freundlich isotherm models are the most common and widely used. In this study, the mentioned models were used to determine the adsorption process by which polyphenols from olive leaf extracts adsorb onto the BC from grapevine pruning residues. BC properties and adsorption capacity were described in our previous works [29,39].

Among all investigated compounds, hydroxytyrosol and the total amount of polyphenols fitted better in the Langmuir model, obtaining the R^2 closest to 1, suggesting the suitability of this model for the mentioned compounds' adsorption. Hydroxytyrosol and total polyphenols obtained the highest values for maximum monolayer adsorption capacity, showing that the adsorption of those compounds was more favorable compared to the others, and suggesting a main monolayer adsorption reaction. Luteolin-7-*O*-glucoside has obtained an R^2 of 0.5492, with the highest K_L indicating a strong interaction between the adsorbent and the adsorbate. The obtained value was higher than in the study by Aliakbarian et al., in which commercial activated carbon (AC; Sigma-Aldrich Chemical Co.) was used in phenolic adsorption from olive mill wastewater [61]. Vanillic acid-4-glucoside, luteolin-7-*O*-rutinoside, apigenin-7-*O*-glucoside, and oleuropein obtained an R^2 coefficient equal to or higher than 0.9179. However, those compounds achieved negative K_L and R_L values. A negative K_L value was also obtained in our previous work with onion peel extracts [39]. The negative K_L value indicates that at high addition of adsorbent mass, adsorption does not follow Langmuir premises and the adsorption capacity reaches a specific limit by increasing the adsorbent mass at a certain point [62]. Moreover, the shape of the isotherm depends on the R_L value. The isotherm is unfavorable ($R_L > 1$), linear ($R_L = 1$), favorable ($0 < R_L < 1$), or reversible ($R_L = 0$) [63]. In this work, the value of R_L for vanillic acid-4-glucoside, luteolin-7-*O*-rutinoside, and apigenin-7-*O*-glucoside was negative, suggesting the inappropriateness of this model for the mentioned compounds' adsorption. As for oleuropein and luteolin-7-*O*-glucoside, the values ranged from 0.00 to 1.32, and 0.00 to 0.91, indicating a reversible and unfavorable adsorption and a reversible and favorable adsorption, respectively. Nonetheless, in all of the other cases it was between 0 and 1, indicating that hydroxytyrosol and total polyphenols adsorption by BC is favorable.

The Freundlich isotherm model was the best-fit isotherm for adsorption for all investigated compounds, ranging the values of the determination coefficient between 0.8538 and 0.9994. Those findings concur with Abid et al. [64] and Göktepeli et al. [65]. The highest R^2 value was obtained by vanillic acid-4-glucoside, and the highest K_f value was achieved by oleuropein. This constant is used to describe the adsorption of solute molecules onto the surface of a solid adsorbent [66], suggesting a greater adsorption of oleuropein. The $1/n$ value was in range between 0 and 1, which indicates that the adsorption capacity increases with concentration, but at a decreasing rate [67], although representing favorable adsorption conditions [68]. Among all investigated compounds, hydroxytyrosol and total polyphenolics adsorptions fitted better with both Langmuir and Freundlich models. This observation was reported by Hadrich et al., who concluded that both the Langmuir and the Freundlich isotherm models fitted the equilibrium data of the adsorption process of hydroxytyrosol from olive leaves using a modified spherical activated carbon [69]. Those findings suggested that monolayer and heterolayer phenolic compounds may exist on the adsorbent surface due to the heterogeneity of the BC's surface [64]. In our previous work [29], BC from grapevine pruning residues was investigated as an adsorbent for polyphenols. In that paper, the standard of oleuropein, among others, was used. The obtained results fitted in both Langmuir and Freundlich models, reaching high adsorption capacity and efficient adsorption by BC, while in this research, oleuropein fitted better with the Freundlich model. These differences between the results may be explained by the concentration of the compound in the solution, and the competition and interaction between the compounds in the extracts. The investigated compounds in this study range from weak to high polar: oleuropein, hydroxytyrosol, vanillic acid-4-glucoside, luteolin-7-*O*-glucoside, apigenin-7-*O*-glucoside, and the most polar compound, luteolin-7-*O*-rutinoside. Considering this data, as well as the adsorption results according to Freundlich's model, the influence of the polarity of the compounds may affect the adsorption potential. Vanillic acid-4-glucoside and luteolin-7-*O*-rutinoside have obtained the lowest K_f values among all investigated compounds. Vanillic acid-4-glucoside and luteolin-7-*O*-rutinoside are more hydrophilic compared to oleuropein, which has obtained the highest K_f value. Furthermore, the structure of oleuropein is more complex and contains many glucose moieties. When compared to vanillic acid-4-O-glucoside and luteolin-7-O-rutinoside, its overall polarity may be reduced by the presence of more extended sugar units and higher complexity. In comparison to the other two compounds, oleuropein may exhibit better interactions with the polar functional groups on the surface of BC.

In regard to the effect of BC dosage on adsorption, the lowest BC dosage of 0.5 g performed the best adsorption capacity per g of BC, which rapidly decreased with increasing dosages, suggesting that compounds in the solution reached adsorption equilibrium. A similar observation was provided by Senol et al. [70] using commercial active carbon and Fseha et al. [71] in the removal of phenols from contaminated municipal wastewater using date palm frond BC. As for the absolute adsorption capacity, there was no visible influence of the dosage on vanillic acid-4-glucoside and luteolin-7-O-rutinoside, as previously reported [39]. Luteolin-7-O-glucoside and apigenin-7-O-glucoside performed similarly, obtaining a zig-zag pattern. However, if the lowest BC dosage, 0.5 g, was compared to the highest (2.5 g), the results would suggest a visible increase in adsorption. The greatest increase of an adsorbed compound was visible in oleuropein; the amount of the compound increased almost threefold, as the BC dosage did. A similar trend was observed in hydroxytyrosol and total polyphenols adsorption. The components that are found in the highest concentrations include oleuropein, hydroxytyrosol, and therefore the total amount of polyphenols, suggesting the influence of the compound concentration in the solution on the adsorption. In addition, it could also be explained by the formation of more adsorption sites as a consequence of the increased surface area [64], but could also be attributed to the nature of the adsorbate, specifically, its functional groups, polarity, molecular weight, and size [72].

There are some limitations to this study. The temperature of the pyrolysis process during the conversion of grape pruning residues could not be controlled, due to the design of the kon-tiki system. This could lead to lower active surface area and subsequently lower adsorption capacity of the investigated biochar. Another limitation of the study is the variation in the phytochemical content of the olive leaves, which is dependent upon genetic and environmental factors, and ultimately has an effect on the reported profile or adsorption kinetics on the biochar's surface. Finally, olive leaf extracts have an abundance of hydrophilic compounds besides polyphenols, which can interfere with the adsorption process and also modify the adsorption kinetics.

5. Conclusions

Olive leaves are rich in valuable phytochemicals with high antioxidant activity. On the other hand, the intensive viticulture practiced today requires the implementation of certain measures in order to achieve a higher yield with better quality. In this paper, these two materials were investigated with the aim of biomass valorization in the agricultural sector. In order to extract bioactive compounds, water was used as a green solvent in three extraction methods, together with modulation of temperature and s/l ratio. The conventional MAC method proved to be more effective compared to the other methods at temperatures between 75 and 90 °C, obtaining higher polyphenol yields, especially oleuropein, as the main compound, with no adverse effects on antioxidant activity. Furthermore, using the Langmuir and Freundlich isotherm models, the potential of BC obtained from grapevine pruning residues in the adsorption of the polyphenolic compounds was tested. The Freundlich isotherm fitted better with all investigated compounds. Hence, a novel approach for a sustainable extraction of polyphenols from olive leaves, fitting with the principles of green chemistry and leading to eco-friendly processes of adsorption, was proposed in this study. The findings suggest the possibility of using water as solvent to obtain non-toxic and environmentally friendly extracts from olive leaves which can be used in the food industry or in other industries. The process could be easily implemented in the industry and has the potential to become an additional source of income for olive and grapevine growers.

Supplementary Materials: The following supporting information can be downloaded at: https://www.mdpi.com/article/10.3390/antiox13010001/s1, Table S1: Olive leaves polyphenolic compounds content (μg/g DW) using MAC, UAE and MAE at different extraction conditions.

Author Contributions: Conceptualization, M.P., N.M. and I.P.; methodology, N.M., Z.U., J.Ć., D.B., M.R. and I.P.; validation, N.M. and J.Ć.; formal analysis, M.P., D.A., D.C., T.K.K. and N.M.; investigation, M.P., D.A., D.C., T.K.K., Z.U., N.M. and I.P.; resources, S.G.B. and D.B.; writing—original draft, M.P.; writing—review and editing, I.P., S.G.B., N.M., J.Ć. and M.R.; supervision, I.P.; project administration, I.P.; funding acquisition, D.B. All authors have read and agreed to the published version of the manuscript.

Funding: This work has been supported by the Croatian Science Foundation under the project "Biochar as a tool for environment-friendly and sustainable grapevine nutrient management in the context of climate change"—BIONUTRIVINE (UIP-2019-04-7370) and the Adris Foundation project BioRecovery.

Institutional Review Board Statement: Not applicable.

Informed Consent Statement: Not applicable.

Data Availability Statement: All data is available within this article.

Acknowledgments: The work of Melissa Prelac, Dominik Anđelini and Tvrtko Karlo Kovačević was supported by the Croatian Science Foundation under the project "Young Researchers' Career Development Project—Training New Doctoral Students" (M.P.—DOK-2021-02-9291, D.A.—DOK-2020- 01-3145 and T.K.K.—DOK-2021-02-5148).

Conflicts of Interest: The authors declare no conflict of interest.

References

1. Lorenz, K.; Lal, R. Environmental Impact of Organic Agriculture. In *Advances in Agronomy*; Donald, L.S., Ed.; Academic Press Inc.: London, UK, 2016; Volume 139, pp. 99–152, ISBN 9780128047736.
2. Chen, Y.-H.; Wen, X.-W.; Wang, B.; Nie, P.-Y. Agricultural Pollution and Regulation: How to Subsidize Agriculture? *J. Clean. Prod.* **2017**, *164*, 258–264. [CrossRef]
3. Ghosh, A.; Misra, S.; Bhattacharyya, R.; Sarkar, A.; Singh, A.K.; Tyagi, V.C.; Kumar, R.V.; Meena, V.S. Agriculture, Dairy and Fishery Farming Practices and Greenhouse Gas Emission Footprint: A Strategic Appraisal for Mitigation. *Environ. Sci. Pollut. Res.* **2020**, *27*, 10160–10184. [CrossRef] [PubMed]
4. Baque, M.A.; Moh, S.H.; Lee, E.J.; Zhong, J.J.; Paek, K.Y. Production of Biomass and Useful Compounds from Adventitious Roots of High-Value Added Medicinal Plants Using Bioreactor. *Biotechnol. Adv.* **2012**, *30*, 1255–1267. [CrossRef] [PubMed]
5. Yen, H.W.; Yang, S.C.; Chen, C.H.; Jesisca; Chang, J.S. Supercritical Fluid Extraction of Valuable Compounds from Microalgal Biomass. *Bioresour. Technol.* **2015**, *184*, 291–296. [CrossRef] [PubMed]
6. EU Eurostat. Available online: https://ec.europa.eu/eurostat (accessed on 13 September 2023).
7. Ahmad, S.; Ahmad Chatha, Z.; Nasir, M.A.; Aziz, A.; Ahmad Virk, N.; Rehman Khan, A. Effect of Pruning on the Yield and Quality of Kinnow Fruit. *J. Agric. Soc. Sci.* **2006**, *2*, 51–53.
8. Albert, T.; Karp, K.; Starast, M.; Paal, T. The Effect of Mulching and Pruning on the Vegetative Growth and Yield of the Half-High Blueberry. *Agron. Res.* **2010**, *8*, 759–769.
9. Ruiz, E.; Romero-García, J.M.; Romero, I.; Manzanares, P.; Negro, M.J.; Castro, E. Olive-Derived Biomass as a Source of Energy and Chemicals. *Biofuels Bioprod. Biorefining* **2017**, *11*, 1077–1094. [CrossRef]
10. Molina-Alcaide, E.; Yáñez-Ruiz, D.R. Potential Use of Olive By-Products in Ruminant Feeding: A Review. *Anim. Feed Sci. Technol.* **2008**, *147*, 247–264. [CrossRef]
11. Araújo, Y.R.V.; de Góis, M.L.; Junior, L.M.C.; Carvalho, M. Carbon Footprint Associated with Four Disposal Scenarios for Urban Pruning Waste. *Environ. Sci. Pollut. Res.* **2018**, *25*, 1863–1868. [CrossRef]
12. da Rosa, G.S.; Martiny, T.R.; Dotto, G.L.; Vanga, S.K.; Parrine, D.; Gariepy, Y.; Lefsrud, M.; Raghavan, V. Eco-Friendly Extraction for the Recovery of Bioactive Compounds from Brazilian Olive Leaves. *Sustain. Mater. Technol.* **2021**, *28*, e00276. [CrossRef]
13. De Marco, E.; Savarese, M.; Paduano, A.; Sacchi, R. Characterization and Fractionation of Phenolic Compounds Extracted from Olive Oil Mill Wastewaters. *Food Chem.* **2007**, *104*, 858–867. [CrossRef]
14. Benincasa, C.; Santoro, I.; Nardi, M.; Cassano, A.; Sindona, G. Eco-Friendly Extraction and Characterisation of Nutraceuticals from Olive Leaves. *Molecules* **2019**, *24*, 3481. [CrossRef]
15. Martín-García, B.; Pimentel-Moral, S.; Gómez-Caravaca, A.M.; Arráez-Román, D.; Segura-Carretero, A. Box-Behnken Experimental Design for a Green Extraction Method of Phenolic Compounds from Olive Leaves. *Ind. Crops Prod.* **2020**, *154*, 112741. [CrossRef]

16. Cruz, R.M.S.; Brito, R.; Smirniotis, P.; Nikolaidou, Z.; Vieira, M.C. Extraction of Bioactive Compounds from Olive Leaves Using Emerging Technologies. In *Ingredients Extraction by Physicochemical Methods in Food*; Grumezescu, A.M., Holban, A.M., Eds.; Academic Press Inc.: London, UK, 2017; Volume 4, pp. 441–461, ISBN 9780128112021.
17. Mourtzinos, I.; Anastasopoulou, E.; Petrou, A.; Grigorakis, S.; Makris, D.; Biliaderis, C.G. Optimization of a Green Extraction Method for the Recovery of Polyphenols from Olive Leaf Using Cyclodextrins and Glycerin as Co-Solvents. *J. Food Sci. Technol.* **2016**, *53*, 3939–3947. [CrossRef]
18. Lama-Muñoz, A.; Contreras, M.d.M.; Espínola, F.; Moya, M.; Romero, I.; Castro, E. Content of Phenolic Compounds and Mannitol in Olive Leaves Extracts from Six Spanish Cultivars: Extraction with the Soxhlet Method and Pressurized Liquids. *Food Chem.* **2020**, *320*, 126626. [CrossRef]
19. Irakli, M.; Chatzopoulou, P.; Ekateriniadou, L. Optimization of Ultrasound-Assisted Extraction of Phenolic Compounds: Oleuropein, Phenolic Acids, Phenolic Alcohols and Flavonoids from Olive Leaves and Evaluation of Its Antioxidant Activities. *Ind. Crops Prod.* **2018**, *124*, 382–388. [CrossRef]
20. European Commission. The EU Chemical Strategy for Sustainability towards a Toxic-Free Environment. *Chim. Oggi Chem. Today* **2020**, *39*, 40–41.
21. Maraulo, G.E.; dos Santos Ferreira, C.; Mazzobre, M.F. β-Cyclodextrin Enhanced Ultrasound-Assisted Extraction as a Green Method to Recover Olive Pomace Bioactive Compounds. *J. Food Process. Preserv.* **2021**, *45*, e15194. [CrossRef]
22. Fernández, M.d.L.; Espino, M.; Gomez, F.J.; Silva, M.F. Novel Approaches Mediated by Tailor-Made Green Solvents for the Extraction of Phenolic Compounds from Agro-Food Industrial by-Products. *Food Chem.* **2018**, *239*, 671–678. [CrossRef]
23. Abd-Elsalam, H.A.H.; Gamal, M.; Naguib, I.A.; Al-Ghobashy, M.A.; Zaazaa, H.E.; Abdelkawy, M. Development of Green and Efficient Extraction Methods of Quercetin from Red Onion Scales Wastes Using Factorial Design for Method Optimization: A Comparative Study. *Separations* **2021**, *8*, 137. [CrossRef]
24. Santillán, D.; Sotés, V.; Iglesias, A.; Garrote, L. Adapting Viticulture to Climate Change in the Mediterranean Region: Evaluations Accounting for Spatial Differences in the Producers-Climate Interactions. *BIO Web Conf.* **2019**, *12*, 01001. [CrossRef]
25. Spinelli, R.; Nati, C.; Pari, L.; Mescalchin, E.; Magagnotti, N. Production and Quality of Biomass Fuels from Mechanized Collection and Processing of Vineyard Pruning Residues. *Appl. Energy* **2012**, *89*, 374–379. [CrossRef]
26. Liang, L.; Xi, F.; Tan, W.; Meng, X.; Hu, B.; Wang, X. Review of Organic and Inorganic Pollutants Removal by Biochar and Biochar-Based Composites. *Biochar* **2021**, *3*, 255–281. [CrossRef]
27. Zhao, L.; Xiao, D.; Liu, Y.; Xu, H.; Nan, H.; Li, D.; Kan, Y.; Cao, X. Biochar as Simultaneous Shelter, Adsorbent, PH Buffer, and Substrate of Pseudomonas Citronellolis to Promote Biodegradation of High Concentrations of Phenol in Wastewater. *Water Res.* **2020**, *172*, 115494. [CrossRef] [PubMed]
28. Komnitsas, K.A.; Zaharaki, D. Morphology of Modified Biochar and Its Potential for Phenol Removal from Aqueous Solutions. *Front. Environ. Sci.* **2016**, *4*, 26. [CrossRef]
29. Prelac, M.; Palcic, I.; Cvitan, D.; Andelini, D.; Repaji'c, M.; Curko, J.; Kova˘cevi´c, T.K.; Goreta Ban, S.; Užila, Z.; Ban, D.; et al. Biochar from Grapevine Pruning Residues as an Efficient Adsorbent of Polyphenolic Compounds. *Materials* **2023**, *16*, 4716. [CrossRef]
30. Wang, J.; Wang, S. Preparation, Modification and Environmental Application of Biochar: A Review. *J. Clean. Prod.* **2019**, *227*, 1002–1022. [CrossRef]
31. Han, Y.; Boateng, A.A.; Qi, P.X.; Lima, I.M.; Chang, J. Heavy Metal and Phenol Adsorptive Properties of Biochars from Pyrolyzed Switchgrass and Woody Biomass in Correlation with Surface Properties. *J. Environ. Manag.* **2013**, *118*, 196–204. [CrossRef]
32. Brand-Williams, W.; Cuvelier, M.E.; Berset, C. Use of a Free Radical Method to Evaluate Antioxidant Activity. *LWT—Food Sci. Technol.* **1995**, *28*, 25–30. [CrossRef]
33. Benzie, I.F.F.; Strain, J.J. The Ferric Reducing Ability of Plasma (FRAP) as a Measure of "Antioxidant Power": The FRAP Assay. *Anal. Biochem.* **1996**, *239*, 70–76. [CrossRef]
34. Ou, B.; Hampsch-Woodill, M.; Prior, R.L. Development and Validation of an Improved Oxygen Radical Absorbance Capacity Assay Using Fluorescein as the Fluorescent Probe. *J. Agric. Food Chem.* **2001**, *49*, 4619–4626. [CrossRef] [PubMed]
35. Langmuir, I. The Adsorption of Gases on Plane Surfaces of Mica. *J. Am. Chem. Soc.* **1938**, *40*, 1361–1403. [CrossRef]
36. Markhali, F.S.; Teixeira, J.A.; Rocha, C.M.R. Olive Tree Leaves—A Source of Valuable Active Compounds. *Processes* **2020**, *8*, 1177. [CrossRef]
37. Rahmanian, N.; Jafari, S.M.; Wani, T.A. *Bioactive Profile, Dehydration, Extraction and Application of the Bioactive Components of Olive Leaves*; Elsevier: Amsterdam, The Netherlands, 2015; Volume 42, ISBN 9190864174.
38. Castro-Puyana, M.; Marina, M.L.; Plaza, M. Water as Green Extraction Solvent: Principles and Reasons for Its Use. *Curr. Opin. Green Sustain. Chem.* **2017**, *5*, 31–36. [CrossRef]
39. Prelac, M.; Palčić, I.; Cvitan, D.; Anđelini, D.; Repajić, M.; Ćurko, J.; Kovačević, T.K.; Ban Goreta, S.; Užila, Z.; Ban, D.; et al. From Waste to Green: Water-Based Extraction of Polyphenols from Onion Peel and Their Adsorption on Biochar from Grapevine Pruning Residues. *Antioxidants* **2023**, *12*, 1697. [CrossRef]
40. Dobrinčić, A.; Repajić, M.; Elez Garofulić, I.; Tuden, L.; Dragović-Uzelac, V.; Levaj, B. Comparison of Different Extraction Methods for the Recovery of Olive Leaves Polyphenols. *Processes* **2020**, *8*, 1008. [CrossRef]

41. Khemakhem, I.; Ahmad-Qasem, M.H.; Catalán, E.B.; Micol, V.; García-Pérez, J.V.; Ayadi, M.A.; Bouaziz, M. Kinetic Improvement of Olive Leaves' Bioactive Compounds Extraction by Using Power Ultrasound in a Wide Temperature Range. *Ultrason. Sonochem.* **2017**, *34*, 466–473. [CrossRef]
42. Goldsmith, C.D.; Vuong, Q.V.; Stathopoulos, C.E.; Roach, P.D.; Scarlett, C.J. Optimization of the Aqueous Extraction of Phenolic Compounds from Olive Leaves. *Antioxidants* **2014**, *3*, 700–712. [CrossRef] [PubMed]
43. Lukić, I.; Pasković, I.; Žurga, P.; Germek, V.M.; Brkljača, M.; Marcelić, Š.; Ban, D.; Grozić, K.; Lukić, M.; Užila, Z.; et al. Determination of the Variability of Biophenols and Mineral Nutrients in Olive Leaves with Respect to Cultivar, Collection Period and Geographical Location for Their Targeted and Well-Timed Exploitation. *Plants* **2020**, *9*, 1667. [CrossRef] [PubMed]
44. Pasković, I.; Lukić, I.; Žurga, P.; Germek, V.M.; Brkljača, M.; Koprivnjak, O.; Major, N.; Grozić, K.; Franić, M.; Ban, D.; et al. Temporal Variation of Phenolic and Mineral Composition in Olive Leaves Is Cultivar Dependent. *Plants* **2020**, *9*, 1099. [CrossRef]
45. Polić Pasković, M.; Vidović, N.; Lukić, I.; Žurga, P.; Majetić Germek, V.; Goreta Ban, S.; Kos, T.; Čoga, L.; Tomljanović, T.; Simonić-Kocijan, S.; et al. Phenolic Potential of Olive Leaves from Different Istrian Cultivars in Croatia. *Horticulturae* **2023**, *9*, 594. [CrossRef]
46. Zakraoui, M.; Hannachi, H.; Pasković, I.; Vidović, N.; Polić Pasković, M.; Palčić, I.; Major, N.; Goreta Ban, S.; Hamrouni, L. Effect of Geographical Location on the Phenolic and Mineral Composition of Chetoui Olive Leaves. *Foods* **2023**, *12*, 2565. [CrossRef] [PubMed]
47. Wang, B.; Qu, J.; Feng, S.; Chen, T.; Yuan, M.; Huang, Y.; Liao, J. Liangshan Olive Leaves and Their Antioxidant and Their Antioxidant and Anticancer Activities. *Foods* **2019**, *8*, 657. [CrossRef] [PubMed]
48. Palmeri, R.; Siracusa, L.; Carrubba, M.; Parafati, L.; Proetto, I.; Pesce, F.; Fallico, B. Olive Leaves, a Promising Byproduct of Olive Oil Industry : Assessment of Metabolic Profiles and Antioxidant Capacity as a Function of Cultivar and Seasonal Change. *Agronomy* **2022**, *12*, 2007. [CrossRef]
49. Şahin, S.; Malik, N.S.A.; Perez, J.L.; Brockington, J.E. Seasonal Changes of Individual Phenolic Compounds in Leaves of Twenty Olive Cultivars Grown in Texas. *J. Agric. Sci. Technol.* **2012**, *2*, 242.
50. Talhaoui, N.; Gómez-Caravaca, A.M.; Roldán, C.; León, L.; De la Rosa, R.; Fernández-Gutiérrez, A.; Segura-Carretero, A. Chemometric Analysis for the Evaluation of Phenolic Patterns in Olive Leaves from Six Cultivars at Different Growth Stages. *J. Agric. Food Chem.* **2015**, *63*, 1722–1729. [CrossRef] [PubMed]
51. Ranalli, A.; Contento, S.; Lucera, L.; Di Febo, M.; Marchegiani, D.; Di Fonzo, V. Factors Affecting the Contents of Iridoid Oleuropein in Olive Leaves (*Olea europaea* L.). *J. Agric. Food Chem.* **2006**, *54*, 434–440. [CrossRef] [PubMed]
52. Clodoveo, M.L.; Crupi, P.; Annunziato, A.; Corbo, F. Innovative Extraction Technologies for Development of Functional Ingredients Based on Polyphenols from Olive Leaves. *Foods* **2022**, *11*, 103. [CrossRef]
53. Xie, P.; Huang, L.; Zhang, C.; You, F. Reduced Pressure Extraction of Oleuropein from Olive Leaves (*Olea europaea* L.) with Ultrasound. *Food Bioprod. Process.* **2013**, *93*, 29–38. [CrossRef]
54. da Rosa, G.S.; Vanga, S.K.; Gariepy, Y.; Raghavan, V. Comparison of Microwave, Ultrasonic and Conventional Techniques for Extraction of Bioactive Compounds from Olive Leaves (*Olea europaea* L.). *Innov. Food Sci. Emerg. Technol.* **2019**, *58*, 102234. [CrossRef]
55. Rafiee, Z.; Jafari, S.M.; Alami, M.; Khomeiri, M. Microwave-Assisted Extraction of Phenolic Compounds from Olive Leaves; A Comparison with Maceration. *J. Anim. Plant Sci.* **2011**, *21*, 738–745.
56. Valinger, D.; Kušen, M.; Benković, M.; Jurina, T.; Panić, M.; Redovniković, I.R.; Kljusurić, J.G.; Tušek, A.J. Enhancement of the Green Extraction of Bioactive Molecules from Olea Europaea Leaves. *Separations* **2022**, *9*, 33. [CrossRef]
57. Vizzarri, V.; Ienco, A.; Benincasa, C.; Perri, E.; Pucci, N.; Cesari, E.; Novellis, C.; Rizzo, P.; Pellegrino, M.; Zaffina, F.; et al. Phenolic Extract from Olive Leaves as a Promising Endotherapeutic Treatment against *Xylella fastidiosa* in Naturally Infected *Olea europaea* (Var. *europaea*) Trees. *Biology* **2023**, *12*, 1141. [CrossRef] [PubMed]
58. Sánchez-Gutiérrez, M.; Bascón-Villegas, I.; Rodríguez, A.; Pérez-Rodríguez, F.; Fernández-Prior, Á.; Rosal, A.; Carrasco, E. Valorisation of *Olea europaea* L. Olive Leaves through the Evaluation of Their Extracts: Antioxidant and Antimicrobial Activity. *Foods* **2021**, *10*, 966. [CrossRef] [PubMed]
59. Guo, X.; Wang, J. Comparison of Linearization Methods for Modeling the Langmuir Adsorption Isotherm. *J. Mol. Liq.* **2019**, *296*, 111850. [CrossRef]
60. Al-Ghouti, M.A.; Da'ana, D.A. Guidelines for the Use and Interpretation of Adsorption Isotherm Models: A Review. *J. Hazard. Mater.* **2020**, *393*, 122383. [CrossRef] [PubMed]
61. Aliakbarian, B.; Casazza, A.A.; Perego, P. Kinetic and Isotherm Modelling of the Adsorption of Phenolic Compounds from Olive Mill Wastewater onto Activated Carbon. *Food Technol. Biotechnol.* **2015**, *53*, 207–214. [CrossRef] [PubMed]
62. Perwitasari, D.S.; Ardian, Y.; Pracesa, Y.; Pangestu, M.A.; Sampe Tola, P. Langmuir and Freundlich Isotherm Approximation on Adsorption Mechanism of Chrome Waste by Using Tofu Dregs. *Nusant. Sci. Technol. Proc.* **2021**, *2021*, 106–112.
63. Abodif, A.M.; Abodif, A.M.; Meng, L.; Ma, S.; Ahmed, A.S.A.; Belvett, N.; Wei, Z.Z.; Ning, D. Mechanisms and Models of Adsorption: TiO2-Supported Biochar for Removal of 3,4-Dimethylaniline. *ACS Omega* **2020**, *5*, 13630–13640. [CrossRef]
64. Abid, N.; Masmoudi, M.A.; Megdiche, M.; Barakat, A.; Ellouze, M.; Chamkha, M.; Ksibi, M.; Sayadi, S. Biochar from Olive Mill Solid Waste as an Eco-Friendly Adsorbent for the Removal of Polyphenols from Olive Mill Wastewater. *Chem. Eng. Res. Des.* **2022**, *181*, 384–398. [CrossRef]

65. Goktepeli, G.; Yildiz, S.; Yel, E. Phenol Adsorption on Magnetic Biochar Derived from Olive Pomace: Equilibrium, Kinetic and Thermodynamics. *Hacet. J. Biol. Chem.* **2021**, *49*, 133–145. [CrossRef]
66. Freundlich, H.M.F. Over the Adsorption in Solution. *J. Phys. Chem* **1906**, *57*, 1100–1107.
67. Ismail, M.G.B.H.; Weng, C.N.; Rahman, H.A.; Zakaria, N.A. Freundlich Isotherm Equilibrium Equastions in Determining Effectiveness a Low Cost Absorbent to Heavy Metal Removal in Wastewater (Leachate) At Teluk Kitang Landfill, Pengkalan Chepa, Kelantan, Malaysia. *J. Geogr. Earth Sci.* **2013**, *1*, 55477126.
68. Anah, L.; Astrini, N. Isotherm Adsorption Studies of Ni(II) Ion Removal from Aqueous Solutions by Modified Carboxymethyl Cellulose Hydrogel. *IOP Conf. Ser. Earth Environ. Sci.* **2018**, *160*, 012017. [CrossRef]
69. Hadrich, F.; Geißen, S.U.; Chamkha, M.; Sayadi, S. Optimizing the Extraction Conditions of Hydroxytyrosol from Olive Leaves Using a Modified Spherical Activated Carbon: A New Experimental Design. *Biomed. Res. Int.* **2022**, *2022*, 6199627. [CrossRef] [PubMed]
70. Senol, A.; Hasdemir, İ.M.; Hasdemir, B.; Kurdaş, İ. Adsorptive Removal of Biophenols from Olive Mill Wastewaters (OMW) by Activated Carbon: Mass Transfer, Equilibrium and Kinetic Studies. *Asia-Pac. J. Chem. Eng.* **2017**, *12*, 128–146. [CrossRef]
71. Fseha, Y.H.; Shaheen, J.; Sizirici, B. Phenol Contaminated Municipal Wastewater Treatment Using Date Palm Frond Biochar: Optimization Using Response Surface Methodology. *Emerg. Contam.* **2023**, *9*, 100202. [CrossRef]
72. Dąbrowski, A.; Podkościelny, P.; Hubicki, Z.; Barczak, M. Adsorption of Phenolic Compounds by Activated Carbon—A Critical Review. *Chemosphere* **2005**, *58*, 1049–1070. [CrossRef]

MDPI AG
Grosspeteranlage 5
4052 Basel
Switzerland
Tel.: +41 61 683 77 34

Antioxidants Editorial Office
E-mail: antioxidants@mdpi.com
www.mdpi.com/journal/antioxidants

www.ingramcontent.com/pod-product-compliance
Lightning Source LLC
Chambersburg PA
CBHW061444210926
51850CB00008B/1613
9783725852475